Minority Health in America

Minority Health in America

Findings and Policy Implications from
The Commonwealth Fund Minority
Health Survey

Edited by

Carol J. R. Hogue, Ph.D., M.P.H.
Martha A. Hargraves, Ph.D., M.P.H.
Karen Scott Collins, M.D., M.P.H.

The Johns Hopkins University Press
Baltimore and London

The Johns Hopkins University Press
2715 North Charles Street
Baltimore, Maryland 21218-4363
www.press.jhu.edu

Library of Congress Cataloging-in-Publication Data will be found at the end of
this book.
A catalog record for this book is available from the British Library.

ISBN 0-8018-6298-1
ISBN 0-8018-6299-X (pbk.)

Contents

Foreword

Minority Americans face serious disparities in health compared with white Americans, including higher infant mortality among African American infants, higher rates of diabetes and heart disease, and overall shorter life spans. The Commonwealth Fund, concerned with the failure in this country to narrow such health gaps, sponsored a comprehensive national health survey in 1994 of more than 3,700 African American, Hispanic, Asian American, and white adults. This survey addressed experiences with health care, including language barriers, perceptions of discrimination, access and utilization of health care services, and health status.

Initial analysis of this survey data revealed significant differences in experiences between minority and white Americans:

- Thirty-one percent of minority Americans did not have health insurance, compared with 14 percent of whites. Minority workers were less likely than white workers to have employer-sponsored coverage (56% vs. 66%).
- Twenty-nine percent of minority adults reported very little or no choice in where they could obtain health care.
- Access to specialty care was a major problem for 18 percent of minority adults, compared with 8 percent of white adults.
- Fifteen percent of minority adults felt they would have received better care if they were of a different race.

Troubling findings such as these, and the uniqueness of a database large enough to examine data on minority populations and ethnic groups, led The Commonwealth Fund to commission a thorough analysis of the survey data. With Fund support, Carol Hogue of Emory University and Martha Hargraves of the University of Texas recruited experts in minority health, health care, and health policy to prepare a set of analyses that together provide a richer understanding of the health care experiences of minority Americans. This volume makes clear some of the most significant barriers to health care: financial limitations, and interpersonal experiences rooted in cultural differences and discrimination all obstruct the pathway to needed health care. Health policy to improve the health outcomes of all Americans will be needed to lower these barriers. As the American population becomes increasingly diverse, with Hispanic and Asian American populations growing most rapidly, shaping a health care system that effectively cares for a diverse patient population and that resolves the historical disparities in health will be as great a challenge as any facing the health care system.

The Commonwealth Fund has a long history of recognizing disparities in access to health care and of creating programs to help lessen those disparities. In the 1920s, the Fund supported the training of black nurse midwives in rural southern towns, where few other providers would care for black patients. The Fund's Rural Hospital program built hospitals in southern communities, with the stipulation that all patients—black and white—and all physicians had to be allowed to use those hospitals. The Fund has continued this focus over the years, with support for minority medical education. Currently, the Fund supports health services research to improve health outcomes among minority populations. Specific issues include assuring access to and quality of care for minorities in managed care; assessing the impact of managed care on safety-net providers; and providing adequate information on disparities in health status, barriers to care, and effective policies and practices to reduce disparities. In addition, The Commonwealth Fund / Harvard University Fellowship in Minority Health Policy invests in the development of a cadre of minority physician-leaders who will undertake key roles in the formulation of minority health policy.

This book provides a significant contribution to such efforts. The work of each author in this volume is greatly appreciated. I also want to commend co-editors Carol Hogue, Martha Hargraves, and Karen Scott Collins for their outstanding work in shaping a volume of analyses that can help guide the development of policies and programs to assure that all Americans can benefit from the strengths of our health care system, in order to lead healthier and more productive lives.

Karen Davis
President, The Commonwealth Fund

Acknowledgments

We wish to recognize Karen Davis for her outstanding leadership in The Commonwealth Fund's ongoing mission to improve minority health. Her personal interest and support were crucial to the success of this project. We are also deeply appreciative of our multidisciplinary team of collaborators. Their expertise and dedication to quality research contributed greatly to the breadth and depth of the discussions in this volume.

Many individuals worked to assure the quality and accuracy of the data. We would like to thank particularly the staff of Louis Harris and Associates, who conducted the survey; Tso-Yu Liao, who prepared the analysis files for all contributors; and Ronald Forthofer and Donna Brogan, who provided invaluable statistical advice regarding analysis of data from a complex sample survey.

Many others provided key help in manuscript preparation. We are grateful for the careful review and comments on every chapter provided by Allyson Hall, program officer at The Commonwealth Fund; by Beth Atkins Clinton, our meticulous text editor; and by the anonymous "outside reviewer," whose thoughtful and incisive comments greatly improved the manuscript. We wish to thank especially Patricia Huckaby, editorial assistant, for her immaculate manuscript preparation as well as her ongoing moral support; Tracy Craft Woods, Emory University; and Charlotte Neuhaus, program assistant at The Commonwealth Fund, for administrative support.

We are also deeply indebted to Wendy Harris, medical editor at the Johns Hopkins University Press. Working behind the scenes, she provided constant and enthusiastic support. We extend our sincere appreciation, as well, to Garland Andersen, Chairman, University of Texas Medical Branch, Department of Obstetrics and Gynecology, for his advice and counsel.

We wish to recognize the considerable financial assistance of The Commonwealth Fund; of the Rollins School of Public Health of Emory University; of the Jules and Deen Terry Maternal and Child Health Endowment; and of the Department of Obstetrics and Gynecology of the University of Texas Medical Branch.

Finally, we wish to thank our patient, loving, and forbearing families—Lynn and Elizabeth Hogue; Sharon Hargraves; and Greg, Lauren, and Austin Collins—to whom we owe thanks and so much more.

Contributors

DOROTHY CHIN, PH.D., Assistant Research Psychologist, Department of Psychiatry and Biobehavioral Sciences, University of California, Los Angeles

SUSAN D. COCHRAN, PH.D., M.S., Professor, Department of Epidemiology, School of Public Health, University of California, Los Angeles

KAREN SCOTT COLLINS, M.D., M.P.H., Assistant Vice President, The Commonwealth Fund, New York

LLEWELLYN J. CORNELIUS, PH.D., Associate Professor and Assistant Dean for Informatics, University of Maryland School of Social Work, Baltimore

CHAMBERLAIN DIALA, PH.D., Director of Consulting Services, Managed Care Assistance Corporation, Rockville, Maryland

SYLVIA GUENDELMAN, PH.D., Associate Professor, Health Policy and Administration, School of Public Health, University of California, Berkeley

ALLYSON G. HALL, PH.D., Program Officer, The Commonwealth Fund, New York

MARTHA A. HARGRAVES, PH.D., M.P.H., Assistant Professor, Department of Obstetrics and Gynecology, University of Texas Medical Branch, Galveston

LISA E. HARRIS, M.D., Assistant Professor of Medicine, Indiana University School of Medicine, and Regenstrief Institute for Health Care, Indianapolis, Indiana

CAROL J. R. HOGUE, PH.D., M.P.H., Terry Professor of Maternal and Child Health, Department of Epidemiology, and Director, Women's and Children's Center, Rollins School of Public Health, Emory University, Atlanta, Georgia

NICOLE C. JARRETT, doctoral candidate, Johns Hopkins School of Hygiene and Public Health, Baltimore, Maryland

VERNA M. KEITH, PH.D., Associate Professor, Department of Sociology, Arizona State University, Tempe

THOMAS A. LAVEIST, PH.D., Associate Professor, Department of Health Policy and Management and Department of Sociology, Johns Hopkins School of Hygiene and Public Health, Baltimore, Maryland

VICKIE M. MAYS, PH.D., Professor, Department of Psychology, University of California, Los Angeles

SIMON MUNGAI, M.A., Biostatistician, Regenstrief Institute for Health Care, Indianapolis, Indiana

DONG W. SUH, M.P.H., Legislative and Governmental Affairs Coordinator, Asian and Pacific Islander American Health Forum, San Francisco, California

J. GREER SULLIVAN, M.D., M.S.P.H., Director, Mental Illness Research, Education, and Clinical Center (MIRECC) for Veterans Integrated Service Network (VISN) 16; Manager, Mental Health Product Line for VISN 16; and Associate Professor, Department of Psychiatry, University of Arkansas for Medical Science, Little Rock

DAVID T. TAKEUCHI, PH.D., Professor of Sociology, Indiana University, Bloomington

WILLIAM M. TIERNEY, M.D., Professor of Medicine, Indiana University School of Medicine, Richard Roudebush VA Medical Center, and Senior Scientist, Regenstrief Institute for Health Care, Indianapolis, Indiana

TODD WAGNER, PH.D., Health Economist, VA HSR&D Health Economics Resource Center, Menlo Park, California, and Consulting Assistant Professor, Stanford University School of Medicine, Stanford, California

DAVID R. WILLIAMS, PH.D., M.P.H., Professor of Sociology and Senior Research Scientist, Institute for Social Research, University of Michigan, Ann Arbor

Minority Health in America

The Commonwealth Fund Minority Health Survey of 1994

An Overview

Carol J. R. Hogue, Ph.D., M.P.H.
Martha A. Hargraves, Ph.D., M.P.H.

African American, Hispanic, and certain Asian minority populations suffer disproportionate burdens of morbidity and mortality in the United States (National Center for Health Statistics 1992). African American babies are twice as likely as white babies to die before reaching their first birthday. For minority adults, excess mortality is as high as or even higher than the excess mortality for infants, especially for the major causes of death, such as cardiovascular disease, certain cancers, and violence.

W. E. B. DuBois first noted these racial and ethnic disparities more than a century ago in his analysis of 1890 census data in Philadelphia (DuBois 1906). He claimed that health disparities reflected "a vast set of problems having a common center [that] must be studied according to some general plan" (Foner 1970). Since then, dramatic overall improvements in health have been the hallmark of medical care and disease prevention. Yet despite a near doubling in life expectancy at birth for the general population, inequities in racial and ethnic death rates remain a national paradox (U.S. Department of Health and Human Services 1985).

Why do such health disparities continue unabated? And what policies should be changed to close the racial and ethnic gap in health? Answers to these questions still require study "according to some general plan" that examines ongoing health problems of racial and ethnic minority populations within the broad context of social, environmental, economic, and, to a lesser extent, cultural factors. In 1994, The Commonwealth Fund commissioned a national survey on minority health with this goal in mind. Specifically, the survey focused on how differences in health insurance coverage, choice in selecting a health care provider, and other health care access barriers might affect how minority populations use health services for needed preventive and curative services. Implicit in this approach is the link between health status and access to health care. Better access to health care means better health and longer life expectancy. The survey made this link explicit by examining both the relationship between health care access and mental distress and the relationship between the need for and the receipt of health promotion advice.

The timing of the survey—a decade after the federal government had established its Office of Minority Health and at the threshold of monumental changes in both health care delivery systems and support systems for the poor—makes the survey results particularly useful. In 1994, most minority populations received medical care in settings without managed care. That year also predated welfare reform, which changed eligibility for publicly funded health insurance among some minority populations, particularly those who were not U.S. citizens and those poor women who no longer received Medicaid benefits.

The Commonwealth Fund Minority Health Survey (CMHS) snapshot of minority health and health care taken in 1994 permits health services researchers to assess (1) what barriers to accessing quality health care still plagued minority populations after a decade of activities designed to eliminate those barriers; (2) whether some minority populations are more or less affected by those barriers; and (3) what benchmarks of health care access and utilization, as well as of the health status of minority populations, help to compare contemporary health care and status indicators now that managed care dominates health care and health care access has been affected by welfare reform.

Preliminary findings of the CMHS confirmed concerns about health care access, especially for particular subgroups within minority populations (Davis 1995). The survey revealed problems with insurance coverage, difficulties related to language problems for some respondents, and problems in obtaining needed services, including specialty care. Based on these preliminary findings, The Commonwealth Fund commissioned several health services researchers to explore these findings in greater depth—examining problems that might pertain only to certain subgroups as well as problems related to minority health status as a whole. For this, researchers examined historical discrimination as reflected in current socioeconomic levels, as well as contemporaneous discrimination as reflected in perceived discriminatory actions within health care practices. This book is a result of these researchers' efforts.

THE SAMPLE

The CMHS was actually two surveys using the same interview instrument. The main survey was intended to be a nationally representative sample of adults 18 years of age and older, residing in households with telephones within the forty-eight contiguous United States. Louis Harris and Associates, Inc., asked potential respondents to self-identify as African American or black, Hispanic or Latino, non-Hispanic white, Asian, or Native American. To increase numbers within minority populations, African Americans and Hispanics were oversampled so that the final main sample included 1,114 non-Hispanic whites, 1,048 African Americans or blacks, and 1,001 Latino Americans or Hispanics (531 Mexican, 155 Puerto Rican, 43 Cuban, and 272 other) (Figure 1.1).

Potential households were chosen for the main sample through random-digit dialing. (For details of the complex, multistage sampling design, see the Technical Appendix.) In each chosen household, the screener selected a household member using a methodology designed to

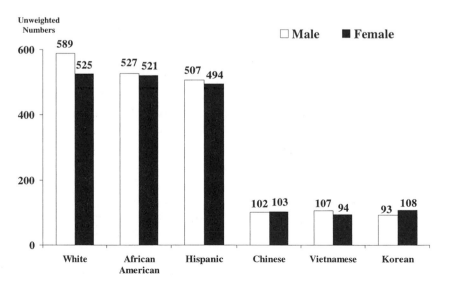

Figure 1.1 *Number of respondents, by gender, race, and ethnicity*
Source: Data from The Commonwealth Fund Minority Health Survey, 1994

assure balance by age and gender. Interviewers telephoned these households on nights and weekends and made callbacks to selected respondents, either by appointment or at different times on nights and weekends, to complete the interviews. For the respondents' convenience, daytime interviews were conducted when requested.

The overall response rate was 60 percent of eligible respondents (see Technical Appendix). This response rate is within the range expected of telephone interview surveys, especially of minority populations, during the 1990s. However, the fact that 40 percent of eligible respondents refused to participate or could not be located does limit confidence in the generalizability of findings from the respondents. Nonrespondents may have been different from respondents in characteristics that would have affected their answers to health status and health care experiences. For example, nonrespondents might have been sicker and therefore unable to participate in an interview, or more healthy and therefore unavailable owing to working or continually being away from home for other reasons.

Postsampling analysis of the data suggested that respondents were similar to the populations from which they were sampled in many respects, but they were also dissimilar. On average the respondents were better educated, had higher incomes, and were more likely to be employed (see Technical Appendix). These differences would be expected from the results of a telephone survey, because people without telephones generally are poorer than people with telephones.

To correct statistically for some of these dissimilarities, authors analyzed data that were weighted to match the concurrent Current Population Survey (CPS) parameters on the basis of gender, race, age, educational attainment, and health insurance status. When possible, researchers in this volume compared the results of their analyses with the results of other national surveys for Hispanics, African Americans, and whites. Finally, the researchers assessed the potential impact of remaining, unmeasurable nonresponse biases that may be related to their specific analyses.

Concerns have also been raised about whether telephone respondents under-report health events and illnesses. However, because telephone surveying affords a greater sense of anonymity, the respondent may be more likely to report socially undesirable responses such as ill health or substance abuse in a telephone interview than in a face-to-face interview. Respondents may accurately report having received health tests, such as a mammogram, but overestimate clinical screening, such as rectal exams (see Technical Appendix). In sum, although there are certain disadvantages associated with telephone surveys, they do produce information comparable to that collected by other means and they do so at a lower cost (Aday 1996).

The second survey sampled three subgroups of Asian Americans— Chinese, Koreans, and Vietnamese. Potential households of people with surnames common to these groups were chosen from telephone lists compiled by Survey Sampling, Inc., for cities with large Asian populations. Interviewers reached a total of 205 Chinese, 201 Vietnamese, 201 Koreans, and 25 other Asians.

For all individuals, interviewers asked questions in the respondents' native language. Interviews, averaging twenty-five minutes in length, were completed between May 13, 1994, and July 28, 1994. Participants described their health status and health-related behaviors, their access to and use of health care services, their attitudes toward care received, and related socioeconomic data.

The analyses of the survey presented in this volume follow a general format. First, authors examined bivariate relationships (e.g., between race/ethnicity and access to health care services) in some detail. Tests of statistical significance contribute to these descriptions but are not meant to be definitive tests of differences. Second, authors developed multivariate models to test associations between race/ethnicity and health care, while adjusting for potentially confounding variables or variables that might modify the effect between race/ethnicity and health care. Models were tested using software designed for analyses of complex sample surveys. Although the sampling was done without replacement (i.e., the individual cannot be chosen for the sample more than once), authors used "with replacement" for sampling design statements. This convention simplifies analysis and provides reasonable estimates when, as with this survey, the sample is small relative to the population being sampled. The rationale was that sampling fractions were small in comparison to the total population in each survey stratum. Authors chose variables to include in their multivariate analyses on the basis of their importance in adjusting for socioeconomic differences (e.g., income and education), the underlying theoretical framework (see, e.g., Chapter 11), or the initial tests of statistical significance in the bivariate analysis (see, e.g., Chapter 8). In the last case, to avoid the problem of multiple comparisons, more stringent criteria for a variable to be included in the final analysis were introduced in the multivariate model. When presenting multivariate analyses, some authors chose to describe the relationship among all variables, rather than just the statistically significant variables, to discuss why certain ones that they had considered a priori to be important were not statistically significant.

The CMHS, although one of the largest samples of African Americans and Hispanics available, is limited in its ability to describe unique health experiences of small subgroups within minority populations (e.g., Cuban Americans or African Americans from the Caribbean). Modest sample size, particularly within particular ethnic/racial groups, presents problems in interpreting nonsignificant findings. The lack of statistical significance may reflect the lesser statistical power of the CMHS to delineate differences for these subgroups rather than a true lack of differences. Conversely, because of small samples, a few responses that are quite different from those of the larger group might lead to a false conclusion that differences exist. Thus, the authors urge caution when interpreting differences among small subgroups.

When appropriate, authors included the Asian sample in their bivariate descriptions. However, owing to the differences in sampling between the Asian sample and the main survey, the Asian sample presented difficulties for analysts performing multivariate comparisons of racial and ethnic subgroups. As a result, multivariate analyses generally omitted the Asian subpopulations.

The differences between the CMHS sample and the CPS suggest some caution in interpreting findings from our survey. In particular, findings that do not control for socioeconomic differences in the analysis are likely to be biased, in that poor and unemployed individuals were underrepresented. Likewise, differences between ethnic groups are likely to be muted, owing to the associations between poverty, unemployment, and minority status. However, in this book, all authors controlled for income and education in their multivariate analyses. Thus, when they examine the complex interrelationships between ethnicity and the access to, availability of, and use of health care, their conclusions should not be unduly affected by the overall sampling biases.

KEY FINDINGS

This volume seeks to use analyses of the CMHS to answer the following questions.

1. What is the experience of health care access and utilization among different minority populations and within minority popu-

lations (by socioeconomic status and ethnic group), and what are the implications for policy change? This objective is addressed in profiles of Hispanics (see Chapter 2), African Americans (see Chapter 3), Asians (see Chapter 4), and minority women (see Chapter 5).

2. What are the barriers to health care access and utilization, and how do these differ across minority populations (by socioeconomic status and ethnic group)? Separate analyses focus on financial barriers (see Chapter 6), particular barriers faced by the uninsured (see Chapter 7), satisfaction with health care (see Chapter 8), source and choice of health care provider (see Chapter 9), and perceived discrimination in the health care system (see Chapter 10).

3. What is the relationship between health care and health status among minority populations, and what are the policy implications of those relationships? These questions are addressed with specific attention to the mental and social well-being of minority populations (see Chapter 11) and the health promotion habits of minority populations (see Chapter 12).

4. The book concludes with a look to the future (see Chapter 13), to begin to answer the question, what can be done in the changing world of health care to ensure continued improvement in the health and health care of minority populations?

Health Care of Minority Populations Is Inadequate to Meet Their Needs

Most respondents reported that they had seen a health care provider at least once during the previous 12 months (Figure 1.2), but this similarity masks some important differences in the need for care and the ease with which the needed care can be obtained. In the CMHS, as in other surveys of perceived or measured health status, the minority groups included higher proportions of individuals in perceived poor or fair health (Figure 1.3). Given their poor health, members of minority groups might be expected to have made more health care visits than the majority population. However, minority populations had fewer—rather than more—such visits (Figure 1.4). Putting these results together, it is not surprising that more minority than white respondents indicated that they did not receive the health care that they felt they needed (Figure 1.5). One reason for poorer health care for minority populations is that they were more

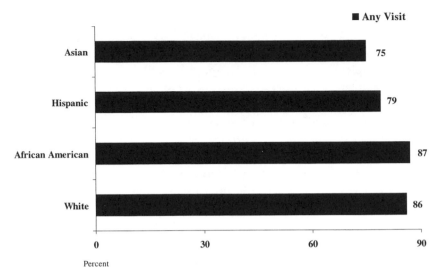

Figure 1.2 *Percentage of respondents with any visit to a doctor in the last twelve months, by race and ethnicity*
Source: Data from The Commonwealth Fund Minority Health Survey, 1994

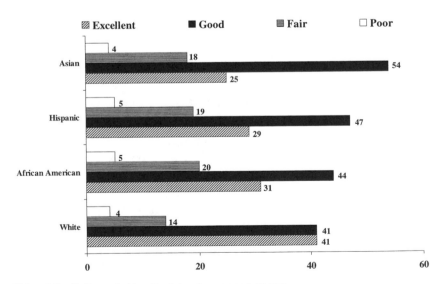

Figure 1.3 *Self-reported health status, by race and ethnicity*
Source: Data from The Commonwealth Fund Minority Health Survey, 1994
Note: Percentages may not add up to 100 because of nonresponse.

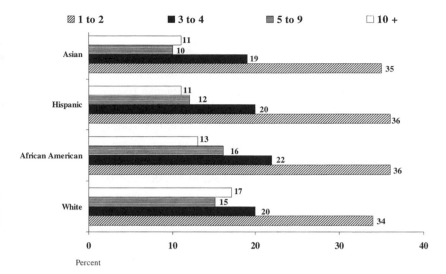

Figure 1.4 *Distribution of health care visits in the last twelve months, by race and ethnicity*
Source: Data from The Commonwealth Fund Minority Health Survey, 1994
Note: Percentages may not add up to 100 because of nonresponse.

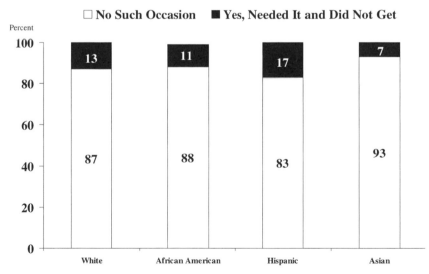

Figure 1.5 *Percentage of respondents who needed medical care but did not get it, by race and ethnicity*
Source: Data from The Commonwealth Fund Minority Health Survey, 1994
Note: Percentages may not add up to 100 because of nonresponse.

likely to have to surmount the barrier of having no regular health care provider (Figure 1.6).

People who lack health insurance face an immediate barrier to getting needed health care (see Chapters 2 through 7). In 1994, almost 25 percent of Asian and African American adults and nearly 40 percent of Hispanic adults lacked insurance, compared with only 12 percent of white adults (Figure 1.7). Part of this discrepancy resulted from differences in employer-sponsored health insurance plans. Even though slightly more minority than white adults were employed (67% vs. 63%), only 45 percent of employed minority adults received health insurance through an employer, compared with 55 percent of white workers. However, this does not tell the whole story. At virtually all levels of income and education, white respondents were more likely than members of minority populations to have health insurance (see Chapters 6 and 7). More minority women than white women lack health insurance, regardless of income (see Chapter 5).

Disruptions in health insurance during the two years prior to the survey were also more common among the minority population respondents (19%) than among the majority population respondents (12%). Among men and women, Chinese Americans were at greatest risk of

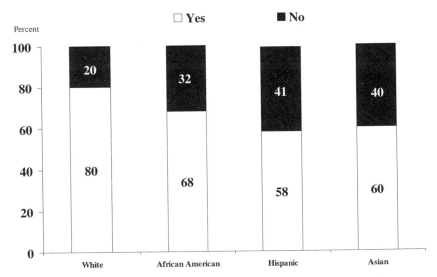

Figure 1.6   *Percentage of respondents with a regular provider, by race and ethnicity*
Source: Data from The Commonwealth Fund Minority Health Survey, 1994
Note: Percentages may not add up to 100 because of nonresponse.

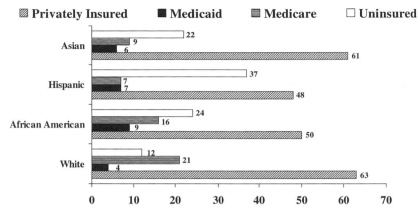

Figure 1.7 *Level of health insurance coverage, by race and ethnicity*
Source: Data from The Commonwealth Fund Minority Health Survey, 1994
Note: Percentages may not add up to 100 because of nonresponse.

lapses in insurance coverage (23%). Even more Latina women—about one-half—experienced problems with health insurance coverage (see Chapter 5).

Problems with health insurance were by far the most common reason given when a respondent indicated having limited health care choices (see Chapter 9). Coupled with financial barriers, which were reported more than twice as frequently by minority groups as by white respondents (see Chapter 9), health insurance barriers contributed to limitations in choices of health care providers. Limited choice is an important reason people postpone seeking needed health care services. More than one-half of those with limited choices reported delays in seeking health care, compared with only about one-third of those whose choice of provider was not limited (see Chapter 9).

Historical Discrimination Explains Some Discrepancies in Minority Health and Health Care

Are disparities in health status and health care related to race and ethnicity because minority populations are poorer than the majority? All the analysts addressed this question. If health and health care disparities can be attributed to socioeconomic status (SES), the relationship between those disparities and race or ethnicity should prove to be a historical one, based on the continuing legacy of racism reflected in socioeconomic disparities (see Chapter 11). Even with the biases toward better-educated and wealthier respondents that are inherent in a telephone sample, it is clear from the CMHS that minority populations are poorer and less educated (Figures 1.8 and 1.9). Among Hispanics and Asian Americans, poverty and lower educational attainment characterize more recent immigrants (see Chapters 2 and 4). But to what extent do these SES differences account for health and health care differences? And, within racial and ethnic groups, are there indications that more advantaged subpopulations have better health and receive better health care?

To answer the first question, analysts used educational attainment and household income as measures of SES differentials, and they compared individuals in minority populations with the white group. Not surprisingly, financial and health insurance barriers were greater for people of limited means (see Chapters 6 through 9). After statistical adjustment for SES, racial and ethnic differences in satisfaction with the quality of health care services were no longer statistically significant. Moreover, when SES variables were held constant, African Americans and Latino Americans were less—not more—likely to delay seeking care (see Chapter 9).

Satisfaction with life was lower, and measures indicating psycholog-

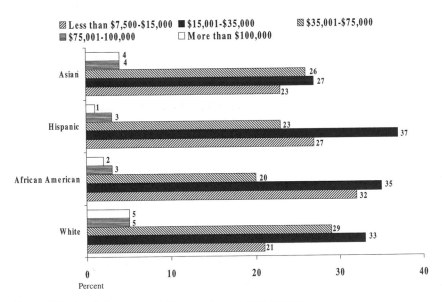

Figure 1.8 *Level of respondents' income, by race and ethnicity*
Source: Data from The Commonwealth Fund Minority Health Survey, 1994
Note: Percentages may not add up to 100 because of nonresponse.

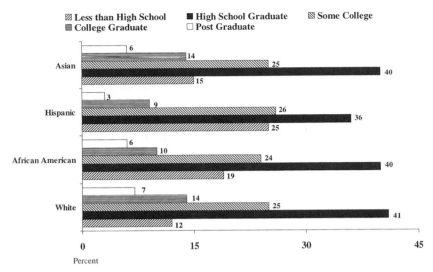

Figure 1.9 *Level of respondents' education, by race and ethnicity*
Source: Data from The Commonwealth Fund Minority Health Survey, 1994
Note: Percentages may not add up to 100 because of nonresponse.

ical distress were higher, for poorer and less-educated individuals (see Chapter 11). With two notable exceptions, adjustments for these SES differences eliminated racial/ethnic differences in psychological distress and life satisfaction. Both black Americans from the Caribbean and Korean Americans expressed less satisfaction with life than did other members of racial and ethnic subgroups. Although not definitive because of small samples, these intriguing findings point to the need for focused research into subgroups at potentially higher risk of ill health than would be predicted, given their income and educational attainment.

Based on these data on financial and health insurance barriers to health care and on mental distress, one can conclude that poverty paves a common pathway from minority status to poor health care and illness, and the root cause of that poverty is the legacy of historical racism and discrimination and its consequences (see Chapter 11). Fortunately, however, many members of minority groups have escaped poverty. About one-half of Latino and African Americans in the CMHS had annual incomes in excess of $25,000 (see Chapters 2 and 3). Proportions of Asians with household incomes greater than $25,000 varied by ethnic group, with more than half of Chinese and Vietnamese and more than three-fourths of Koreans above this income level (see Chapter 4). High school graduates constituted more than three-fourths of the Latino,

African American, and Korean groups, and more than 70 percent of the Chinese and Vietnamese groups. These within-group differences in SES enabled the analysts to further test the hypothesis that SES deficits explain the higher rate of health care problems among minority groups. By focusing within minority groups, the analysts examined other barriers to high-quality care that might have been masked when minority groups were compared with the majority population. Further, because women represent a discriminated population within all racial and ethnic groups, a separate analysis focused on women in all groups (see Chapter 5).

Separate CMHS analyses of Hispanic, African American, and Asian subgroups reveal that SES does play a role in access to and use of health care services within each subgroup. However, the role is generally indirect, in that wealthier and more-educated individuals are better insured and are also more likely to have a regular health care provider. Those two structural variables were highly correlated with whether the person had seen a health care provider in the past twelve months, and, if so, how many visits were made in the year. In some instances, having a regular health care provider was so important to health care utilization that uninsured individuals with a regular provider were just as likely to receive care as were insured individuals with a regular provider.

These within-group analyses also reveal important factors in health care access factors that are unique to minority populations. For example, Hispanics in the survey were less likely to have been seen by a provider if English was not their native language or if they felt that the quality of their health care would have been better had they been of a different race or ethnicity (see Chapter 2). African Americans, on the contrary, did not vary their care-seeking behaviors because of feelings about the quality of their health care being different owing to their race or ethnicity, but they were less satisfied with their care when they did share those feelings (see Chapter 3). Also, African Americans were more satisfied with their care when their provider was also African American (see Chapter 3). Thus, it appears that racial and ethnic discrimination is a potent barrier to receiving health care.

Ongoing Discrimination Is a Major Health and Health Care Problem for Minority Populations

Almost one-fourth of African Americans and one-sixth of Hispanics felt that they would have received better care if they had been of a different race or ethnicity (see Chapter 10). Such feelings are one indication of perceived discrimination within the health care system. Perceived discrimination has been hypothesized to be a barrier to obtaining needed health care, in that disparaged people will avoid disparaging circumstances. The CMHS inquired explicitly about respondents' experiences of discrimination, with some surprising findings. Experiences of discrimination were common in all minority groups. However, these experiences were more common if the individuals had had more, rather than fewer, visits to the health care system within the twelve months leading up to the survey (see Chapters 2 through 4).

Although at first glance this finding seems to refute the hypothesis of discrimination as a barrier, it may well be that more exposure to the health care system creates more risk for discriminatory acts. Those acts, in turn, may discourage further visits for ill patients who should be seen more frequently. For example, virtually all Hispanic individuals who reported that they had been treated badly within the last year were dissatisfied with their care, and dissatisfied individuals were nearly four times as likely as satisfied individuals to postpone getting needed care (see Chapter 2). Further, people in poor health were far more likely to report experiencing discrimination (see Chapter 10). Finally, after adjusting for SES, health status, and other variables, those individuals—with or without health insurance—who reported having been discriminated against in the health care system were more than twice as likely to postpone needed care as those reporting no such experiences (see Chapter 9).

A related barrier is dissatisfaction with services received. With respect to health care quality, access, and impact, recording an individual's satisfaction with care is not a "trivial pursuit" (Kravitz 1998). Rather, a record of dissatisfied patients may be the most important indicator of a system in need of change—whether or not the patients decide to act on their feelings by switching providers (Zapka et al. 1995; Patrick et al. 1997).

Discrimination can cause dissatisfaction, but among minority respondents, perceived racial discrimination was not associated with perceived dissatisfaction with services when patients felt that their regular providers had strong interpersonal skills and spent adequate time with them. This finding points to the need to recognize behaviors that are perceived to be discriminatory and to offer enhanced training in interpersonal skills to health care practitioners. Among CMHS respondents of all races and ethnicities, dissatisfaction also came from a variety of other sources, such as system unresponsiveness, lack of a regular source of care, lack of access to specialty care, and inappropriate behavior by the doctor. Respondents were more satisfied with their doctors if they received preventive services, including advice on lifestyle issues. They were more dissatisfied with both providers and services if they did not receive the care they felt they needed (see Chapter 8).

By asking patients to provide details about their experiences, providers can learn how to improve their behaviors, reduce their discriminatory practices, and better adapt themselves to the needs of their clients (Kravitz 1998). Actions to address clients' concerns are particularly called for in the current environment that stresses cutbacks in the very aspects of care that make a difference to clients, including choice of provider and site, ease in making appointments, and the length of time the patient can spend with the doctor.

Studying Minority Populations Sheds Light on Health and Health Care Issues for All Populations

Because of the burdens of historical and ongoing discrimination, minority populations are not as healthy as the majority population. Nonetheless, minority populations are not as sick as one might suppose, given those burdens. Both smoking and stress are associated with poor health and increased health care visits. Compared with the white population, minority groups smoke less (see Chapter 12) and exhibit less of a relationship between stress and mental distress (see Chapter 11). Why is this? One hypothesis is that minority cultures nurture coping mechanisms (such as spirituality) that could conceivably work to improve health for all populations. Exploring this hypothesis would necessitate new and culturally sensitive measures of coping skills.

Some health problems identified in the CMHS span diverse populations and are universal. This is apparent, for example, concerning the lack of exercise (see Chapter 12). Regardless of race or ethnicity, most men and even more women do not practice routine, vigorous, heart-healthy exercise. Neither do they receive counseling or advice from their health care providers about changing their behaviors. Given the rising prevalence of morbid obesity in the United States, the medical community should address this universal problem directly.

FUTURE DIRECTIONS

Directions for Developing Policy and Research

Chapter 13 concludes with some directions for developing policy to improve minority health and for further research. Now, of course, addressing access and quality of care for minority populations must be considered largely within a managed care system. At the same time, expanding insurance coverage, maintaining a safety net, and increasing the diversity of the health care workforce require continued attention in policy discussions. Health services research can contribute to these discussions by focusing on (1) evaluations of ways to assure ensure that clients have regular providers, particularly within Medicaid managed care; (2) evaluations of different approaches to reducing discriminatory practices within health care settings; (3) research and policy recommendations to optimize the benefits of diversity in provider characteristics; (4) options for securing insurance coverage for the working poor; and (5) the impact of changes in safety net providers on access and utilization of health care. Epidemiologic and sociologic research is needed to improve our understanding of the special needs of subpopulations within minority populations and to delineate the coping strategies among minority populations that inure them to some of the ill effects of discrimination.

Planning for Healthier Minority Populations

Our analysts provide many suggestions for improving the health care system. Prominent among these are (1) implementing universal health insurance incrementally, beginning with assured coverage for the working poor (see Chapter 7); (2) assuring access to a regular health care provider—the key component of a health care team (with numerous examples in various chapters); and (3) eliminating discriminatory practices in health care settings (with numerous examples in various chapters). Implicit in many of the analyses (see Chapters 2 through 5, 8, and others) is the call for a better organization of health care services to reduce transportation, language, and perceived discriminatory barriers. Aday and colleagues (1998) proposed a model framework for accomplishing these goals; this framework includes the components of a distributive system with basic minimum services for all. Chapter 13 discusses other approaches, including major social change to eliminate socioeconomic disparities between the majority and minority populations.

The overall conclusion of this study is that issues of equity continue to haunt our current health care system. When we focus exclusively on cost containment and market competition, a sense of the common good seems to escape our vision of efficiency and effectiveness. Finally, inequities in access to high-quality and sufficient health care are rooted in the lack of universal health care insurance. Insurance is the principal tool for obtaining access to sufficient health care in the United States. Based on our findings, we propose that policymakers at both the state and national levels embrace a broader framework of distributive justice. This framework would value the histories and the contributions made to this country's development by individuals representing the diversity on which our country was built.

References

Aday, L. A. 1996. *Designing and Conducting Health Surveys: A Comprehensive Guide.* San Francisco: Jossey-Bass.

Aday, L. A., Begley, C. E., Lairson, D. R., and Slater, C. H. 1998. *Evaluating the Health Care System: Effectiveness, Efficiency, and Equity.* 2d ed. Ann Arbor: Health Administration Press.

Davis, K. 1995. *Minority Americans Do Not Have Equal Health Opportunities. A Briefing Note from The Commonwealth Fund.* New York: The Commonwealth Fund.

DuBois, W. E. B. 1906. *Negro Health and Physique.* New York: Octagon Books.

Foner, Philip S. (ed.). 1970. *W.E.B. DuBois Speaks: Speeches and Addresses 1890–1919.* New York: Pathfinder Press.

Kravitz, R. 1998. Patient satisfaction with health care: critical outcome or trivial pursuit? (Editorial). *Journal of General Internal Medicine* 13:280–282.

National Center for Health Statistics. 1992. *Health, United States, 1991.* DHHS Publication No. (PHS) 92-1232. Hyattsville, Md.: U.S. Department of Health and Human Services, Public Health Service, Centers for Disease Control.

Patrick, D. L., Martin, D. P., Madden, C. W., Diehr, P., Cheadle, A., and Skillman, S. M. 1997. Dissatisfaction and disenrollment in a subsidized managed care program. *Medical Care Research and Review* 54(1):61–79.

U.S. Department of Health and Human Services. 1985. *Report of the Secretary's Task Force on Black and Minority Health, Margaret M. Heckler, Secretary.* Vol. 1, Executive Summary. DHHS Publication No. (PHS) 86-52-P. Washington, D.C.: U.S. Department of Health and Human Services.

Zapka, J. G., Palmer, R. H., Hargraves, J. L., Nerenz, D., Frazier, H. S., and Warner, C. K. 1995. Relationships of patient satisfaction with experience of system performance and health status. *Journal of Ambulatory Care Management* 18(1):73–83.

2

Hispanics' Experience within the Health Care System

Access, Utilization, and Satisfaction

Sylvia Guendelman, Ph.D.
Todd Wagner, Ph.D.

In 1990 Hispanics represented approximately 9 percent of the total U.S. population (National Council of LaRaza 1991). Estimated at 22.4 million, excluding the residents of the Commonwealth of Puerto Rico and undocumented workers, Hispanics are a community of different national origin groups (U.S. Bureau of the Census 1991). The majority (63%) identify themselves as Mexican Americans, 11 percent as Puerto Rican, 4.9 percent as Cuban, and the remaining as Central and South American or "Other Hispanic." More than 70 percent of Hispanics were born in the United States; only 29 percent are immigrants. Hispanics are a young population. Both high fertility and immigration account for population growth among Hispanics, which is five times faster than the rate of the total U.S. population (Molina and Aguirre-Molina 1994). Hispanics are projected to become the largest population group in several states, including California, New Mexico, and Texas. These demographic trends have major implications for planning health services.

Three decades of research underscore the problems that Hispanics face accessing health services. Early research considered health care behavior to be a consequence of cultural beliefs and demographic traits (Madsen 1964; Nall and Speilberg 1967), but more recent research emphasizes low socioeconomic status, lack of or insufficient health insurance coverage, and barriers to care placed by the health delivery system itself (Andersen et al. 1981; Freeman et al. 1990; Giachello 1994). Studies consistently show that Hispanics are less likely than any other group to be linked to a regular source of care (Robert Wood Johnson Foundation 1987; Lieu et al. 1993).

Moreover, this situation seems to have worsened in recent years. A 1986 national survey found that the percentage of Hispanics without a regular source of care had almost tripled since 1982, and was nearly twice that of whites (30% versus 16%) (Robert Wood Johnson Foundation 1987). In the same period, the proportion of uninsured Hispanics increased by half to 21.7 percent. Valdez et al. (1993) found that, by 1989, 39 percent of Hispanics under the age of 65 were uninsured, compared with 14 percent of whites and 24 percent of African Americans. These high rates of uninsured Hispanics reflect weaknesses in employment-based insurance and lower rates of Medicaid coverage, particularly among Mexican Americans and Hispanics of Central and South American origin (Valdez et al. 1993; Trevino et al. 1991; Berk et al. 1996). This difference is important because uninsured individuals are more likely to lack a regular source of care and less likely to access the health care system.

GAPS IN THE SYSTEM

In our rapidly changing health care system, health insurance does not ensure access to health care. Health care providers increasingly are choosing which insurance they will accept, and many plans, even if accepted, do not cover preventive care (Valdez et al. 1993; Committee on Small Business 1994; Himmelstein and Woolhandler 1995). Furthermore, gatekeeper arrangements and utilization review practices in managed care both restrict and alter the use of services. Consequently, poor and uninsured Hispanics pay high out-of-pocket fees; experience long waits in crowded, underfunded clinics; and face problems being admitted to charity and public hospitals, many of which are closing (Giachello 1994; Committee on Small Business 1994).

There are also indications that the health care system is not responsive to patients who have different cultural practices or languages (Andersen et al. 1981; Solis et al. 1990). Hispanics value personal touch, good treatment, and trust in the physician-patient relationship (Giachello 1994). Yet the actual quality of the relationship they experience may be jeopardized by prejudices that reinforce the social distance between patients and providers.

Empirical models indicate that health need and financial factors, including income level and whether there is insurance coverage, are the strongest determinants of entry into health care for Hispanics (Andersen et al. 1981; Giachello 1994; Guendelman and Schwalbe 1986). Nonetheless, when individuals are in the system, language, institutional, and discrimination barriers tend to discourage further use of services.

Ultimately, Hispanics' use of health services, and the satisfaction with the services that they receive, reflect the degree of their access to care (Andersen et al. 1981; Giachello 1994; Bashshur et al. 1994). Several studies show that Hispanics use fewer services than non-Hispanics (Andersen et al. 1981; Freeman et al. 1990; Giachello 1994; Robert Wood Johnson Foundation 1987; Lieu, Newacheck and McManus 1993; Committee on Small Business 1994; Guendelman and Schwalbe 1986; Bashshur et al. 1994; Trevino and Moss 1984). Studies also show that Hispanics are not satisfied with the medical care they receive (Andersen et al. 1981; Trevino et al. 1991). Yet Hispanic subpopulations also differ in their use of medical care (Trevino et al. 1991; Schur et al. 1987; Markides et al. 1985). Puerto Ricans and Cubans are the highest users, whereas Mexicans are the lowest (Schur et al. 1987). The degree of satisfaction reflected by each Hispanic subpopulation is not known.

The most recent large representative survey of access to care comparing Hispanic subpopulations was conducted in 1982–84. The proliferation of managed care programs and the heavy influx of newcomers into the United States in recent years, however, makes a new assessment of the health system's responsiveness to diverse Hispanic groups very timely.

This chapter assesses the patterns of health care utilization and satisfaction in the representative sample of Hispanics of diverse national origins in The Commonwealth Fund Minority Health Survey (CMHS). In addition, we examine the effects of perceived experiences with health services and of socioeconomic, structural, cultural/migratory, behavioral, and health status differentials on the use of and satisfaction with health services. Through a better understanding of these subpopulations and their experiences in the health system, we can plan better services to prevent Hispanics from losing further ground.

METHODS OF ANALYSIS

Sample and Data Collection Procedures

The analytic sample for this study was restricted to the 1,001 subjects of Hispanic origin in the survey, which included 552 (55.1%) Mexican Americans, 146 (14.6%) Puerto Ricans, and 303 (30.3%) "Other Hispanics." Although individuals in the latter group originated from various Latin American countries, such as Cuba, Costa Rica, and the Dominican Republic, separate analysis by country of origin was precluded because of small sample sizes.

Telephone interviews of approximately twenty-five minutes' duration were conducted in English or Spanish with an adult who answered the call in a selected household. Interview calls were made at different times of day, and the interviews took place either by appointment or at the time of the call. (See Technical Appendix for more details.)

Variables

The outcomes were three dimensions of health care utilization: (1) the probability of gaining entry into health care over the last 12 months prior to the interview; (2) the number of visits (volume) among users in the last 12 months; and (3) satisfaction with the health care provider. "Entry" is a measure of achievement in getting into the health care system, and "volume" is a measure of use of services after entry. This distinction allows for a separate analysis of the barriers that influence patient-initiated entry into care, which tends to reflect discretionary use, and barriers to follow-up care, which is generally introduced by the provider (Schur et al. 1987; Newhouse et al. 1980). "Satisfaction" is a measure of perceived quality of care. We measured satisfaction with a four-point Likert scale ranging from very satisfied to very dissatisfied and later dichotomized to minimize problems of unreliability and measurement error (Ross et al. 1995).

Three types of independent variables were considered to be potential influences on the outcomes: need-related, enabling, and predisposing variables (Andersen et al. 1981). Variables were selected based on previous literature (Andersen et al. 1981; Giachello 1994; Markides et al. 1985; Robert Wood Johnson Foundation 1987; Ross et al. 1994; Schur et al. 1987; Solis et al. 1990; Thamer et al. 1997; Valdez et al. 1993) or on whether they were at least moderately associated with an outcome. We assessed health need by perceived health status, which is a subjective measure of overall health described as excellent, good, fair, or poor, and by the extent of current satisfaction with life, which is a proxy for quality of life and well-being (Guyatt et al. 1993), ranging from very satisfied to very dissatisfied.

Financial factors and structural factors were the enabling variables examined. The financial factors were income; receipt of food stamps, Aid to Families with Dependent Children (AFDC), or Supplemental Securities

Income (SSI); employment status; and health insurance coverage. The health insurance variable included "any private insurance," "only public," and "none," and was further categorized into coverage through a private health maintenance organization (HMO), private non-HMO, public HMO, and public non-HMO. Structural factors, which assess availability of services, included having a regular source of care, the amount of time spent with the doctor, and having a choice of where to get care. We also assessed subjective experiences, including measuring perceptions of any barrier to care; whether the quality of care received was lower owing to the person's ethnicity; whether the individual was refused or postponed health care during the past year; and whether the individual was treated badly, distrusted doctors, or felt welcome by the doctor.

Predisposing factors refer to the demographic, behavioral, and acculturation variables that antecede an illness episode. The demographic variables examined were age, gender, level of education, number of people in the household, and marital status. The behavioral variables included current smoking status, daily number of cigarettes consumed, and the use of any herbal medicine. Acculturation indicators included generational status (first versus second or beyond), number of years in the United States (categorized into less than 5 years and 5 years or more for the foreign born), use of English as the primary language, and the use of an interpreter to interact with the health care system. National origin was the key stratifying variable used to assess differences across Hispanic subpopulations.

Analytic Techniques

We examined differences in perceptions and sources of care and demographic, behavioral, and health characteristics among Mexican Americans, Puerto Ricans, and "Other Hispanics" by using bivariate analyses. We tested statistical significance across the three subgroups by performing a chi-square test for categorical variables and a one-way analysis of variance (ANOVA) for continuous variables.

Next, the relationship between each outcome and each independent variable was examined using bivariate analyses. Logistic regression analyses were performed to determine which variables in the data set predicted entry into care and satisfaction with the provider. Linear regression was used to examine volume of care. Standardized odds-ratios, beta coefficients, and their 95 percent confidence intervals (CIs) were calculated.

We constructed the multivariate models independently for each outcome by using a four-step approach. First, we examined the effects of predisposing and enabling factors exclusive of health status. Next, we added health status and examined changes in the first step's covariates. We then forced in cultural factors, including national origin and generational status, to determine whether the three Hispanic subpopulations differed with respect to these outcomes after controlling for all the other variables in the model. In the final step we examined numerous interaction terms, none of which proved significant. At every step, checks for colinearity were performed. Because the models were not altered much after adjusting for health status, we report only our results that include health status in the model. To assess goodness-of-fit, the Pregibon link test (Pregibon 1979) was generated for the logistic regression models, and an R^2 and an F-test were calculated for volume of care.

Considering that the survey used a multistage, stratified probability sample, weighting was taken into account for all estimation and statistical testing procedures. The original survey weights were corrected for an over-representation of Hispanics in the survey by gender, race, age, educational attainment, and health insurance status (see Technical Appendix). We calculated new weights for this analysis to maintain parity between the original weights and the sample sizes of each subpopulation. Complex design effects were considered using SUDAAN, version 6.34 (Shah et al. 1992).

RESULTS OF ANALYSIS

Demographic and Health Characteristics

The majority of the Hispanic respondents were between 18 and 44 years of age, married, born in the United States, and employed (Table 2.1). The median household income category was $25,001 to $35,000, with 11.3 percent of households receiving public assistance. Reported education levels tended to be low; 25.2 percent of the respondents had less than a high school education. Although most (76.4%) perceived their health as excellent or good, barriers to health care were prevalent. Some 41.4 percent of the respondents reported having no regular source of health care. More than one-third (36.7%) had no health insurance coverage, and 11.3 percent of those covered at the time of the survey had had a lapse in health insurance in the last 2 years. Furthermore, 31.3 percent felt somewhat or not at all welcome by their doctor.

Table 2.1 Demographic and Health Characteristics among Hispanics

	Total		Mexican Americans (N = 552)		Puerto Ricans (N = 146)		Other Hispanics (N = 303)		Adjusted p value[a]
	%	SE	Weighted Mean or %	SE	Weighted Mean or %	SE	Weighted Mean or %	SE	
					Weighted Proportions				
Age									0.30
18–29	33.5	1.80	35.6	2.1	35.2	4.6	29.1	3.2	
30–44	36.1	1.68	36.0	2.1	38.0	4.7	35.4	3.0	
45–64	25.0	1.45	23.2	2.1	23.3	3.2	28.9	2.5	
65+	5.4	0.80	5.2	0.9	3.5	1.9	6.7	1.6	
Female	50.3	1.78	51.4	2.5	48.9	4.4	49.0	2.9	0.79
Has a regular doctor	58.6	2.10	56.2	2.7	62.5	4.6	61.0	3.8	0.35
Household Income									0.44
$7,500 or less	13.4	1.20	12.7	1.5	18.1	3.9	12.4	1.9	—
$7,501–$15,000	14.4	1.37	15.4	1.9	9.5	3.1	15.1	2.6	—
$15,001–$25,000	22.0	1.77	20.8	2.2	22.4	4.2	23.8	3.1	—
$25,001–$35,000	17.5	1.16	18.8	1.6	19.2	3.2	14.3	1.8	—
$35,001–$50,000	17.4	1.37	18.6	1.5	15.3	2.7	16.1	2.6	—
$50,001+	15.4	1.32	13.7	1.5	15.6	3.3	18.3	2.6	—

(continues)

Table 2.1 (*Continued*)

	Total		Mexican Americans (N = 552)		Puerto Ricans (N = 146)		Other Hispanics (N = 303)		Adjusted p value[a]
	%	SE	Weighted Mean or %	SE	Weighted Mean or %	SE	Weighted Mean or %	SE	
					Weighted Proportions				
Receives food stamps, AFDC, or SSI	11.3	1.27	11.8	1.9	19.3	3.1	6.5	1.6	0.04
Education[b]									0.02
Less than high school	25.2	1.80	29.0	2.2	29.3	3.8	16.6	3.3	—
High school graduate	36.2	1.66	39.3	2.5	30.9	3.8	33.2	3.9	—
Some college	26.7	1.35	21.8	1.9	29.5	4.1	32.3	2.7	—
College graduate/ graduate school	12.4	0.74	10.0	0.9	10.3	2.4	17.9	1.9	—
Marital status									0.78
Single	24.0	1.78	23.1	2.3	24.5	3.9	25.3	3.6	—
Married or cohabitating	58.4	1.68	60.3	2.2	54.0	4.8	57.1	3.5	—
Divorced, widowed, separated	17.6	1.34	16.6	1.9	21.5	4.4	17.6	2.4	—
Employment status									0.82
Labor force: employed	68.5	1.65	69.1	2.7	70.5	3.5	66.4	2.7	—
Labor force: unemployed	8.7	1.14	8.7	1.6	6.1	2.7	9.9	2.0	—
Not in labor force	22.8	1.45	22.2	2.0	23.4	3.6	23.7	2.4	—

									P value
Health Insurance[b]									0.49
Private HMO	16.3	1.21	15.4	1.8	20.5	3.1	15.9	1.8	—
Private non-HMO	33.1	1.72	34.0	2.4	34.2	3.7	30.7	2.7	—
Only public HMO	2.2	0.33	1.7	1.0	1.3	0.8	2.2	0.8	—
Only public non-HMO	12.2	0.45	11.8	1.5	16.2	2.8	11.2	2.0	—
None	36.7	2.08	37.4	2.7	27.9	4.0	40.0	4.1	—
Lacked health insurance in past 2 years	11.3	0.93	10.6	1.2	14.7	2.6	11.1	2.0	0.41
Health status									0.28
Excellent	28.8	1.60	26.6	1.9	29.5	4.0	32.2	3.4	—
Good	49.6	2.00	48.6	3.0	44.4	4.1	47.1	3.3	—
Fair	19.0	1.60	18.6	2.2	21.5	3.5	18.4	2.8	—
Poor	4.8	0.70	6.2	1.4	4.6	1.7	2.3	0.7	—
Feels welcome by doctor									0.12
Very welcome	68.7	2.07	70.5	3.0	57.9	3.9	70.4	2.8	—
Somewhat welcome	28.2	1.75	27.1	2.6	40.0	4.0	24.7	2.7	—
Not at all welcome	3.1	0.80	2.4	1.0	2.1	0.9	4.8	1.4	—
Current smoker	20.1	1.32	18.8	1.7	29.5	4.3	20.8	2.5	0.10
First generation	32.6	3.29	30.5	3.6	6.2	2.5	49.0	4.9	<0.01
Years in U.S.									0.02
≤5	2.9	0.73	3.3	1.2	0.0	0.0	3.6	1.1	—
6+	29.7	2.83	27.4	2.9	6.2	2.5	45.2	4.8	—
Born in U.S.	67.5	3.30	69.4	3.6	93.8	2.5	51.2	5.0	—
Needs interpreter	10.9	1.65	13.9	2.2	5.3	1.7	8.3	2.5	0.06

(continues)

Table 2.1 (Continued)

	Total		Mexican Americans (N = 552)		Puerto Ricans (N = 146)		Other Hispanics (N = 303)		Adjusted p value[a]
	%	SE	Weighted Mean or %	SE	Weighted Mean or %	SE	Weighted Mean or %	SE	
					Weighted Means				
People in household	3.6	0.07	3.77	0.09	3.25	0.13	3.32	0.11	<0.01
Children in household	1.4	0.05	1.59	0.07	1.32	0.12	1.22	0.08	<0.01
Mental health score	11.47	0.15	11.30	0.21	12.32	0.34	11.37	0.31	0.09
Cigarettes per day (smokers)	11.63	0.81	9.77	0.96	11.71	1.12	14.57	1.68	0.04

Source: Data from The Commonwealth Fund Minority Health Survey, 1994.
[a]Corrected for complex design effects.
[b]N = 545.

Overall, the three Hispanic subpopulations had similar sociodemo-graphic and health profiles. Nonetheless, Mexican Americans and Puerto Ricans were more likely than "Other Hispanics" to have less than a high school education (p = 0.02). Compared to the other two subpopula-tions, Mexican Americans were the most likely to have large households with numerous children (p < 0.01), and they were the least likely to smoke (p = 0.10) (data not shown). Among smokers, Mexican Ameri-cans consumed the least number of cigarettes (p = 0.04). "Other His-panics" were the most likely to be recent immigrants (p < 0.01), and these were the least likely to receive public assistance (p = 0.04).

Experience with Health Care Providers

Approximately 78 percent of the Hispanic respondents had entered the health care system in the past year (Table 2.2). Acculturation, financial factors, availability of care, and perceptions of barriers to care were as-sociated with entry into care in the past 12 months. Hispanics born in the United States were more likely than immigrants to have used health services (p = 0.05). Those Hispanics who had a regular source of care, experienced no barriers to care, and felt welcome by the doctor were more likely to use health care when compared to Hispanics who had no regular source of care (p < 0.01), experienced barriers to care (p < 0.01), and felt somewhat welcome or not at all welcome by the doctor (p = 0.02). Perceived health status was significantly related to entry (p < 0.04), such that worse health increased the likelihood of health ser-vices utilization.

In addition, Hispanics with health insurance, particularly insurance through an HMO, were more likely to use services than those without insurance (see Table 2.2; p = 0.01). In our sample, membership in an HMO varied by geographic region. HMO membership was twice as high for Hispanics in urban (26.2%) or suburban areas (28.9%) com-pared to rural areas (14%). HMO membership also varied by ethnicity: 62 percent of the Hispanics had health insurance, and of these, 29 per-cent reported being a member of an HMO; in comparison, 23 percent of the 88 percent of whites covered by any insurance were enrolled in HMOs. Similarly, a recent study of a representative sample of 18- to 64-year-old California residents reports a higher representation of Hispanics in HMOs than in indemnity plans, whereas the reverse pattern is ob-served for whites (Gordon et al. 1997).

Using multivariate logistic regression, we found that among CMHS

Table 2.2   Characteristics of Entry and Satisfaction of Care among Hispanics in the Last Twelve Months

	Entry to Care				Satisfaction with Care			
	N^a	No (%)	Yes (%)	Adjusted p value[b]	N^a	Satisfied (%)	Dissatisfied (%)	Adjusted p value[b]
Total	991	21.7	78.3		983	85.5	14.5	
Ethnicity	990				983			
Mexican	547	22.2	77.8	0.79	542	89.1	10.9	0.06
Puerto Rican	142	19.3	80.7		144	79.5	20.5	
Other Hispanic	301	21.6	78.4		297	81.9	18.1	
English as primary language	985				978			
Yes	577	18.9	81.1	0.13	574	83.2	16.8	0.06
No	408	25.4	74.6		404	88.7	11.3	
Generations in U.S.	988				981			
First generation	321	27.1	72.9	0.05	317	89.4	10.6	0.07
Second generation or later	667	19.0	81.0		664	83.9	16.1	
Years in U.S.	990				983			
≤5	29	36.0	64.0	0.12	29	97.3	2.7	0.09
6+	292	26.3	73.7		288	88.6	11.4	
Born in U.S.	669	18.9	81.1		667	83.7	16.3	
Use of herbal medicine	984				978			
Yes	231	25.9	74.1	0.21	229	77.7	22.3	0.01
No / not sure	753	20.4	79.6		749	88.0	12.0	
Quality of care less owing to ethnicity	976				972			
Yes	137	18.3	81.7	0.50	137	74.9	25.1	0.03
No	839	21.6	78.4		835	87.1	12.9	
Choice of where to get care	967				956			
A great deal	414	14.8	85.2	0.05	412	96.8	3.2	<0.01
Some	250	19.0	81.0		247	88.6	11.4	
Very little	212	33.8	66.2		210	71.9	28.1	
No choice	91	23.5	76.5		86	59.9	40.1	
Regular source of care	987				980			
Yes	577	8.6	91.4	<0.01	576	93.8	6.2	<0.01
No / not sure	410	39.5	60.5		405	74.0	26.0	
Barriers to care	990				983			
One or more	840	23.6	76.4	<0.01	834	83.0	17.0	<0.01
None	150	10.2	89.8		149	99.5	0.5	
Feels welcome by doctor	970				968			
Very	666	15.9	84.1	0.02	668	92.3	7.7	<0.01
Somewhat	274	31.2	68.8		271	76.1	23.9	
Not at all	30	34.8	65.2		30	43.8	56.2	

(continues)

Table 2.2 (*Continued*)

		Entry to Care				Satisfaction with Care		
	N^a	No (%)	Yes (%)	Adjusted p value[b]	N^a	Satisfied (%)	Dissatisfied (%)	Adjusted p value[b]
Trusts doctors	978				972			
Very much	485	16.2	83.8	0.02	485	91.4	8.6	0.04
Somewhat	404	26.7	73.3		393	82.8	17.2	
Not very much	56	24.8	75.2		58	67.3	32.7	
Not at all	33	23.2	76.8		36	68.5	31.5	
Time spent with doctor in last visit	968				961			
<5 minutes	37	28.0	72.0	0.92	37	65.9	34.1	0.10
5–15 minutes	344	21.0	79.0		346	82.0	18.0	
16–30 minutes	393	19.7	80.3		388	87.4	12.6	
31 minutes–1 hour	147	19.4	80.6		142	91.2	8.8	
>1 hour	47	21.6	78.4		42	93.3	6.7	
Postponed getting care in past 12 months	984				978			
Yes	322	22.2	77.8	0.70	316	71.2	28.8	<0.01
No	663	20.8	79.2		662	92.6	7.4	
Refused care in past 12 months	987				980			
Yes	22	10.6	89.4	0.19	22	41.8	58.2	0.04
No	965	21.7	78.3		959	86.5	13.6	
Treated badly in past 12 months	975				969			
Yes	104	20.5	79.5	0.81	103	10.3	89.7	<0.01
No	871	19.2	80.8		867	46.5	53.5	
Welfare	990				983			
AFDC, SSI, or food stamps	110	23.9	76.1	0.68	112	79.2	20.8	0.17
None	879	21.3	78.7		871	86.3	13.7	
Insurance	991				983			
Private HMO	163	8.6	91.4	<0.01	161	92.5	7.5	<0.01
Private non-HMO	328	13.7	86.3		329	91.8	8.2	
Only public HMO	17	5.9	94.1		17	82.4	17.6	
Only public non-HMO	120	19.2	80.8		120	88.3	11.7	
None	363	36.4	63.6		357	75.6	24.4	
Gender	990				983			
Male	489	18.9	81.1	0.15	499	83.4	16.6	0.15
Female	501	24.4	75.6		485	87.6	12.4	
Age (continuous variable)								
Mean in years	989	37.2	41.2	0.03	983	41.8	34.9	<0.01

(*continues*)

Table 2.2 (Continued)

		Entry to Care				Satisfaction with Care		
	N^a	No (%)	Yes (%)	Adjusted p value[b]	N^a	Satisfied (%)	Dissatisfied (%)	Adjusted p value[b]
Number of people in household								
Mean number	988	3.68	3.54	0.32	982	3.60	3.27	0.13
Health status	986				979			
Excellent	283	26.3	73.7	0.04	281	89.0	11.0	0.13
Good	471	21.8	78.2		463	86.7	13.3	
Fair	187	17.3	82.7		189	82.9	17.1	
Poor	44	10.0	90.0		46	69.5	30.5	
Overall satisfaction with life	985				978			
Very satisfied	498	20.7	79.3	0.80	494	91.8	8.2	0.01
Somewhat satisfied	386	21.6	78.4		385	85.6	14.4	
Somewhat dissatisfied	75	27.0	73.0		72	53.4	46.6	
Very dissatisfied	26	24.4	75.6		26	58.1	41.9	
Cigarettes smoked per day Mean number								
(all persons)	989	3.1	2.1	0.17	983	1.9	4.5	0.02
Mean number (among smokers)	195	12.0	11.6	0.84	196	10.8	13.3	0.28

Source: Data from The Commonwealth Fund Minority Health Survey, 1994.
[a]May not add exactly owing to rounding.
[b]Adjusted for complex survey design.

respondents, the model for entry into the health care system was significantly determined by availability of care, financial factors, and perceived experiences with the health care system (Table 2.3). Individuals who had a regular source of care were four times as likely to enter the health care system than those who did not. Also, those who felt very welcome by the doctor and who felt that the quality of care they received was not lessened because of their ethnicity were 2.4 and 3.2 times, respectively, as likely to utilize health care as those who did not feel welcome by the doctor and those who felt they received poorer quality care because of their ethnicity.

In this multivariate model, insurance coverage significantly increased the likelihood of entry into care. Compared with individuals with no health insurance, those covered by private insurance in an HMO were

Table 2.3   Predictors of Entry into Health Care for Hispanics in the Last Twelve Months
($N = 947$)

	Adjusted Odds Ratio[a]	95% Confidence Interval
Health need		
Health status		
Excellent	0.28	0.06,1.23
Good	0.42	0.10,1.83
Fair	0.76	0.20,3.03
Enabling factors		
Health Insurance		
Private HMO	4.61	2.19,9.17
Private non-HMO	2.70	1.62,4.49
Only public HMO	5.61	1.34,23.48
Only public non-HMO	1.48	0.79,2.78
Regular source of care	4.24	2.75,6.26
Feels welcome by doctor		
Very	2.35	1.09,5.45
Somewhat	1.09	0.48,2.47
Quality of care less owing to ethnicity	3.23	1.52,7.02
Predisposing factors		
Ethnicity		
Puerto Rican	1.17	0.59,2.33
Other Hispanic	1.10	0.67,1.79
First generation	0.81	0.53,1.31
Use of herbal medicine	0.68	0.38,1.17
Age (continuous variable)	1.00	1.00,1.01

Source: Data from The Commonwealth Fund Minority Health Survey, 1994.

Note: Dependant variable: 0, did not visit doctor; 1, visited doctor. Referent categories: poor health status, no insurance, no regular source of care, feels not at all welcome, quality of care is not less owing to ethnicity, Mexican American, second or later generation, no use of herbal medicine.

[a]Adjusted for complex survey design.

4.6 times as likely to use the health care system. Those with private in-surance but who did not belong to an HMO were approximately 2.7 times as likely to enter. Less than 2 percent had public insurance through an HMO. Compared to the uninsured, this public HMO group was 5.6 times as likely to enter into care. Individuals with publicly funded insur-ance who were not enrolled in an HMO were not significantly more likely to enter the health care system than individuals without insurance. Compared to the uninsured, those with public non-HMO insurance were over the age of 65, received other forms of public assistance, were either unemployed or not in the work force, or were single. After adjusting for other factors, health status and cultural factors (such as national origin and generational status) did not predict entry. The Pregibon link goodness-of-fit test did not indicate that there were any problems with the model.

On average, Hispanics had made 5.3 visits to the health care system in the past year (data not shown). An analysis of the log of the volume, which gives a more normal distribution by controlling for outliers, indicated that Puerto Ricans made slightly more visits than the other two subgroups (data not shown; $p = 0.06$). The volume of visits for people with at least one visit was significantly higher for English-speaking than Spanish-speaking Hispanics ($p = 0.05$) and was higher for those living in the country for five years or less than those who had lived in the country longer than five years ($p = 0.02$). Females experienced a higher volume of visits than males ($p < 0.01$), regardless of whether they were of reproductive age or older than 45 years. Volume was also significantly higher for individuals with a regular source of care, compared to those without a regular source of care ($p = 0.01$); for individuals who had been refused care at some time in the past year ($p < 0.01$); for those receiving some type of public assistance ($p < 0.01$); and for individuals suffering from ill health ($p < 0.01$) (data not shown).

After adjusting for other variables in a multivariate model, the strongest predictors of volume were (1) health status; (2) public insurance, particularly those with HMO coverage; (3) having a regular source of care; (4) having been refused care; and (5) having experienced bad treatment in the past year. Demographic variables, such as being female, of younger age, and living in a larger household size, were also strong determinants (Table 2.4). National origin was not an important predictor of volume. The use of English as a primary language and a newcomer immigrant status significantly increased the volume of visits, after adjusting for other variables. Overall, the model accounted for 20 percent of the variance in volume of care ($F_{19,\ 743} = 77.69$; $p < 0.01$).

Levels of Health Care Satisfaction

Most Hispanics (85.5%) were satisfied with their regular doctor or health care professional (see Table 2.2). Satisfaction was positively associated with the lack of herbal medicine usage ($p = 0.01$), an absence of feelings that the quality of care received was lower because of the respondent's ethnicity ($p = 0.03$), having a regular source of care ($p < 0.01$), perceiving no barriers to care ($p < 0 .01$), not having postponed getting care (p < 0.01), and feeling very welcome by the doctor (p < 0.01). Not being refused care (p = 0.04) and having insurance, particularly private insurance through an HMO (p < 0.01), were also significantly associated with satisfaction.

The multivariate model (Table 2.5) identified several predictors of satisfaction. Compared to individuals who had no choice of where to get care, those individuals who reported having a great deal of choice were

Table 2.4   Predictors of Volume of Health Care Utilization in the Last Twelve Months for Hispanics ($N = 764$)

	Beta[a]	95% Confidence Interval
Health need		
Health status		
Excellent	−0.98	−1.29,−0.66
Good	−0.42	−0.73,−0.10
Fair	−0.19	−0.52,0.14
Enabling factors		
Health Insurance		
Private HMO	0.21	0.01,0.40
Private non-HMO	0.15	−0.01,0.31
Only public HMO	0.54	−0.01,1.09
Only public non-HMO	0.27	0.09,0.45
Regular source of care	0.20	0.04,0.35
Treated badly in past 12 months	0.28	0.07,0.50
Predisposing factors		
Ethnicity		
Puerto Rican	0.15	0.03,0.33
Gender (0 − male, 1 − female)	0.31	0.198,0.42
Age (continuous variable)	−0.0009	0.001,0.0003
Number of people in household	0.05	0.01,0.09
Years in U.S.		
≤5 and foreign born	0.52	0.23,0.82
6+ and foreign born	0.19	0.10,0.49
First generation	−0.05	0.20,0.11
English as primary language	0.17	0.02,0.33

Source: Data from The Commonwealth Fund Minority Health Survey, 1994.

Note: Dependent variable: natural log number of visits to doctor in last year. Referent categories: poor health status, no insurance, no regular source of care, feels not at all welcome, quality of care is not less owing to ethnicity, Mexican American, second or later generation, no use of herbal medicine, not treated badly in last 12 months, not refused care in last 12 months, male, born in U.S., English not primary language.

[a]Adjusted for complex survey design.

$R^2 = 0.20$.

$F_{19,743} = 77.69; p < .01$.

7.3 times as likely to be satisfied with their doctor. Availability of a regular source of care increased satisfaction approximately fivefold, compared to having no regular source of care. In addition, a lack of any barrier to care, in contrast to one or more barriers, increased satisfaction significantly. Whereas the amount of time spent with the doctor was positively associated with satisfaction in the initial multivariate analysis ($p = 0.006$), it no longer remained significant after correcting for complex design effects.

Perceptions of the quality of personal interactions with the health care provider also predicted satisfaction with the care received. Individuals treated badly were more likely to be dissatisfied than those treated well, and those who trusted doctors were four times as likely to be satisfied with the care received as those who did not trust doctors.

Although perceived health status was not a significant predictor of satisfaction, mental health and smoking behavior were strong predictors. Compared to individuals who were very dissatisfied with life, those who expressed high satisfaction with life were almost ten times as likely to be satisfied with the health care provider. The more cigarettes consumed by smokers, the more likely they were to be dissatisfied with the provider.

Satisfaction with the provider was higher among "Other Hispanics" than Mexican Americans. Satisfaction was 2.8 times as high among first-generation compared to second-generation Hispanics. Interestingly, after controlling for other factors, financial factors did not appear to be significant predictors of satisfaction. The Pregibon link goodness-of-fit test indicated that there were no problems with the model's fit.

PATTERNS OF VULNERABILITY IN HEALTH CARE ACCESS

Our findings indicate that 78 percent of the adult Hispanics surveyed had gained entry into the health care system in the past year, making 5.3 visits on average. In comparison, 87 percent of white non-Hispanics and 89 percent of African Americans had gained entry in that same period (Louis Harris and Associates 1994). These findings for Hispanics are alarming, given the rapid growth of the U.S. Hispanic population, the recent cutbacks in health services because of cost-containment efforts, and legislation resulting in reduced services to immigrants.

Who among the Hispanics are the most vulnerable to health access problems? The study shows that patterns of use among the three Hispanic subpopulations are similar. This is not surprising because the groups do not differ much in the distribution of characteristics corre-

Table 2.5 Predictors of Satisfaction with Care among Hispanics ($N = 919$)

	Adjusted Odds Ratio[a]	95% Confidence Interval
Health need		
Health status		
Excellent	1.59	0.47,5.36
Good	1.81	0.66,4.91
Fair	1.32	0.44,3.96
Overall satisfaction with life		
Very satisfied	9.88	2.76,35.32
Somewhat satisfied	8.76	2.65,28.96
Somewhat dissatisfied	1.82	0.46,7.19
Enabling factors		
Choice of where to get care		
A great deal	7.32	2.75,19.49
Some	3.59	1.51,8.50
Very little	1.39	0.63,3.04
Postponed getting care in past 12 months	0.46	0.21,1.02
Treated badly in past 12 months	0.17	0.08,0.39
Regular source of care	5.36	2.76,10.45
Any barriers versus none	0.14	0.02,0.93
Trusts doctors		
Very much	3.83	0.94,15.73
Somewhat	4.32	1.31,14.27
Not very much	3.46	0.72,16.58
Amount of time spent with doctor in last visit		
<5 minutes	0.27	0.03,2.63
5–15 minutes	0.23	0.04,1.28
16–30 minutes	0.37	0.06,2.35
31 minutes–1 hour	0.78	0.10,6.14
Predisposing factors		
Ethnicity		
Puerto Rican	0.59	0.27,1.30
Other Hispanic	0.48	0.26,0.90
Cigarettes smoked per day (all persons)	0.94	0.90,0.97
English as primary language	0.69	0.34,1.40
First generation (0 = second or later, 1 = first)	2.76	1.24,6.17

Source: Data from The Commonwealth Fund Minority Health Survey, 1994.

Note: Dependent variable: 1, satisfied; 0, dissatisfied. Referent categories: poor health, very dissatisfied, no choice, did not postpone care, not treated badly, no regular source of care, no barriers, does not trust doctors at all, >1 hour spent with doctor, Mexican American, English not primary language, second or later generation.

[a]Adjusted for complex survey design.

lated with health services utilization in other studies. Similarities among the Hispanic subgroups in this study may be a result of the sampling approach, because only households with telephones were surveyed. After adjusting for other cultural, financial, structural, perceptual, behavioral, and health status characteristics, we found no differences in entry, volume, or satisfaction among the three Hispanic subpopulations. The only exception was a higher level of satisfaction among "Other Hispanics" than Mexican Americans, perhaps because "Other Hispanics" were more likely to be newcomer immigrants.

The findings suggest that acculturation variables, other than national origin, may be sensitive determinants of patterns of health care use among Hispanic adults. After controlling for other variables in the model, familiarity with the English language and having lived in the United States for no more than 5 years increased the volume of visits to providers. Moreover, first-generation Hispanics were almost three times as likely to be satisfied with their health care providers as U.S.-born, second-generation Hispanics. Acculturation variables did not affect entry into care, however.

Prediction of Usage and Satisfaction

Structural factors that measure availability of care were stronger than cultural factors as determinants of use. Consistent with other studies, having a regular source of care strongly predicted all three outcomes. After controlling for other factors, this one factor increased the probability of entering the health care system by 4.2 times and the probability of being satisfied with the health care provider by 5 times. Furthermore, having a choice of where to get care increased satisfaction 7.3 times. A regular source of care was also positively correlated with the number of visits.

Because more than 40 percent of the survey respondents lacked a regular source of care, making large improvements in health care system responsiveness and satisfaction with care would require greatly increasing access to a regular source of care. Unfortunately, political and welfare reforms that cap health insurance benefits constrain these opportunities for many Hispanics. Nonetheless, the expansion of managed care programs and the freedom to choose among plans may increase the opportunity for Hispanics to have a regular source of care.

Insurance status and HMO membership strongly affected entry into care. Belonging to an HMO with either public or private insurance increased the likelihood of entry, while lack of health insurance decreased entry. For example, people with private insurance through an HMO were approximately 5 times as likely to enter the health care system as people without insurance. Those with HMO coverage were more likely than individuals with non-HMO coverage to enter health care, probably because an HMO facilitates entry through cost sharing, and the cost is typically less than for private fee-for-service–based insurance plans. Lower premiums and copayments may partially influence low-income individuals in their decision to seek care. We found that insurance coverage also influenced the volume of care—a situation that reflects stronger decision making by the provider than by the consumer.

Public insurance correlated more strongly with volume than private insurance, especially among those individuals who did not belong to an HMO. Perhaps this is because poorer people tend to be sicker and because non-HMO providers are less likely than HMOs to limit follow-up visits to contain costs. These findings corroborate other studies (Valdez et al. 1993; Giachello 1994; Schur et al. 1987; Halfon et al. 1997) indicating that health insurance coverage significantly influences the ability of Hispanics to obtain needed services. Because 37 percent of the Hispanic survey respondents were uninsured, this lack of coverage depresses Hispanic utilization rates. Legislative changes in Medicaid and social service provisions to immigrants further restrict access to care for newcomer and undocumented Hispanics. If the traditional safety net disappears—which has been delivering health care to the uninsured—this population will have nowhere to turn.

Subjective Experiences Predict Satisfaction

Interestingly, financial factors do not influence satisfaction with the provider, after adjusting for other factors. Instead, in addition to availability of care, subjective experiences with both the health care system and the provider are significant determinants of satisfaction. Our analysis found that Hispanics are more likely to be dissatisfied if they feel they have been treated badly by providers and staff, and if they do not trust doctors. First-generation Hispanics were more likely to be satisfied with the health care system than second-generation Hispanics, perhaps owing to lower expectations.

Perceived experiences with the health care system are also important predictors of entry and volume. Findings from the multivariate models indicate that the individuals who felt welcome by their doctors were 2.3 times as likely to gain entrance to care. Those who felt that the quality of care they received was not inferior because of their ethnicity were 3.2 times as likely to gain entry. In contrast, people who were refused care or who felt that the health care system treated them badly were actually more likely to have more visits. Unfortunately, from these cross-sectional data we could not ascertain whether more exposure to the system increased negative perceptions, or alternatively, whether bad treatment from providers increased an individual's health care needs. However, the former seems more probable. The logical extension is that sicker individuals risk exposure to more insults, and this leads them to pull back from the health care system. If this is true, then the health care system needs to be more sensitive to get them back into the system.

Past studies have shown that socioeconomic factors are the strongest determinants of health care utilization for Hispanics, and that structural, gender, language use, and social discrimination predict volume among those individuals using health care (Giachello 1994). Our findings show that subjective experiences with the health care system strongly influence entry, volume, and satisfaction. Given the rapid changes in the organization and delivery of care, experiences with quality care may be gaining far more influence as determinants of utilization.

The health status of Hispanics is a weak predictor of entry into care, but it strongly influences the number of visits after controlling for other factors. Other health indicators, such as satisfaction with life and tobacco use, positively influence satisfaction, although they are not predictors of satisfaction.

Sampling Cautions

Our results must be interpreted cautiously because of some limitations in the study design. Because the survey only sampled households with telephones, it may under-represent Hispanic households without telephones, such as those of seasonal migrants, undocumented immigrants, and newcomers. The sample may also be biased toward more educated, wealthier, and employed individuals, which could have a significant impact on some estimates and comparisons (U.S. Bureau of the Census 1994).

Most likely, this survey under-represents more vulnerable and less-educated Hispanics, suggesting that the findings are conservative. Second, the cross-sectional design does not allow a determination of the temporal sequence of the independent variables relative to the outcomes. Third, self-reporting of insurance and HMO status may be inaccurate because of the multiple changes in health care organization. Last, methodological research on Hispanics has documented problems that are likely to attend in administering surveys to this group, such as acquiescence or providing more "socially desirable" responses and related skewedness in the distribution of responses to Likert scales such as the ones used in this study (Marin and Marin 1991).

Despite these shortcomings, the findings suggest that access to care for Hispanics remains a major problem in the United States. They also suggest that significant differentials exist by structural and financial availability, experiences with the health care system, and migratory history. Further research would help distinguish the specific barriers that affect inpatient and outpatient care. In the meantime, entry into care may be facilitated by policies that ensure basic insurance benefits and increase Hispanic enrollment in low-cost HMOs.

POLICY IMPLICATIONS

The high rate of uninsurance among Hispanics limits their access to health care services. As previous studies have shown, a lack of insurance for Hispanics is associated with lower income, educational attainment, and occupational status, as well as with illegal immigration status, foreign birth, and a U.S. residency of less than 5 years (Freeman et al. 1990; Giachello 1994; Valdez et al. 1993; Thamer et al. 1997). Welfare reforms that seek to curtail the use of public benefit programs by legal and undocumented immigrants will likely swell the uninsured rates among Hispanics. For this reason, policy solutions that address the health service needs of the uninsured would greatly benefit Hispanics. Because the Hispanic population is diverse and because uninsured rates differ by Hispanic subpopulations, multiple strategies may be needed. These could include expanding employer-based coverage, providing subsidies for purchasing affordable coverage, provision of affordable coverage, and expansion of the federal initiative known as the Children's Health Insurance Program (CHIP) through state governments to cover parents of children.

Immigration policies and politics further impede access to health insurance for much of this population. Recent welfare and immigration reforms place a ban on providing federal public benefits to undocumented aliens, with the exception of benefits to meet emergency needs. Federal law allows states to provide public health assistance to the undocumented population for immunizations and for testing for communicable diseases as well as treatment of communicable disease symptoms. However, states are prohibited from using Medicaid funds to either provide these services or to offer prenatal care. Under the welfare reform law, state and local governments are permitted to provide their own benefits to undocumented people only if state legislatures enact new laws affirming an intent to do so. Furthermore, undocumented individuals on welfare rolls can be systematically reported to the Immigration and Naturalization Service and can run the risk of deportation. In California, checks on documentation will occur four times a year (California Department of Social Services 1997). In addition, in 1994 California voters passed Proposition 187, a ballot initiative that required publicly funded health care facilities to deny care to illegal immigrants and to report them to government officials. Although currently partially held up in the courts, access to care for the undocumented population will probably decline, especially in rural areas, owing to this threat (Halfon et al. 1997).

The shift toward Medicaid managed care also means that local health departments and other safety net providers will lose the Medicaid reimbursements that have helped them subsidize care for the uninsured. Consequently, the large proportions of Hispanics who lack insurance coverage are likely to face increasing barriers to accessing health care in the public sector. The Balanced Budget Act, enacted a year after the 1996 welfare reform law, falls short of restoring all the cuts mandated by welfare reform. Immigrants are facing cutbacks in food stamps, and legal residents arriving after October 1996 are ineligible for disability insurance and other assistance.

The growth of managed care represents opportunities and challenges for the Hispanic population. As the findings from this nationally representative sample indicate, belonging to an HMO increases the odds of entry into care for Hispanics. After adjusting for health status, gender, and age, our findings show that Hispanics with private HMO insurance are more likely to access care than those with private insurance (but not covered by an HMO). Similarly, controlled analyses showed that Hispanics with public HMO insurance are more likely to access care than those with non-HMO public insurance. One factor that may explain the improved utilization among the insured with an HMO plan is the reduced burden of cost sharing in managed care, particularly for people with low incomes.

HMOs Must Change to Reflect Diverse Population Needs

Improving Hispanics' access to managed care would appear to be a step toward improved access and health care utilization, but it is also necessary to ensure that these plans can serve diverse populations. HMOs have traditionally catered to white, middle-class populations. As a result, they have little experience in delivering services to minorities. For services to be successful, interventions have to be tailored to the cultural idiosyncrasies of different Hispanic groups and to economic conditions, and these efforts must extend beyond marketing. For instance, evidence suggests that less-acculturated Mexican Americans interpret health symptoms differently, compared to those who are more acculturated (Angel and Thoits 1987). This may suggest that different attitudes toward health and health care, and different levels of family supports, must be considered when designing behavioral change interventions for the varying acculturation levels of Hispanics. The vast experience gained by community clinics in promoting healthy behaviors among diverse Hispanic groups can contribute to the design of culturally sensitive, preventive service HMOs.

Managed care plans also must be made more accountable. HMOs have the potential for improving Hispanic health outcomes through prevention and health promotion (Miller and Luft 1994). HMOs have practice guidelines, clinical protocols, and reminder systems that promote wellness and deliver preventive services (Thompson 1996). Moreover, an HMO can be held accountable for the delivery of services to multiethnic groups (Centers for Disease Control and Prevention 1995). Such accountability has been reinforced by the work of groups like the Committee for Quality Assurance, which accredits and measures the performance of plans (National Committee for Quality Assurance 1995).

The extent to which managed care increases participation, quality of care, and healthy outcomes for Hispanics must be monitored. A recent study suggests that HMOs work better for younger, healthier, and more affluent members (Ware et al. 1996). If this is true, poor, elderly, and ill Hispanics might be at risk for deteriorated physical health in HMOs when compared to fee-for-service plans. This raises the issue of whether more regulation will be necessary or whether market incentives, such as reputational assets and improved consumer information, will improve the quality of HMO care. In the meantime, the monitoring of health outcomes for Hispanics should be greatly facilitated by efforts from prominent organizations such as Kaiser-Permanente, who until recently viewed itself as "color-blind" but is now considering ethnic/racial data collection (Kaiser-Permanente Division of Research 1997). This will enable researchers to better discern the differences in access to managed care between Hispanics and non-Hispanics.

Finally, the findings of this study strongly indicate that personal experiences with the health care system matter. Our findings highlight the importance of personal interactions—such as the extent to which a person is treated badly by providers and staff, experiences discrimination, or is unable to develop trust with the provider—in determining ongoing use of the health care system. These subjective aspects of care require increasing attention as our health care system functions in a competitive managed care environment. Culturally appropriate personal interactions may serve as the basis for monitoring satisfaction with health care plans in the future and for assessing patient-provider communication. The extent to which Hispanics report having inadequate or bad experiences with the health care system further suggests areas on which health providers will have to focus if we are to improve quality of care for diverse Hispanic populations.

References

Andersen, R., Lewis, S. Z., Giachello, A. L., Aday, L. A., and Chiu, G. 1981. Access to medical care among the Hispanic population of the southwestern United States. *Journal of Health and Social Behavior* 22:78–89.

Angel, R., and Thoits, P. 1987. The impact of culture on the cognitive structure of illness. *Culture, Medicine and Psychiatry* 2:465–494.

Bashshur, R., Homan, R., and Smith, D. 1994. Beyond the uninsured: problems in access to care. *Medical Care* 32:409–419.

Berk, M., Albers, L., and Schur, C. 1996. The growth in the U.S. uninsured population: trend in Hispanic subgroups, 1977 to 1992. *American Journal of Public Health* 86:572–576.

California Department of Social Services (CDSS). 1997. *The California Temporary Assistance Program: Questions and Answers.* Sacramento, Calif.: CDSS.

Centers for Disease Control and Prevention. 1995. Prevention and managed care: opportunities for managed care organizations, purchases of health care, and public health agencies. *Morbidity and Mortality Weekly Report* 44:1–12.

Committee on Small Business. 1994. *Health Care Issues Affecting the Hispanic Population at the Time of Health Care Reform.* Washington, D.C.: U.S. Congress, House of Representatives.

Freeman, H. E., Aiken, L. H., Blendon, R. J., and Corey, C. R. 1990. Uninsured working-age adults: characteristics and consequences. *Health Services Research* 24:811–823.

Giachello, A. 1994. Issues in access and use. In C. Molina and M. Aguirre-Molina, eds., *Latino Health in the U.S.: A Growing Challenge.* Washington, D.C.: American Public Health Association.

Gordon, N., Rundall, T., Parker, L., and Perkins, C. 1997. *A Comparison of the*

Sociodemographic and Health Characteristics of "Working Age" Adults in California Covered by HMOs versus other Types of Private Health Insurance. Berkeley, Calif.: University of California, Berkeley.

Guendelman, S., and Schwalbe, J. 1986. Medical care utilization by Hispanic children: how does it differ from black and white peers? *Medical Care* 24:925–940.

Guyatt, G. H., Feeny, D. H., and Patrick, D. L. 1993. Measuring health-related quality of life. *Annals of Internal Medicine* 118:622–629.

Halfon, N., Wood, D., Burciaga-Valdez, R., Pereyra, M., and Duan, N. 1997. Medicaid enrollment and health services access by Latino children in inner-city Los Angeles. *Journal of the American Medical Association* 277:636–641.

Himmelstein, D., and Woolhandler, S. 1995. Care denied: U.S. residents who are unable to obtain needed medical services. *American Journal of Public Health* 85:341–344.

Kaiser-Permanente Division of Research. 1997. Collecting data on race/ethnicity and social class: implications for health care delivery and research. Symposium. March 7, 1997. Oakland, Calif.: Kaiser-Permanente.

Lieu, T., Newacheck, P., and McManus, M. 1993. Race, ethnicity, and access to ambulatory care among U.S. adolescents. *American Journal of Public Health* 83:960–965.

Louis Harris and Associates. 1994. *Health Care Services and Minority Groups: A Comparison Survey of Whites, African Americans, Hispanics and Asian Americans.* New York: Louis Harris and Associates.

Madsen, N. 1964. *Mexican Americans of South Texas.* Chicago: Holt, Rinehart and Winston.

Marin, G., and Marin, B. 1991. *Research with Hispanic Populations.* Thousand Oaks, Calif.: Sage.

Markides, K. S., Levin, J. S., and Ray, L. A. 1985. Determinants of physician utilization among Mexican-Americans: a three-generations study. *Medical Care* 23:236–246.

Miller, R. H., and Luft, H. S. 1994. Managed care plan performance since 1980: a literature analysis. *Journal of the American Medical Association* 271:1512–1519.

Molina, C., and Aguirre-Molina, M. 1994. *Latino Health in the U.S.: A Growing Challenge.* Washington, D.C.: American Public Health Association.

Nall, F. C., and Speilberg, J. 1967. Social and cultural factors in the responses of Mexican-Americans to medical treatment. *Journal of Health and Social Behavior* 8:299–308.

National Committee for Quality Assurance. 1995. Medicaid HEDIS, Version 2.0/2.5. Washington, D.C.

National Council of La Raza. 1991. *State of Hispanic America 1991: An Overview.* Washington, D.C.: National Council of La Raza.

Newhouse, J., Phelps, C., and Marquis, M. 1980. On having your cake and eating it too: econometric problems in estimating the demand for health services. *Journal of Econometrics* 13:365.

Pregibon, D. 1979. *Data Analytic Methods for Generalized Linear Models*. Toronto: University of Toronto.

Robert Wood Johnson Foundation. 1987. *Access to Health Care in the United States: Results of a 1986 Survey*. Princeton, N.J.: Robert Wood Johnson Foundation.

Ross, C., Steward, C., and Sinacore, J. 1994. A comparative study of seven measures of patient satisfaction. *Medical Care* 33:392–406.

Schur, C., Bernstein, A., and Berk, M. 1987. The importance of distinguishing Hispanic sub-populations in the use of medical care. *Medical Care* 25: 627–641.

Shah, B. V., Barnwell, B. G., Hunt, P. N., and Lavange, L. M. 1992. *SUDAAN User's Manual*. Research Triangle Park, N.C.: Research Triangle Institute.

Solis, J., Marks, G., Garcia, M., and Shelton, D. 1990. Acculturation, access to care, and use of preventive services by Hispanics: findings from HHANES, 1982–84. *American Journal of Public Health* 80:11–19.

Thamer, M., Richard, C., Waldman-Casebeer, A., and Fox-Ray, N. 1997. Health insurance coverage among foreign-born U.S. residents: the impact of race, ethnicity, and length of residence. *American Journal of Public Health* 87:96–102.

Thompson, R. 1996. What have HMOs learned about clinical prevention services? An examination of the experience at Group Health Cooperative of Puget Sound. *Milbank Quarterly* 74:469–510.

Trevino, F. M., and Moss, A. J. 1984. Health indicators for Hispanic, black, and white Americans. *Vital and Health Statistics* Series 10:148.

Trevino, F. M., Moyer, M. E., Valdez, R. B., and Stroup-Benham, C. A. 1991. Health insurance coverage and utilization of health services by Mexican Americans, mainland Puerto Ricans, and Cuban Americans. *Journal of the American Medical Association* 265(2):233–237. (Erratum appears in *JAMA* 265[8]:978.)

U.S. Bureau of the Census. 1991. *The Hispanic Population in the United States: March 1991*. Washington, D.C.: U.S. Bureau of the Census.

U.S. Bureau of the Census. 1994. *CPS Annual Demographic Survey, March Supplement*. Washington, D.C.: U.S. Bureau of the Census.

Valdez, R. B., Giachello, A., Rodriguez-Trias, H., Gomez, P., and de la Rocha, C. 1993. Improving access to health-care in Latino communities. *Public Health Reports* 108:534–539.

Ware, J., Bayliss, M., Rogers, W., Kosinski, M., and Tarlov, A. 1996. Differences in 4-year health outcomes for elderly and poor, chronically ill patients treated in HMO and fee-for-services systems: results from the medical outcomes study. *Journal of the American Medical Association* 276:1039–1047.

3

A Profile of African Americans' Health Care

Subgroup Differences in Need and Access

Verna M. Keith, Ph.D.

The ability to use health services in a timely and appropriate manner remains more of a problem for African Americans than for whites. After two decades of movement in the 1960s and 1970s toward more equitable access (Aday, Fleming, and Andersen 1984), research in the 1980s suggested a reversal in the trend toward racial convergence. Blendon and colleagues (1989), for example, found that African Americans were less likely to visit a physician and that they reported fewer visits on average, even when accounting for the poorer health status of African Americans. The largest racial disparity in African Americans' contact with physicians occurred among those in fair or poor health, which is the subpopulation in greatest need of services (Blendon et al. 1989; Cornelius 1993).

Long-standing racial inequities in unmet need, financial barriers to access, and quality of care also persisted into the 1980s (Davis et al. 1987; Hayward et al. 1988). Perhaps most distressing is that several studies indicate that the intensity of medical treatment varies by race, with African Americans being significantly less likely to receive cardiovascular and other diagnostic procedures, even when clinically warranted (e.g., Escarce et al. 1993; Wenneker and Epstein 1989).

LIFE CHANCES OF AFRICAN AMERICANS DIFFER FROM THOSE OF WHITES

Given the economic disadvantage of the African American population, a common explanation for racial differences in health services usage focuses on socioeconomic status (SES) and its correlates, such as insurance coverage and health status. However, in most of the studies cited, racial differences remain even when considering these factors. Increasingly, researchers acknowledge that the life chances of African Americans and Anglo Americans of similar socioeconomic status are not comparable.

Krieger et al. (1993) point to a body of literature demonstrating that the economic returns for the same level of educational attainment are lower for African Americans, and that African Americans hold lower-paying positions within the same job classifications. Similarly, Williams and Collins (1995) note that conventional measures of socioeconomic status do not adequately capture racial differences in wealth. In 1988, African American households had a median net worth of $3,700, compared to $43,800 for white households. Also, substantial racial differences in wealth occur across education, occupation, and income levels (Oliver and Shapiro 1995).

The argument that African Americans and whites at similar SES levels face different life chances is also relevant when examining issues related to health services research. For example, African Americans at all income levels are more likely to live in medically underserved areas than their white counterparts (Schlesinger 1987). This stems in part from persistent patterns of racial segregation that relegate middle-class African Americans to less affluent neighborhoods that have fewer services and amenities than other neighborhoods (Krieger et al. 1993; Massey, Condran, and Denton 1987). Furthermore, compared to poor whites, poor African Americans are more likely to live in neighborhoods where poverty is more highly concentrated (Krieger et al. 1993; Wilson 1987).

Emerging research on morbidity and mortality patterns points to the fruitfulness of examining class-based differences within racial groups. These studies indicate that the relationship between SES and health varies within racial groups. The relationship is stronger for African Americans in some studies (Krieger 1990; Hogue et al. 1987) than others (Miller and Korenman 1994). With some exceptions (e.g., Kleinman, Gold, and Makuc 1981), however, most studies of health care use have not systematically assessed the effects of socioeconomic status within racial groups. This approach may be particularly useful for providing insight on African Americans' use of services, given the growing economic diversity among African Americans.

Variations in Health Care Use within Population Groups

A decade ago Wilson (1987) forcefully argued that economic growth in the 1960s, coupled with civil rights legislation, resulted in expanded opportunities for skilled and educated African Americans. At the same time, the shift from manufacturing to service sector jobs, and the movement of industries out of central cities, resulted in fewer economic opportunities for unskilled and untrained African Americans. Thus, while the life chances and resources available to African Americans at all SES levels are considerably less than those available to their white counterparts, the situation has improved for higher-status African Americans while it has worsened for those of a lower status.

Raw figures show that low-income African Americans make more health care visits than their more affluent counterparts (Reed, Darity, and Roberson 1993), but lower-income individuals have lower utilization rates relative to their need for health care (Blendon et al. 1989; Muller 1986). Income differences in health care are especially notable for preventive services. Among African American women, for example, those with incomes above the poverty line are more likely to have breast examinations and Pap smears (Makuc, Freid, and Kleinman 1989). Lower-income women are still less likely to have adequate prenatal care than more affluent women (LaVeist, Keith, and Gutierrez 1995; Ingram, Makuc, and Kleinman 1986).

Socioeconomic status is also associated with several factors predictive of access to health care, such as insurance coverage and structural barriers, that may help us understand class-based differences among African Americans. The poor are more likely to be uninsured and to have Medicaid coverage rather than private insurance coverage. The uninsured report fewer physician visits (Newacheck 1988), tend to be sicker at the time of hospitalization, and are more likely to die before being discharged (Hadley, Steinberg, and Feder 1991). These findings indicate serious delays in seeking medical attention. Medicaid recipients, while being more advantaged than the uninsured (Braveman et al. 1991), encounter limitations on covered services (Muller 1988). In addition, African Americans are disproportionately represented in states that have comparatively less generous Medicaid programs.

Structural Barriers to Health Care

Structural barriers that impede access to health care also vary by socioeconomic status. Having a regular source of medical care, for example, is associated with increased visits for illness and preventive care (Berki and Ashcraft 1979; Baker, Stevens, and Brook 1994). Low-income individuals are less likely to have a regular source of care, and, when they do, that source is likely to be an emergency room or other site for their usual care, as opposed to office-based physicians or health maintenance organizations (HMOs) (Andersen, Aday, and Lyttle 1987). Attitudinal barriers, such as belief in the efficacy of medical care, also vary by class (e.g., Berkanovic and Reeder 1974), usually to the detriment of the lower classes. One exception is that people who are better educated are more likely than others to be skeptical of medical care (Haug and Lavin 1983).

Entry into the health care system is only the first step toward adequate health care. The quality of medical care accessed is a critical issue for individuals with few economic resources. While studies indicate that Americans generally have high levels of satisfaction with their own physicians (Blendon and Taylor 1989), establishing effective communication between physicians and patients remains a barrier to quality care (Waitzkin and Stoeckle 1987; Gibbs, Gibbs, and Henrich 1987). SES and racial differences between a physician and a patient may exacerbate communication problems. Blendon et al. (1989) found that African Americans are more likely than whites to report that their physicians did not inquire sufficiently about pain, did not explain the seriousness of the illness or injury, and did not discuss test or examination findings during their last ambulatory visit. The combination of low-income and minority group status may intensify these problems.

This study investigates the relationship between socioeconomic status and African Americans' health care. A major goal is to determine the extent to which the use of ambulatory services and perceptions of quality vary by status groups. A second goal is to examine the extent to which class-based differences are modified by demographic characteristics, structural and attitudinal barriers, and other factors that affect use of care and perceptions of quality. The results should yield insight into which specific groups within the African American population encounter the greatest difficulties in negotiating the health care system.

METHODS OF ANALYSIS

Dependent Variables

The analyses presented in this study are based on the 1,048 African Americans who participated in The Commonwealth Fund Minority Health Survey (CMHS) in 1994. We analyzed three dependent variables: (1) entry into care within the last 12 months, (2) volume of visits, and (3) satisfaction with provider.

"Entry into care" is a dichotomous variable that compares respondents who visited a provider or medical facility in the past year with those who did not. A provider visit demonstrates the extent to which respondents were successful in gaining access to the health care delivery system. "Volume of visits" measures how many times respondents visited a provider or facility within the last year among those who entered the health care system. To avoid giving disproportionate weight to a small number of higher users, this variable was truncated at twelve visits or higher. "Satisfaction with provider" is a dichotomous variable comparing those who were "very satisfied" with a combined category of those reporting "somewhat satisfied," "somewhat dissatisfied," or "very dissatisfied."

Independent Variables

"Household income" and "educational attainment" indicate SES. Measures of SES such as net assets and poverty status were unavailable. We recoded income from seven original categories into five—less than $7,501; $7,501–$15,000; $15,001–$25,000; $25,001–$50,000; and greater than $50,000. Three categorical variables measure education: "less than high school," "high school graduate," and "some college or more."

"Insurance coverage" is measured using three dummy variables that indicate whether a respondent has "private insurance only," "any public insurance," or is "uninsured." The "any public" category combines Medicare beneficiaries with and without private coverage as well as Medicaid recipients, making the measurement less than ideal. However, the small numbers of cases hampered finer distinctions. "Regular provider" indicates whether respondents have a regular physician or other health care provider. "Barriers to care" measures whether respondents had a major problem when seeking care with having to pay too much, transportation, getting an appointment, waiting too long, or being nervous or afraid. "Trust providers" is a dichotomous variable that measures whether respondents trust providers "very much" to help with their medical problems. "Quality of care less due to ethnicity" indicates whether respondents have ever felt that they would have received better medical care if they were not a member of an ethnic minority.

Health status and stress are measures of need for health care. "Health status" is an ordinal measure of self-perceived health as being "excellent," "good," "fair," or "poor." "Stress" is measured by an eleven-item index asking respondents to indicate if they were affected by any of the following in the last year: problems with money, aging parents, spouse, or children; death of a family member; trouble balancing work and family demands; hassle at work; loss of job or spouse's job; treated badly because of race or cultural background; fear of crime or violence in the community; and knowing someone who was a victim of violence. Responses were coded on a three-point scale from "not affected," to "affected somewhat," to "affected strongly." Possible scores ranged from 11 to 33.

Lower-income individuals, especially lower-status African Americans, are generally exposed to more stressful life events and chronic strains than others (Ulbrich, Warheit, and Zimmerman 1989). Environmental stressors often find expression in the form of somatic symptoms that may bring individuals to ambulatory care physicians (see Schurman, Kramer, and Mitchell 1985). While health status may mediate the effects of stress (Elliot and Eisdorfer 1982), some individuals with high levels of stress may not define themselves as being in poor health.

The analyses of provider satisfaction include additional predictors. "Choice in place of care" measures whether or not respondents have some or a great deal of choice in where they go for medical care. "Time spent with provider" measures whether or not respondents spent more than 15 minutes with their provider during the most recent visit. Provider ethnicity, nonblack versus black, is also assessed.

Demographic variables that affect health care use are controlled in the multivariate analyses—age, gender, marital status (formerly married contrasted with married or single), place of residence, and household size (truncated at ten or more members to avoid the disproportionate weighting of large households). Caribbean heritage is also controlled because language and other cultural differences may affect experiences with the health care delivery system.

Weighted Data Analysis

Our analysis of data in the CMHS is based on weighted data that take into account different probabilities of selection from primary sampling units. The two-tailed chi-square test of significance is used to describe the bivariate relationships between categorical variables, and the F-test is used to describe the bivariate relationships between categorical and noncategorical variables. We use logistic regression in the analysis of entry into care and satisfaction with provider. Ordinary least-squares regression is used in the analyses of volume of care. Variables are entered hierarchically in both types of regression models. This technique permits an evaluation of how various effects change as other variables enter the model. The first model enters demographic characteristics and educational attainment. The second model adds household income. The third model considers the effects of various structural and subjective factors that may hinder entry and volume or that may affect satisfaction with provider. The final model assesses the effects of need for health care.

RESULTS OF ANALYSIS

Demographic and Health Status Variables

The demographic characteristics of the sample, and their distribution by socioeconomic status (Table 3.1, last column) indicate that 63.6 percent of African American respondents are under 45 years of age (mean age 41.4 years), 54.4 percent are female, and 10.7 percent are of Caribbean heritage. Just under one-fifth (19.6%) reside in rural areas, and 26.5 percent are either divorced or widowed. The average household size is 2.9 persons (data not shown), with 22.1 percent of respondents living alone, 24.1 percent residing in two-person households, and 15.1 percent living in households with five people or more. Some 16.4 percent of respondents (Table 3.1, first row) are in the lowest-income category (<$7,501), and 14.7 percent are in the highest-income category (>$50,000). Less than 20 percent of respondents have not completed high school, 40.1 percent have a high school education, and 40.6 percent have attended or completed college. The youngest and oldest respondents, females, people formerly married, rural residents, and smaller households have lower incomes.

The distribution of access and health status variables for the total sample, by household income and education (Table 3.2), shows that 23.4 percent of the African American respondents are uninsured, and that 31.3 percent report having no regular health care provider. Just over half the sample have experienced one or more barriers to care. Almost 55 percent report that they trust their provider very much, and 71.5 percent report either a great deal of, or some, choice in the place of care. Three-fourths of African American respondents have a nonblack provider, just over a third spent 15 minutes or less time with their provider at the last visit, 17.1 percent experience high levels of stress, and 25.6 percent report fair or poor health.

Table 3.1 Percentage Distribution of Demographic Characteristics by Socioeconomic Status—African Americans

	Household Income						Education				Total (N)	% of Total
	<$7,501	$7,501–$15,000	$15,001–$25,000	$25,001–$50,000	>$50,000	p value	<High School	High School	Some College	p value		
Total	16.4	15.6	21.5	31.8	14.7		19.2	40.1	40.6		1043	
Age						0.00				0.00		
18–29	17.4	18.1	25.5	26.2	12.8		11.7	43.5	44.8		299	28.7
30–44	11.0	13.7	21.7	34.9	18.7		8.5	43.7	47.8		364	34.9
45–64	14.3	14.7	18.2	39.5	10.7		26.2	39.8	34.0		256	24.6
65+	34.4	17.2	17.2	20.5	10.7		56.1	22.0	22.0		123	11.8
Gender						0.00				0.24		
Female	19.2	15.9	24.2	28.6	12.2		17.5	40.5	42.0		474	54.4
Male	12.8	15.4	18.1	36.0	17.7		21.5	39.7	38.8		566	45.6
Ethnicity						0.25				0.49		
Caribbean	12.4	21.2	24.8	30.1	11.5		15.3	40.5	44.1		111	10.7
Non-Caribbean	16.8	15.0	21.0	32.2	13.4		19.8	40.4	40.2		929	89.3

						p				p	N	%
Marital status						0.00				0.00		
Formerly married	24.3	21.4	18.5	28.6	7.2		30.4	38.8	30.8		276	26.5
Married/single	13.4	13.6	22.5	33.2	17.4		15.3	40.7	44.1		765	73.5
Residence						0.00				0.00		
Rural	25.4	16.1	20.5	31.2	6.8		27.0	47.5	25.5		204	19.6
Urban	14.1	15.5	21.7	32.0	16.7		17.6	38.2	35.5		837	80.4
Household size						0.00				0.00		
1	26.5	13.0	23.0	29.6	11.8		28.6	29.4	42.0		230	22.1
2	13.5	20.3	17.1	32.3	16.7		19.3	23.7	24.2		251	24.1
3	13.5	14.3	21.1	35.9	15.2		12.6	45.9	21.8		223	21.4
4	11.5	18.1	23.6	29.3	17.0		17.7	47.5	34.8		182	17.4
≥5	15.9	10.8	24.2	14.8	18.3		16.7	39.7	15.0		157	15.1

Source: Data from The Commonwealth Fund Minority Health Survey, 1994.

Table 3.2 Percentage Distribution of Access and Health Status Variables by Socioeconomic Status—African Americans[a]

		Household Income						Education			
	Total	<$7,501	$7,501–$15,000	$15,001–$25,000	$25,001–$50,000	>$50,000	p value	<High School	High School	Some College	p value
Insurance	N = 1041	N = 170	N = 163	N = 223	N = 332	N = 153	<0.01	N = 202	N = 417	N = 422	<0.01
Private only	51.4	15.3	29.4	54.3	69.6	71.2		26.2	50.4	64.2	
Any public	25.2	52.4	31.3	16.1	17.5	18.3		48.0	24.3	15.2	
Uninsured	23.4	32.4	39.3	29.6	13.0	10.5		25.7	25.4	20.6	
Regular provider	N = 1040	N = 170	N = 163	N = 222	N = 332	N = 153	<0.01	N = 201	N = 417	N = 422	<0.01
Yes	68.7	58.8	60.7	67.6	74.4	77.1		64.7	64.5	74.4	
No	31.3	41.2	39.3	32.4	25.6	22.9		35.3	35.5	25.6	
Barriers to care	N = 992	N = 154	N = 155	N = 217	N = 320	N = 146	<0.01	N = 184	N = 402	N = 404	0.53
≥1	50.2	53.9	59.4	56.2	46.6	35.6		53.8	49.0	49.5	
None	49.8	46.1	40.6	43.8	53.4	64.7		46.2	51.0	50.5	
Trust providers	N = 1034	N = 168	N = 162	N = 222	N = 329	N = 153	0.32	N = 196	N = 416	N = 420	<0.01
Some / not much / not at all	45.3	43.5	39.5	43.7	48.3	49.0		31.1	45.7	51.7	
Very much	54.7	56.7	60.5	56.3	51.7	51.0		68.9	54.3	48.3	
Quality less due to ethnicity	N = 1009	N = 163	N = 155	N = 219	N = 323	N = 149	0.04	N = 187	N = 410	N = 411	0.16
Yes	20.2	28.4	14.8	27.4	19.2	19.5		21.9	17.3	22.4	
No	79.8	81.6	85.2	72.6	80.8	80.5		78.1	82.7	77.6	

							P value				P value
Choice of place of care	N = 1025	N = 167	N = 158	N = 221	N = 328	N = 151	<0.01	N = 195	N = 410	N = 419	<0.01
None / very little	28.5	42.5	37.3	31.7	20.7	15.9		43.1	26.6	23.6	
Great deal / some	71.5	57.5	62.7	68.3	79.3	84.1		56.9	73.4	76.4	
Provider's ethnicity[b]	N = 683	N = 96	N = 93	N = 144	N = 236	N = 114	0.73	N = 118	N = 262	N = 301	0.74
Black	24.5	25.0	22.6	27.8	22.0	26.3		27.1	24.0	23.6	
Not black	75.5	75.0	77.4	72.2	78.0	73.7		72.9	76.0	76.4	
Time spent with provider	N = 1026	N = 166	N = 162	N = 221	N = 327	N = 150	0.22	N = 194	N = 415	N = 418	<0.01
≤15 minutes	33.9	41.0	30.2	34.4	33.6	30.0		25.8	39.3	32.5	
>15 minutes	66.1	59.0	69.8	65.6	66.4	70.0		74.2	60.7	67.5	
Stress	N = 1040	N = 171	N = 163	N = 222	N = 331	N = 153	0.03	N = 136	N = 725	N = 178	<0.01
Low (<12)	13.0	18.1	9.8	9.5	13.9	13.7		22.5	10.8	10.9	
Medium (12–20)	69.9	64.3	71.2	67.6	71.9	73.9		61.0	74.3	69.4	
High (21–33)	17.1	17.5	19.0	23.0	14.2	12.4		16.5	14.9	19.7	
Health status	N = 1041	N = 170	N = 162	N = 223	N = 333	N = 153	<0.01	N = 322	N = 453	N = 209	<0.01
Excellent	30.9	20.6	22.8	30.9	36.6	38.6		22.8	30.5	35.5	
Good	43.5	32.9	39.5	45.3	45.3	52.9		27.2	46.3	48.8	
Fair	20.3	32.9	29.0	21.1	15.0	7.2		37.6	18.9	12.9	
Poor	5.3	13.5	8.6	2.7	3.0	1.3		12.4	4.3	2.9	

Source: Data from The Commonwealth Fund Minority Health Survey, 1994.

[a] Column percentages add to 100 (except for rounding errors) for each income and education category.

[b] Provider ethnicity ascertained only from respondents with a regular provider.

Both insurance coverage and access to a regular provider vary by income and education. Generally, people with higher incomes and education levels are more likely to have private insurance, less likely to be uninsured, and more likely to have a regular provider (Table 3.2). Higher-income respondents are less likely to experience barriers to care, and higher SES is positively associated with having greater choice. Consistent with Haug and Lavin (1983), trust in providers varies inversely with education in this study. Less-educated respondents spend more time with their doctors, perhaps indicating more severe health problems related to lower incomes. Income and education also have positive effects on stress levels, although these relationships are not linear. High levels of stress are more prevalent among those in the middle-income categories ($7,501–$15,000 and $15,001–$25,000). On the other hand, high levels of stress are more prevalent among those who have not finished high school and those who have attended college. As expected, poor health is more prevalent among the low-income respondents and those with less education.

Overall, about 87.3 percent of the sample have entered the health care system (Table 3.3). Females are more likely to enter care than males, while high school graduates are less likely to enter care than other educational groups. Having a regular source of care and poorer health status increase the likelihood of entry into the health system. Overall, respondents who have seen a provider in the last twelve months averaged 4.42 visits. Females and formerly married people report more visits. High school graduates report slightly fewer visits than groups with other educational attainments.

Insurance also has a significant relationship with the volume of visits. The uninsured have the fewest average number of visits (3.77), followed by those with private insurance (4.32). Those with public insurance report the highest average number of visits (5.23). This finding may reflect the inclusion of Medicare recipients who are older and in greater need of health care in the "any public" insurance coverage group. Having a regular provider and worsening health are also associated with increased volume of care. The proportion of respondents who report being very satisfied with their provider is high (78.8%). Satisfaction with provider increases with increasing age. Being very satisfied is also inversely associated with education. Those who have experienced one or more barriers, who have a low level of trust in providers, and who feel that the quality of care is lower due to their ethnicity, are less likely to report being very satisfied. Being very satisfied is more common among

Table 3.3 Entry into Care, Volume of Care, and Satisfaction with Provider, by Demographic Characteristics, Socioeconomic Status, Other Access Variables

	Entry into Care			Volume of Care			Satisfaction Provider—Very Satisfied		
	N	%	p value	N	Mean	p value	N	%	p value
Total	1031	87.3		915	4.42		707	78.8	
Age	1031		0.79	915		0.07	708		<0.01
18-29	296	89.5		265	4.09		163	71.2	
30-44	362	87.3		316	4.29		245	73.9	
45-64	252	89.3		225	4.77		205	84.9	
65+	121	89.3		108	4.91		95	90.5	
Gender	1031		0.00	915		<0.01	707		.25
Female	559	91.9		514	4.74		427	80.1	
Male	472	85.0		401	4.03		280	76.4	
Ethnicity	1031		0.66	915		0.12	708		0.09
Caribbean	110	90.0		816	4.96		80	71.3	
Non-Caribbean	921	88.6		99	4.36		628	79.6	
Marital Status	1030		0.29	915		<0.01	707		0.02
Formerly married	269	87.0		234	5.00		203	84.7	
Married/single	761	89.4		680	4.23		504	76.2	
Residence	1031		0.37	915		0.10	706		0.03
Rural	199	86.9		173	4.02		155	72.3	
Urban	832	89.2		742	4.52		551	80.6	
Household size	1031		0.16	915		0.09	707		0.01
1	228	84.2		192	4.59		154	82.5	
2	248	90.7		225	4.11		180	83.9	
3	220	89.5		197	4.96		145	76.6	
4	180	88.9		160	4.10		119	79.0	
≥5	155	91.0		141	4.33		109	67.0	
Education	1025			912		0.04	704		0.02
<High school	194	88.1	<0.01	171	4.96		125	88.0	
High school	411	85.6		352	4.13		267	78.3	
Some college	420	92.9		390	4.46		312	75.3	
Household Income	1025		0.34	914		0.35	706		0.70
<$7,501	163	87.7		143	4.91		100	80.0	
$7,501-$15,000	161	89.4		144	4.28		97	81.4	
$15,001-$25,000	222	89.6		199	4.27		149	81.2	
$25,001-$50,000	327	87.5		286	4.50		243	77.4	
>$50,000	152	93.4		142	4.12		117	75.2	
Insurance	1031		0.08	915		<0.01	706		0.37
Private only	528	87.1		460	4.32		407	77.4	
Any public	254	92.5		235	5.23		177	82.5	
Uninsured	249	88.4		220	3.77		122	77.9	

(*continues*)

Table 3.3 (*Continued*)

	Entry into Care			Volume of Care			Satisfaction Provider—Very Satisfied		
	N	%	p value	N	Mean	p value	N	%	p value
Regular provider	1031		<0.01	915		<0.01			
Yes	783	95.3		670	4.78		NA		
No	328	74.7		245	3.46				
Barriers to care	985		0.29	883		0.21	676		<0.01
≥1	493	50.1		447	4.61		291	65.3	
None	492	49.9		436	4.31		385	88.3	
Trust providers	1024		0.69	909		0.49	703		<0.01
Some / not much / not at all	463	88.3		409	4.34		288	60.4	
Very much	561	89.1		500	4.5		415	91.3	
Choice of place of care	NA			NA			694		<0.01
None / very little							175	71.4	
Some / great deal							519	80.9	
Quality less due to ethnicity	999		0.53	885		0.22	689		<0.01
Yes	798	88.6		178	4.72		120	69.2	
No	201	88.6		707	4.34		569	80.8	
Provider's ethnicity[a]	NA			NA			679		<0.01
Black							164	87.2	
Not black							515	75.8	
Time spent with provider	NA			NA			700		<0.01
≤15 minutes							208	64.4	
>15 minutes							492	84.6	
Stress	1028		0.29	913		0.07	NA		
Low (<12)	131	86.5		186	4.21				
Medium (12–20)	719	88.7		564	4.33				
High (21–33)	178	91.6		163	5.01				
Health status	1031		0.03	915		<0.01	707		0.20
Excellent	323	86.1		278	3.80		231	83.5	
Good	451	88.2		398	4.08		298	76.5	
Fair	205	91.7		188	5.23		138	76.1	
Poor	52	98.1		51	7.41		40	77.5	

Source: Data from The Commonwealth Fund Minority Health Survey, 1994.
[a] Provider ethnicity ascertained only from respondents with a regular provider.

African Americans who report having a great deal of or some choice in the place of care, having a black provider, and spending more time with their provider during the last visit.

Predictors of Entry into Care

Concerning SES, the major emphasis of this chapter, model 1 (Table 3.4) indicates that those African Americans who did not attend college are less likely to enter care even when background characteristics are controlled. In model 4, educational differences remain after all other factors are entered. However, the p values are modest for both groups (.03). African Americans who attended or completed college are 2.38 times as likely as those with less than a high school education to have obtained care (inverse of odds ratio = $1 \div 0.42 = 2.38$), and 2.04 times as likely as high school graduates to have obtained care (inverse of odds ratio = $1 \div 0.49 = 2.04$).

Because the probability of entering care remains significantly different by gender across all models, separate analyses for males and females (data not shown) reveal that the relationship between education and entry differs by gender. Among males, the relationship is not significant after income is considered. Among females, those with some college or higher educational attainment are five times as likely to enter health care as those with less than a high school education (inverse of odds ratio = $1 \div 0.20 = 5.00$)—and eight times as likely to enter care as those with only a high school education (inverse of odds ratio = $1 \div 0.12 = 8.33$). Thus, the relationship between education and entry into care appears to reflect differences among females. This finding suggests that African American working-class women are especially at risk of having insufficient access to health care.

Models 3 and 4 (Table 3.4) indicate that African American respondents with public insurance are more likely to have had a physician visit than those with private insurance only. This may reflect the inclusion of Medicare beneficiaries with supplemental policies in the "any public" insurance group. Surprisingly, there are no significant differences (p = 0.10) between the uninsured and those with private insurance. It is important to note, however, that insurance status is strongly correlated with having a regular provider which is, in turn, strongly associated with entry into care. In this study, those respondents with a regular provider are 13.89 times as likely to enter care as those without a provider. The findings reflected in models 3 and 4 suggest that when the uninsured have a regular

Table 3.4 Predictors of Entry into Health Care—African Americans

	MODEL 1		MODEL 2		MODEL 3		MODEL 4	
	Adjusted Odds Ratio	95% Confidence Interval	Adjusted Odds Ratio	95% Confidence Interval	Adjusted Odds Ratio	95% Confidence Interval	Adjusted Odds Ratio	95% Confidence Interval
Age (in years)	1.02[a]	1.00,1.03	1.02[a]	1.00,1.03	1.01	0.99,1.03	1.01	0.99,1.03
Female	2.46[a]	1.54,3.94	2.49[a]	1.53,4.04	2.02[a]	1.07,3.81	1.99[a]	1.05,3.79
Caribbean	0.85	0.39,1.86	0.85	0.39,1.85	0.51	0.20,1.29	0.49	0.19,1.27
Formerly married	0.75	0.41,1.37	0.74	0.40,1.36	0.68	0.33,1.38	0.59	0.28,1.22
Rural	0.83	0.47,1.46	0.87	0.50,1.51	0.65	0.30,1.40	0.70	0.32,1.51
Household size	1.14	0.97,1.34	1.13	0.97,1.33	1.14	0.95,1.27	1.15	0.96,1.38
Education								
<High school	0.53[b]	0.28,1.00	0.56[b]	0.28,1.10	0.45[a]	0.21,0.96	0.42	0.19,0.92
High school	0.47[c]	0.29,0.77	0.47[c]	0.28,0.78	0.54[a]	0.28,1.02	0.49	0.25,0.94
Household income								
<$7,501			0.57	0.23,1.39	0.65	0.21,1.98	0.52	0.17,1.63
$7,501-$15,000			0.81	0.32,2.04	1.33	0.39,4.56	1.08	0.31,3.76
$15,001-$25,000			0.65	0.30,1.42	0.66	0.27,1.61	0.62	0.26,1.52
$25,001-$50,000			0.54	0.27,1.07	0.57	0.24,1.34	0.58	0.24,1.38
Insurance								
Any public					3.06[c]	1.46,6.44	3.23[c]	1.49,7.02
Uninsured					2.73[b]	0.97,7.68	2.55[b]	0.93,7.01

Regular provider	13.53[a]	6.82,26.83	13.89[a]	7.16,26.94
Barriers	1.89	0.99,3.61	1.68	0.88,3.20
Trust providers				
Very much	1.55	0.62,3.90	1.76	0.71,4.34
Quality of care less due to ethnicity	0.97	0.47,2.02	0.75	0.35,1.62
Stress			1.05	0.98,1.13
Health status[d]			1.57	1.03,2.37
−2 log likelihood	35.54	39.62	150.91	160.57

Source: Data from The Commonwealth Fund Minority Health Survey 1994.

Note: Referent categories: male, non-Caribbean, married/single, urban/suburban, some college, income >50,000, private insurance only, trust providers some / little / not at all, quality of care not less due to ethnicity, low stress, better health.

[a]p ≤ .05.

[b]p ≤ .10.

[c]p ≤ .01.

[d]Higher levels of stress and worsening health status associated with entry into care.

provider, they are just as likely to enter the health care system as the privately insured. However, multivariate analyses (data not shown) clearly demonstrate that the uninsured are far less likely to have a regular provider because they are more likely to seek care in community and public health clinics. Finally, as expected, entry into the system becomes more likely as an individual's health status worsens.

Predictors of Volume of Care

Volume of care was analyzed with the same variables in four models as presented for predictors of entry into health care. These analyses indicate that neither education nor income predicts the volume of visits (data not shown). Having public insurance versus private insurance is associated with a greater number of visits (beta = .10; p = .01), and the uninsured have significantly fewer visits than those with private insurance (beta = -0.09; p = .05). Thus, while the uninsured and privately insured are about equally as likely to enter the health system, a lack of insurance limits a person's later visits. Those individuals without a regular provider make fewer visits than others, and this relationship remains significant after health status is considered in model 4 (beta = -0.19; p = 0.001). Unexpectedly, experiencing barriers to care is positively associated with volume of visits. Perhaps experiences with the health care system increase the opportunity for barriers to be realized rather than anticipated barriers acting as deterrents to access. Both stress and poorer health increase the volume of visits. Gender differences, unlike the findings about entry into care, become only marginally significant once all variables enter the model. Further analyses indicate that SES is not significant for either males or females.

Predictors of Satisfaction

Provider satisfaction was also analyzed with four models, according to the pattern presented for health care entry in Table 3.4. Concerning provider satisfaction, while education has no effect on the probability of being very satisfied with a provider, significant variations do occur by income (data not shown). Generally, individuals with incomes of $50,000 or less are more likely to report being very satisfied than are those with incomes above $50,000, although in model 4 the difference is significant only for the $15,001–$25,000 (odds ratio = 2.06) and the $25,001–$50,000 (odds ratio = 1.97) groups. These relationships become stronger as access and health status variables are added in subsequent models.

African Americans who experience barriers to care are less satisfied with their providers, whereas those who trust providers very much and who spend more time with their providers are more likely to be very satisfied (not shown). As health status moves from excellent to poor, however, satisfaction decreases. Age remains significant across models, confirming previous studies that show high levels of satisfaction among the elderly. Interestingly, gender differences become significant when structural and subjective aspects of access are controlled and when health status is controlled. The African American women in this CMHS sample are less trustful, spend less time with their providers, and face fewer barriers than men. Although gender differences in these variables are not statistically significant individually, they may have combined to suppress the relationship between gender and satisfaction observed in earlier models.

SUMMARY AND DISCUSSION

The purpose of this study was to investigate SES differences in utilization and quality of health care among African Americans. Overall, the findings indicate some support for SES differences, and they highlight the impact of structural and subjective access variables on entry into health care, volume of care, and satisfaction with the provider.

Education and Income Differences

Initial findings reveal that, compared to African Americans who attended or graduated from college, high school graduates and those with less than a high school education are less likely to have contact with a health care provider. Further analyses, however, indicate that these educational differences pertain to African American women but not to African American males, who have less access than females regardless of SES. Women who attend or complete college are five times as likely to receive medical attention as those with less than a high school education, and eight times as likely as those who graduated from high school. The lower-status women in this study are less likely to receive preventive care than others; these women might be well served by programs that aggressively target them as a high-risk group. The volume of visits, on the other hand, does not vary significantly by either educational attainment or income. Thus, while less-educated African American females are less likely to gain entry into the health care system, those who do tend to have a similar number of visits to those with higher education levels. This finding may indicate that patient discretion plays a larger role in the decision to enter care, while provider discretion plays a larger role in volume of visits. In other words, after an initial visit, return visits are largely determined by the provider.

It is surprising to observe educational differences among women but not men. Women should have more uniform access to health care because they are far more likely to be eligible for Medicaid than men. One explanation is that the educational differences among women are owing to differences in the use of female-specific screening exams such as breast examinations and Pap smears. Whether an African American woman participates in a preventive screening may be less dependent on ability to pay for this service and more dependent on knowledge of the efficacy of the test and on fear of the test results. African American women with lower levels of education are less knowledgeable regarding the benefits of early detection, have more misconceptions regarding screening examinations, and are more likely to believe that a cancer diagnosis is an automatic death sentence (Dignan et al. 1990; Sylvester 1998). This explanation is supported by our finding that lower-educated African American women in the CMHS were less likely to receive preventive care than their better-educated counterparts. Further support is suggested by the failure to find a relationship between income and entry into care, which would be more indicative of ability to pay. The education gradient may not exist for males because male-specific screening examinations, such as for prostate cancer, are just beginning to emerge. Fewer sex-specific examinations among males may also contribute to their lower levels of entry into care generally.

Income has a significant effect on the likelihood of being very satisfied with one's regular health provider. When access variables and health status are controlled, those respondents with incomes in the $15,001–$25,000 range, and those with incomes in the $25,001–$50,000 range, are more likely than those with incomes greater than $50,000 to report being very satisfied. One explanation for this finding is that higher-income African Americans have higher expectations regarding the patient-physician relationship. Some researchers (e.g., Haug and Lavin 1983) argue that higher-status individuals are becoming less accepting of the traditional patient-physician relationship and are demanding a more active role in health care decisions. Bringing this consumer approach to health care relationships may change expectations about the quality of communications and result in lower levels of satisfaction.

Access Predicts Usage of Health Care

Perhaps the most prominent finding in this research is that access to a regular provider is predictive of both measures of health care use—entering the system and having a series of visits. Individuals who have a regular provider are more likely to enter the health care system and to have more visits on average. Perhaps an established relationship with a provider encourages individuals to seek the recommended annual physical and other routine care, and this in turn facilitates follow-up visits for more serious health problems.

However, approximately 31 percent of respondents, which is a significant minority, report no regular source of health care. Multivariate analyses (not presented) reveal that these people without a regular provider tend to be younger, male, less educated, uninsured, and have lower incomes. Respondents were asked to provide reasons for why they did not have a regular provider. Of the total who report no regular provider, 25 percent give financial reasons as barriers to care. Further, the probability of having a regular provider varies with usual place of care. The percentage who have a regular provider is 84.9 percent for those whose usual place is a private physician, HMO, or group practice; 42 percent for those who go to hospital emergency or outpatient departments; and 43.8 percent for those using other sites, such as public clinics. Overall, having a regular provider has the strongest effect on entry into care and second strongest effect on volume of care, and the most economically vulnerable individuals are those least likely to have an established relationship with a regular provider.

Insurance coverage is also associated with entry into and volume of care, although some results are unanticipated. Compared with African American respondents who have private insurance only, respondents with any public insurance are more likely to enter care and to have a higher number of visits. As noted previously, this finding may reflect measurement error in that Medicare beneficiaries, some of whom have private supplemental coverage, appear in the "any public" category. Another possible explanation is that differences in health care use between people with private insurance and those with public insurance have narrowed because of private coverage restrictions.

When we compare uninsured respondents to the privately insured, findings indicate no difference in entry into care. However, the uninsured have fewer visits. Uninsured individuals are just as likely as insured individuals to gain access to the system, perhaps via emergency departments and public clinics, but they may be unable to afford needed follow-up care. These findings differ from previous findings from a national study (Keith and LaVeist 1996), which showed that while the uninsured are less likely to enter the health care system, the volume of services once they gain entry is similar to that of the privately insured. The Keith and LaVeist study is based on a nonelderly sample, however, and this may account for the different findings. Further analyses show that uninsured respondents tend to be younger, male, and have lower household incomes and poorer health than insured respondents. And when compared to individuals with private insurance, the uninsured and those with public insurance are more likely to seek care in community clinics and public health clinics, which may not offer the same continuity of care levels that private sites offer.

Another major finding is that subjective aspects of health care access contribute to an individual's level of satisfaction with a provider. Respondents who experience barriers to care are less likely to report being very satisfied with their regular provider, while those who trust that providers are generally able to assist with medical problems are more likely to report being very satisfied. Similarly, respondents who have spent more time with their provider at their last visit reported enhanced satisfaction. Respondents appear to have more positive evaluations when they perceive that providers are giving them sufficient time.

It is also possible that perceptions of barriers, trust, and estimates of time spent with a provider are dependent on level of satisfaction. Without longitudinal data, this remains a viable alternative. African Americans are less likely to be satisfied when their provider is not African American. This finding suggests that when patients and providers differ in their racial backgrounds, the patient-provider relationship may be hampered. Both patients and physicians may feel less comfortable in asking questions, and physicians may feel less comfortable making treatment recommendations. This finding reinforces the notion that care could be improved if there were more African American physicians.

Subgroups Face Difficulties

Our research suggests that some African Americans have more difficulty than others in seeking health care. In this study, three such groups stand out: less-educated women, men, and individuals without a regular source of care. The evidence also indicates that less-educated, lower-income, and uninsured African Americans have more difficulty than others seeking care because they are the least likely to have a regular provider, which is the strongest predictor of health care access. All things being equal, lower-status people are equally likely to use the health care system if they have a regular provider. But all things are not equal; many lower-status African Americans do not have a regular provider of health care.

The major conclusion we suggest is that social class operates through lack of insurance to undermine access to health care. The uninsured are less likely to have a regular provider and may be unable to afford the number of visits warranted by their medical condition. While research on racial differences in access to health care continues to be important to the policy debate, this study indicates that further assessment of differences within racial groups may yield useful insights. The findings offered here are tentative and are merely a first step. They should be replicated, using more robust measures of SES, and they should incorporate measures that capture the social class of geographic divisions, such as neighborhoods. In addition, SES differences within other groups should be evaluated and then compared with the findings for African Americans to determine whether class differences are similar. This might explain why race/ethnic differences in health care use often remain, even when SES is controlled.

POLICY IMPLICATIONS IN THE ERA OF MANAGED CARE

Managed care is well on the way to becoming the principal method of financing and delivering health care in the United States. The great expectation is that managed care will deliver health care to all groups at a reasonable cost, without sacrificing access and quality. But there are ongoing concerns about whether managed care can meet this expectation, especially as it pertains to vulnerable populations—the poor, people with public insurance, and the uninsured. Because African Americans are over-represented in these vulnerable populations, it important to briefly review these concerns in light of the current research findings about access and satisfaction with one's regular provider.

Managed care can potentially improve access to health care for a substantial number of African Americans, especially those without a regular provider. A major finding of this study is that African Americans who lack an established relationship with a health care provider are less likely to enter the system in a given year, and they tend to have fewer visits on average. But managed care plans, especially fully capitated plans, place an emphasis on primary care provider management. For this reason, the expansion of managed care could increase usage by facilitating ongoing patient-physician relationships.

In this study, as noted previously, African American women with lower levels of education have fewer overall health care visits than more highly educated women. Fewer visits result, in part, because these women are less likely to receive preventive care. Because managed care plans emphasize prevention, it is likely that less-educated women would benefit from managed care expansion. Low-income individuals in general are likely to benefit as well, because they are the group least likely to have a regular provider. In this study, 41.2 percent of respondents with incomes below $7,500 did not have a regular provider, compared to 22.9 percent of those with incomes above $50,000. African American males may also benefit from the emphasis placed on prevention by managed care.

Managed Care and Medicaid

It is not a foregone conclusion that African Americans will derive enhanced access to quality care from managed care. First, managed care is being extended rapidly to the Medicaid population, but it is not clear whether managed care will be entirely beneficial for these recipients, many of whom, by virtue of their higher poverty rate, are African Americans. Although some studies find that Medicaid managed care improves utilization and cost over fee-for-service arrangements (e.g., Hurley, Freund, and Paul 1993), others do not support these findings (Rowland et al. 1995).

In this study, African Americans with public insurance used more health services than those with private insurance, even when health status was controlled. Under managed care this may no longer be the case. As Perloff (1996) notes, Medicaid managed care plans generally have little experience with high-risk, poor populations beset by many health care problems. They are not accustomed to providing ancillary services such as the outreach and transportation that the poor require. In addition, as Perloff and others point out, many managed care organizations, especially those with full capitation arrangements, face strong financial pressure to limit utilization. As Blendon et al. (1993) argue, Medicaid beneficiaries have trouble paying for the basic necessities of life and have more health problems than other groups. By their estimates, a reduction in services may present a severe financial hardship for 25 to 50 percent of Medicaid beneficiaries.

A second area of concern is that managed care does not directly address the access problems faced by Americans who are uninsured. Perhaps because they are in poorer health, uninsured African Americans are as likely to enter the health care system as the privately insured. However, they may not be getting as much care as they need; when other relevant factors are controlled they make fewer total visits relative to their medical needs.

Several health care reform proposals suggest the expansion of Medicaid to cover at least a portion of uninsured populations. But states are not moving rapidly to embrace these plans. There are fears that the costs will be prohibitive (Holahan and Zedlewski 1991). Moreover, some analyses indicate that only a small fraction of the uninsured population would be covered under such extensions unless accompanied by changes in Medicaid's strict income and categorical eligibility requirements (Capilouto, Thorpe, and Dailey 1992).

The uninsured are also more likely to enter the system via hospital outpatient and emergency departments and community and public health clinics, sites that do not facilitate established provider-patient relationships or continuity of care, and that are experiencing financial strains in the concomitant move toward cost containment. Many researchers and policymakers are also concerned that managed care, especially Medicaid managed care, will actually have adverse effects on access to care among the uninsured. Traditionally, and consistent with the findings in this study, uninsured individuals seek care in hospital emergency and outpatient departments and public clinics—the so-called safety-net providers. Safety-net providers use funds from the privately insured as well as state and local government sources to offset financial losses from the provision of uncompensated care. Medicaid's disproportionate share payments, provided to hospitals who care for a large share of poor and uninsured persons, have heretofore subsidized care for those unable to afford it (Lipson and Naierman 1996). But Medicaid managed care is shifting patients away from some safety-net providers, leading these providers to rely less on disproportionate share payments. As a consequence, the ability of these providers to treat the uninsured may be jeopardized.

While some safety-net providers are prepared to compete successfully in the managed care environment, others are not. Many of these providers are not attractive to managed care organizations because they are undercapitalized, inefficiently managed, and generally in poor financial condition (Perloff 1996). Even when these organizations enter into managed care arrangements, there is no guarantee that patients will be referred, and reimbursement rates may not be adequate to ensure profit (Lipson and Naierman 1996). Managed care could indeed make it even more difficult for the uninsured population to find medical care.

The impact of managed care on provider satisfaction is also likely to yield mixed results. In this study, the probability of being very satisfied is greater for African Americans who encounter fewer barriers to access, have high levels of trust, spend more time with their provider, and have an African American physician. While managed care may reduce a patient's out-of-pocket costs, which might contribute to provider satisfaction as well as to overall satisfaction, managed care may not be as effective in reducing other barriers, such as transportation, getting appointments, and waiting time for appointments. Further, providers in many medical settings are often unable to spend as much time in medical encounters as they and their patients might desire.

The demand for more efficient processing of patients may be even greater in managed care organizations, given their emphasis on cost containment, than in other settings. This situation is likely to lower client satisfaction levels. Managed care organizations serving African American patients do have the potential for promoting higher levels of satisfaction by employing African American physicians, but their ability to do so may be limited by various structural constraints, including the availability of African American physicians. Although significant progress has been made in expanding medical education to African Americans and in overcoming discriminatory behavior aimed at black physicians, African American physicians remain in short supply (Nager and Saadatmand 1991). The shortage is likely to worsen, given the current attack on corrective policies such as affirmative action. It will be to the economic advantage of managed care organizations with significant African American enrollments to support policies that will foster medical education among African Americans.

In summary, managed care offers hope and potential for addressing the health care needs of African Americans. However, policymakers must be cautious in their planning. Detailed assessments of the advantages and disadvantages should be ascertained, especially with regard to vulnerable population subgroups. The federal government should continue to take a leadership role by encouraging states, through financial incentives, to go forward in providing for the uninsured, and through continued support of safety-net providers.

References

Aday, L., Fleming, G. V., and Andersen, R. M., 1984. *Access to Medical Care in the U.S.: Who Has It, Who Doesn't.* Chicago: Pluribus Press.

Andersen, R., Aday, L., and Lyttle, C. 1987. *Ambulatory Care and Insurance Coverage in an Era of Constraint.* Chicago: Pluribus Press.

Baker, D., Stevens, C., and Brook, R. 1994. Regular source of ambulatory care and medical care utilization by patients presenting to a public hospital emergency department. *Journal of the American Medical Association* 271 (24):1909–1912.

Berkanovic, E., and Reeder, L. 1974. Can money buy the appropriate use of services? Some notes on the meaning of utilization data. *Journal of Health and Social Behavior* 15:93–109.

Berki, S., and Ashcraft, M. 1979. On the analysis of ambulatory utilization: an investigation of the roles of need, access and price as predictors of illness and preventive visits. *Medical Care* 17:1163–1181.

Blendon, R., and Taylor, H. 1989. Views on health care: public opinion in three nations. *Health Affairs* 8:149–157.

Blendon, R., Aiden, L., Freeman, H., and Corey, C. 1989. Access to medical care for black and white Americans: a matter of continuing concern. *Journal of the American Medical Association* 261(2)278–281.

Blendon, R., Donelan, K., Hill, C., Scheck, A., Carter, W., Beatrice, D., and Altman, D. 1993. Medicaid beneficiaries and health care reform. *Health Affairs* (Spring):132–143.

Braveman, P., Egerter, S., Bennett, T., and Showstack, J. 1991. Differences in hospital resource allocation among sick newborns according to insurance coverage. *Journal of the American Medical Association* 226(23):3300–3308.

Capilouto, E., Thorpe, K., and Dailey, T. 1992. How restrictive are Medicaid's categorical eligibility requirements? A look at nine southern states. *Inquiry* 29:451–456.

Cornelius, L. 1993. Ethnic minorities and access to medical care: where do they stand? *Journal of the Association for Academic Minority Physicians* 4: 16–25.

Davis, K., Lillie-Blanton, M., Lyons, B., Mullan, F., Powe, N., and Rowland, D. 1987. Health care for black Americans: the public sector role. *The Milbank Quarterly* 65(Suppl. 1):213–247.

Dignan, M., Michielutte, R., Sharp, P., Bahnson, J., Young, L., and Beal, P. 1990. The role of focus groups in health education for cervical cancer among minority women. *Journal of Community Health* 15(6):369–375.

Elliot, G., and Eisdorfer, C. 1982. *Stress and Human Health*. New York: Springer.

Escarce, J., Epstein, K., Colby, D., and Schwartz, J. 1993. Racial differences in the elderly's use of medical procedures and diagnostic tests. *American Journal of Public Health* 87(3):948–954.

Gibbs, R., Gibbs, P., and Henrich, J. 1987. Patient understanding of commonly used medical vocabulary. *Journal of Family Practice* 25:176–178.

Hadley, J., Steinberg, E., and Feder, J. 1991. Comparison of uninsured and privately insured hospital patients: conditions on admission, resource use, and outcome. *Journal of the American Medical Society* 265:374–379.

Haug, M., and Lavin, B. 1983. *Consumerism in Medicine*. Beverly Hills, Calif.: Sage Publications.

Hayward, R., Shapiro, M., Freeman, H., and Corey, C. 1988. Inequities in health services among insured Americans. *New England Journal of Medicine* 318:1507–1512.

Hogue, C. R., Buehler, J., Strauss, L., and Smith, J. 1987. Overview of the national infant mortality surveillance (NIMS) project: design, methods, results. *Public Health Reports* 102:126–138.

Holahan, J., and Zedlewski, S. 1991. Expanding Medicaid to cover uninsured Americans. *Health Affairs* (Spring):45–61.

Hurley, R., Freund, D., and Paul, J. 1993. *Managed Care in Medicaid: Lessons for Policy and Program Design*. Ann Arbor, Mich.: Health Administration Press.

Ingram, D., Makuc, D., and Kleinman, J. 1986. National and state trends in use of prenatal care, 1970–1983. *American Journal of Public Health* 76 (4): 415–423.

Keith, V. M., and LaVeist, T. A. 1996. Social, economic, and health determinants of health care service use: a comparative analysis of whites, African Americans, and Mexican Americans. In *Achieving Equitable Access: Studies of Health Care Issues Affecting Hispanics and African Americans*. Joint Center for Political and Economic Studies. Washington, D.C.: University Press of America.

Kleinman, J., Gold, M., and Makuc, D. 1981. Use of ambulatory medical care by the poor: another look at equity. *Medical Care* 19:1011–1129.

Krieger, N. 1990. Social class and the black/white crossover in the age-specific incidence of breast cancer: a study linking census-derived data to population-based registry records. *American Journal of Epidemiology* 131:804–814.

Krieger, N., Rowley, D., Herman, A., Avery, B., and Phillips, M. 1993. Racism, sexism, and social class: implications for studies of health, disease, and well-being. *American Journal of Preventive Medicine* 9(Suppl.):82–122.

LaVeist, T., Keith, V. M., and Guiterrez, M. L. 1995. Black-white differences in prenatal care utilization: an assessment of predisposing and enabling factors. *Health Services Research* 30(1):45–60.

Lipson, D., and Naierman, N. 1996. Effects of health system changes on safety-net providers. *Health Affairs* 15(2):33–48.

Makuc, D., Freid, V., and Kleinman, J. 1989. National trends in the use of preventive health care by women. *American Journal of Public Health* 79(10)21–26.

Massey, D., Condran, G., and Denton, N. 1987. The effect of residential segregation on black social and economic well-being. *Social Forces* 64:306–371.

Miller, J., and Korenman, S. 1994. Poverty and children's nutritional status in the United States. *American Journal of Epidemiology* 140:233–243.

Muller, C. 1986. Review of twenty years of research on medical care utilization. *Health Services Research* 21(2)129–144.

Muller, C. 1988. Medicaid: the lower tier of health care for women. *Women and Health* 14(2):81–103.

Nager, N., and Saadatmand, F. 1991. The status of medical education for black Americans. *Journal of the National Medical Association* 83(9)787–792.

Newacheck, P. 1988. Access to ambulatory care for poor persons. *Health Services Research* 23:401–419.

Oliver, M., and Shapiro, T. 1995. *Black Wealth/White Wealth: A New Perspective on Racial Inequality.* New York: Routledge.

Perloff, J. 1996. Medicaid managed care and urban poor people: implications for social work. *Health and Social Work* 21(3):189–195.

Reed, W., Darity, W., Sr., and Roberson, N. 1993. *Health Care of African-Americans.* Westport, Conn.: Auburn House.

Rowland, D., Rosenbaum, S., Simon, L., and Chait, E. 1995. *Medicaid and Managed Care: Lessons from the Literature.* Washington, D.C.: Kaiser Commission on the Future of Medicaid.

Schlesinger, M. 1987. Paying the price: medical care, minorities, and the newly competitive health care system. *Milbank Quarterly* 65(Suppl. 2):270–296.

Schurman, R., Kramer, P., and Mitchell, J. 1985. The hidden mental health network: treatment of mental illness by nonpsychiatrist physicians. *Archives of General Psychiatry* 42:89–94.

Sylvester, J. L. 1998. *Directing Health Messages Toward African Americans: Attitudes Toward Health Care and the Mass Media.* New York: Garland.

Ulbrich, P., Warheit, G., and Zimmerman, R. 1989. Socioeconomic status and psychological distress: an examination of differential vulnerability. *Journal of Health and Social Behavior* 30:131–146.

Waitzkin, H., and Stoeckle, J. 1976. Information control and the micropolitics of health care: summary of an ongoing research project. *Social Science and Medicine* 10:263–276.

Wenneker, M., and Epstein, A. 1989. Racial inequalities in the use of procedures for patients with ischemic heart disease in Massachusetts. *Journal of the American Medical Association* 261:253–257.

Williams, D., and Collins, C. 1995. U.S. socioeconomic and racial differences in health: patterns and explanations. *Annual Review of Sociology* 21:349–386.

Wilson, W. 1987. *The Truly Disadvantaged: The Inner City, the Underclass, and Public Policy.* Chicago: University of Chicago Press.

4

Access to Health Care among Chinese, Korean, and Vietnamese Americans

Dorothy Chin, Ph.D.
David T. Takeuchi, Ph.D.
Dong Suh

Health professionals and policymakers identify access to health care as one of the more pressing health issues confronting Asian Americans. Empirical studies consistently document that Asian Americans do not make adequate use of the health care system even when an illness reaches a critical stage (Mayeno and Hirota 1994). For example, in a review of the National Ambulatory Medical Care Survey, Asian Americans had the lowest rate of physician visits compared to other racial/ethnic groups (Yu and Cypress 1982). More recent investigations of specific Asian American groups support this pattern (Korean Health Survey Task Force 1989; Lew and Chen 1989; Rumbaut et al. 1988). Studies on access to mental health services indicate that Asian Americans do not use services as much as other ethnic groups (Sue et al. 1991). Asian Americans are under-represented in both outpatient and inpatient mental health facilities, a finding that has remained relatively stable over the past three decades (Sue et al. 1991; Snowden and Cheung 1990).

Researchers generally advance three hypotheses to explain the pattern of health care utilization among Asian Americans. In the first, because of lifestyle and other sociocultural factors, Asian Americans have lower morbidity and better health status than other ethnic groups; thus, the low use of health services reflects Asian Americans' healthier profile. The second hypothesis argues that the health status of Asian Americans and other ethnic groups is not that different; instead, social, cultural, and institutional barriers prevent Asian Americans from using health services when there is a pressing need. The last hypothesis, similar to the second, suggests that Asian Americans disproportionately belong to high-risk groups (such as the poor, elderly, and uninsured) that typically do not access health services.

The low-morbidity hypothesis has generally not been supported, especially when a wide range of illnesses is considered (Zane, Takeuchi, and Young 1994). Even when statistical analyses control for the effects of health status, Asian Americans report a lower use of health services than whites report (Mayeno and Hirota 1994). Accordingly, recent studies have favored testing the last two hypotheses to understand access issues for Asian Americans.

DIVERSE ETHNICITIES AMONG ASIAN AMERICANS

Despite the theories advanced to explain the low rates of health care utilization among Asian Americans, empirical studies to test these theories have been lacking. In part, the limited number of studies can be attributed to the unique characteristics of the Asian American ethnic category. Because the category "Asian American" encompasses many diverse ethnic groups, which are rapidly undergoing demographic shifts at different rates and trajectories, the Asian American population has been difficult to target. For example, more than twenty ethnic groups speaking thirty different languages may be included in the Asian American category (O'Hare and Felt 1991). In addition, the population of Asian Americans in the United States has grown phenomenally in recent years. In the 1980 U.S. Census, the population of Asian Americans exceeded 3.7 million, easily doubling the 1.5 million figure in 1970. By 1990 the population nearly doubled again, surpassing 7.1 million. The three largest Asian American ethnic groups are Chinese, Japanese, and Filipinos. Koreans and Southeast Asians (such as Vietnamese, Cambodians, and Laotians) also represent a significant number within the Asian American population (Lee 1998).

The diverse characteristics of Asian Americans are meaningful because the combining of different Asian American ethnic groups can lead to misleading conclusions. Uehara, Takeuchi, and Smukler (1994) compared the effects of placing Asian American groups into a single ethnic category versus separate ethnic groups when they examined "client function" in publicly funded mental health programs. When treated as a single ethnic category, Asian Americans demonstrated a lower level of client functioning than whites. However, when Asian Americans were divided into more specific ethnic categories, this lower level of functioning was true only for only one out of five Asian American ethnic groups.

Despite increasing awareness about the differences among Asian American ethnic groups, information about specific groups is still lacking. Conducting large-scale health studies on any single Asian American ethnic group can be quite costly. For example, in a recent study of the mental health of Chinese Americans in the greater Los Angeles area, a large-scale screening of nearly 17,000 households achieved a sample size of only 1,747 respondents because Chinese Americans constitute less than 3 percent of the population in the greater Los Angeles area. This large screening effort was necessary despite a relatively low refusal rate of 18 percent (Takeuchi et al. 1998).

Taking into consideration the many issues involved in conducting research on Asian Americans, The Commonwealth Fund Minority Health Survey (CMHS) included a supplemental sample of three specific Asian American ethnic groups—Chinese, Koreans, and Vietnamese—in addition to samples of African Americans and Hispanics. These Asian samples provide an excellent opportunity for exploring the effects of various social and cultural factors on our understanding of their access to health services. Moreover, the inclusion of these three Asian American ethnic groups, two with a substantial proportion of immigrants and one composed primarily of refugees, provides a rare chance to see how social and cultural factors may operate.

In this chapter, we examine two issues using the Asian American sample of the CMHS: first, what factors are associated with the use of health services, and second, what factors are associated with the frequency of health service use. We examine five separate sets of factors: (1) ethnicity; (2) sociodemographic variables typically found to be associated with the use of health services, including age, gender, marital status, and immigration status; (3) socioeconomic status (SES) factors, as indicated by employment status, education, income, and household size; (4) health status and health insurance coverage; and (5) perceived barriers to access—factors that may constrain or enhance service use.

BACKGROUND OF ASIAN ETHNIC GROUPS

A brief background of the ethnic groups included in the analyses will contribute to our understanding.

Chinese Americans

The first significant migration of the Chinese to the United States began with the California Gold Rush in 1849 (Lee 1998). Between 1849 and

1882, over 275,000 Chinese entered the United States, of whom more than 90 percent were male. Initially, these Chinese immigrants worked primarily in mines, on the transcontinental Central Pacific Railroad, and in agriculture and service trades. Most intended their stay in the United States to be temporary, working only to earn money to return to their homeland. However, daunted by a pervasive anti-Chinese sentiment and discriminatory labor practices, few managed to struggle out of poverty. They remained, creating "bachelor societies." The Chinese Exclusion Act of 1882, the first instance of a legal bar to the immigration of an ethnic group, resulted in a decline in the Chinese population until the 1920s.

The advent of World War II marked a change in U.S. policy toward the Chinese. Because China and the United States were allies, a movement began in the United States to reverse Chinese exclusionary policies, which were ultimately repealed by the Magnuson Act of 1943. A Chinese immigration quota of 105 per year was set (Hing 1993). Despite the quota, subsequent acts of Congress allowed the legal entry of a large influx of Chinese immigrants.

The second significant wave of Chinese immigration occurred after 1965, when family reunification policies allowed Chinese Americans to sponsor their relatives for resettlement in the United States (Hing 1993). By 1990, the Chinese American population surpassed 1.6 million and comprised the largest group of Asian Americans, representing 23 percent of the Asian and Pacific Islander American population and 0.7 percent of the U.S. population (Lee 1998). The greatest number of Chinese Americans came to reside in urban areas in Western and Northeastern states such as California, Washington, New York, and Massachusetts.

Reflecting the two separate waves of immigration, Chinese Americans as a group are diverse in acculturation, educational attainment, income, and employment. Third- and fourth-generation Chinese Americans, descendants of the first wave of immigrants, tend to be highly acculturated and have higher educational attainment and income, whereas recently immigrated Chinese face a host of economic hardships and cultural adjustments.

Korean Americans

Korean Americans are currently the fifth largest Asian American ethnic group, totaling nearly 800,000 in 1990. There have been three waves of immigration of Koreans to the United States. In the late 1800s and early

1900s, several events caused unstable conditions in Korea—including the Tonghak Rebellion, the Sino-Japanese War, the Russo-Japanese War, a cholera epidemic, a drought, a locust plague, and famine—prompting displaced Koreans to migrate to Hawaii to work on plantations (Daniels and Kitano 1970). The first Korean immigrants were primarily male, although some Korean "picture brides" immigrated to the United States before U.S. policy barred Korean immigration in 1924 (Kitano 1991). Between 1951 and 1964, the second wave of Korean immigration consisted of wives of Americans fighting in the Korean War, Korean children orphaned by the Korean War who were adopted by American families, and students (Kitano 1991). The largest wave of Korean immigration, which continues today, followed the 1965 Immigration and Naturalization Act. Recent Korean immigrants tend to come in family units, and the adults in these families are generally highly educated.

Most Korean immigrants live in Koreatowns, isolated from other ethnic groups. A large proportion of Koreans own or work in small businesses. To illustrate, in 1984 there were 7,000 Korean-owned businesses in Los Angeles County (Daniels and Kitano 1970). A current major concern in the Korean community is the growing tension between Korean Americans and other ethnic minority groups. In major cities such as Los Angeles and New York, owing to perceived competition and cultural misunderstanding, conflict between immigrant Korean Americans and other ethnic minority groups, particularly African Americans and Latinos, has escalated into violence.

Vietnamese Americans

Unlike Chinese and Korean Americans, the Vietnamese are largely involuntary immigrants to the United States, prompted by the social upheavals caused by the Vietnam War. Since 1960, two distinct waves of Vietnamese immigrants have relocated to the United States. The first consisted of mainly upper- and middle-class families who, from 1960 to 1975, had the resources to move when it became clear that the war would not quickly end. The second and larger wave came between 1975 and 1994 under very different circumstances, desperate to leave under the threat of political persecution and genocide. Many boarded boats without a clear destination, hoping to reach the United States eventually by way of Hong Kong, Malaysia, or other nearby countries (Lee 1998). Furthermore, many experienced the trauma of pirate attacks en route as well as the overcrowded and often unsanitary conditions of refugee camps. Under the Refugee Assistance Act of 1980, large numbers were accepted into the country, bringing the U.S. Vietnamese population to 1.2 million in 1989 (O'Hare and Felt 1991).

As a group, Vietnamese refugees have lower incomes than all other ethnic minority groups in the United States. They earn significantly less than Chinese or Japanese Americans, who generally have incomes at the higher end of the spectrum (O'Hare and Felt 1991). The largest Vietnamese American communities are in California, Texas, and Florida.

The needs of Vietnamese American refugees are significant. Yet those needs have put them at odds with other ethnic groups, such as African Americans and Latinos, who may resent the special assistance given to refugees and who may perceive that resources to their communities diminished as a result (Lee 1998). Furthermore, racial tensions between Vietnamese Americans and whites have also been documented (United States Commission on Civil Rights 1992), where perceived competition is a source of conflict. For instance, in recent years Vietnamese and white fishermen in Louisiana have clashed over territory and fishing methods.

METHODS OF ANALYSIS

While this CMHS survey oversampled African Americans, Latinos, and Asian Americans within the sampling strata (see the Technical Appendix), the Asian American sample was selected using a different procedure altogether. Asian Americans were selected based on a telephone list of surnames common to three different ethnic groups: Chinese, Korean, and Vietnamese. Post-stratification weights were applied to the samples to equalize their representation in the survey.

The analyses that follow attempt to explore the associations among different factors to Asian Americans' access to and utilization of health services. These exploratory analyses, while not sufficiently robust to allow for generalizations, are a type of analysis that has never before been conducted on three major Asian American ethnic groups. Our analyses seek to answer the following questions: (1) How do the Asian American subgroups differ with respect to sociodemographic characteristics, health status, insurance coverage, and use of health care services? (2) How do demographic characteristics, health status, insurance coverage, and perceived barriers affect entry into and utilization of health care? and (3) What barriers to health care do Asian Americans report?

Two major dependent variables are considered in these analyses: access to care and utilization of health care services. The same source question provides the measures for both dependent variables. Respondents were asked how often they had visited a doctor in the past twelve months prior to the interview. "Access to care" is a dichotomous variable that categorizes respondents into those who had at least one visit versus others who had no visits to the doctor during the time frame. For respondents who had at least one visit, a utilization variable was constructed of the actual number of visits made during the past twelve months. Because utilization is skewed (i.e., generally low number of visits with a few individuals having many visits), this variable was logarithmically transformed.

Five types of predictor variables are explored in the following analyses: ethnicity, sociodemographic, socioeconomic, insurance and health status, and perceived barriers. Sociodemographic variables include age (18-29, 30-44, 45-64, 65+), gender, marital status (married, unmarried, other), and years of residence in the United States (≤5 years, ≥6 years, U.S. born). SES factors consist of household income ($25,000 or less, $25,001-$50,000, $50,001+), education (less than high school, high school graduate, some college, college graduate, postgraduate), and employment status (employed, unemployed, and other). We control for household size when the analyses include income. Health status and insurance coverage are considered together in one set of analyses. Health status is a single variable indicator rated on a four-point scale (excellent, good, fair, poor). Insurance coverage is treated as two separate dummy variables; having private insurance (yes or no) and having any type of public insurance (yes or no). These groups are contrasted with those who are uninsured.

Perceived barriers to care comprise the final set of variables. Eight types of barriers are rated on a three-point scale (major problem, minor problem, or not a problem), which we then coded dichotomously into having a problem versus not having a problem. These barriers include lack of access to specialty care, difficulty getting appointments, high cost of services, language differences, being nervous or afraid, lengthy time waiting for appointments, transportation problems, and too much paperwork. For each dependent variable, we first assess four models that include ethnicity, demographic, socioeconomic, and insurance and health status predictors, each set entered successively by block. Then we consider two models that include barriers and insurance and health predictors.

RESULTS OF ANALYSIS

Description of Sample

A majority of respondents within the three ethnic groups were between the ages of 30 and 64, had completed at least high school, had incomes of less than $50,000, and had resided in the United States for at least six years (Table 4.1). More than half had some type of health insurance and reported their health to be excellent or good.

Ethnic group differences were found for some characteristics. Vietnamese were more likely to be recent immigrants, while the Chinese were less likely to be foreign born. Educational attainment was unevenly distributed for all three groups; the Chinese showed a bimodal profile, with large numbers of people who did not finish high school as well as college and post-college graduates, which is consistent with the diversity expected from two distinct waves of immigration. The Vietnamese had greater numbers in the lower end of educational attainment, consistent with their backgrounds as recent refugees in this country. Koreans demonstrated greater numbers in the middle categories; most had graduated from high school or attended or graduated from college. Income levels also differed by ethnicity, with Koreans less likely to be poor. Koreans were less likely to have public or private health insurance, and the Chinese more likely to have private insurance. About 60 percent of all three groups stated that they had a regular health care provider, and about three-quarters reported visiting a physician at least once in the past year. In terms of health status, Vietnamese reported poorer health than the Chinese or Koreans.

In sum, the demographic profiles of the three groups in the sample reflect their varying histories in the United States. The Vietnamese are more likely to be recent immigrants, with lower education, income, and health status. The Chinese show greater diversity in all demographic characteristics, reflecting their longer history in the United States as well as continued immigration. The Koreans appear to be more middle-class, with higher education and income than the other two groups.

Access to Care

We conducted a series of logistic regression analyses with health care access as the criterion variable. First, we assessed four separate models using four sets of predictors (ethnicity, demographic characteristics, SES,

Table 4.1   Percentage Distribution of Demographic and Health Characteristics among Chinese, Vietnamese, and Korean Americans

	Chinese (N = 205)		Vietnamese (N = 201)		Korean (N = 201)		
	%	Standard Error	%	Standard Error	%	Standard Error	Adjusted p value
Age							0.09
18–29	22.7	2.4	30.9	3.6	29.1	4.2	
30–44	42.1	2.8	42.4	3.8	32.5	4.3	
45–64	26.5	2.5	23.2	3.3	29.9	4.2	
≥65	8.8	1.6	3.6	1.5	8.5	2.6	
Female	51.5	2.8	50.3	3.9	57.0	4.5	0.49
Married	66.4	2.6	61.2	3.8	56.2	4.5	0.12
Time in U.S.							<0.01
≤5 years	20.6	2.4	33.1	3.8	30.7	4.3	
≥6 years	50.2	3.0	52.6	4.0	51.8	4.7	
Born in U.S.	29.3	2.7	14.3	2.8	17.5	3.6	
Employed	63.1	2.7	66.7	3.7	57.4	4.5	0.27
Education							<0.01
<High school	29.9	2.6	33.8	3.8	14.7	3.4	
High school graduate	24.4	2.4	27.6	3.6	32.1	4.5	
Some college	9.3	3.2	19.9	3.2	12.8	3.2	
College graduate	24.1	2.4	15.3	2.9	30.3	4.4	
Postgraduate	12.5	1.8	3.8	1.5	10.1	2.9	
Income							0.02
≤$25,000	36.5	2.7	40.6	3.8	22.3	3.8	
$25,001–$50,000	41.2	2.7	39.4	3.8	50.4	4.5	
>$50,000	22.3	2.3	19.4	3.3	27.3	4.1	
Insurance							<0.01
Public	15.7	2.0	21.8	3.2	9.0	2.6	
Private	67.3	2.6	58.8	3.8	52.9	4.5	
Uninsured	17.2	2.1	19.9	3.1	38.0	4.4	
Health status							<0.01
Excellent	25.8	2.4	12.7	2.6	34.4	4.3	
Good	54.9	3.9	57.9	3.9	46.7	4.5	
Fair	14.2	1.9	26.2	3.4	16.4	3.4	
Poor	4.9	1.2	3.0	1.3	2.5	1.4	
Regular provider	60.3	2.7	57.2	3.8	59.0	4.5	0.58
Physician visit last year	78.6	2.3	72.2	3.5	71.3	4.1	0.15

Source: Data from The Commonwealth Fund Minority Health Survey, 1994.

insurance, and health status) entered hierarchically (Table 4.2). We then assessed two models in which perceived barriers and insurance and health status predictors were entered hierarchically (Table 4.3). This analytic strategy allowed us to consider various explanations for health care access.

As shown in Table 4.2, model 1 assessed ethnicity as a predictor of access to care, with Chinese as the contrast group. Ethnicity was not associated with access to care.

Model 2, which included ethnicity and demographic predictors, significantly predicted access to care. In this model, Koreans were less likely than Chinese to have accessed health care in the previous year. Among the demographic predictors, age was significantly associated with access; those who were 65 years or older were almost eight times more likely to have accessed health care.

In model 3, socioeconomic factors were added to ethnicity and demographic variables as predictors. In this model, both ethnicity and age remained significant, with Koreans less likely and the elderly more likely to access care. In addition, those who were employed accessed health care less than the unemployed. Income was also positively associated with access, with those in the middle income range 1.75 times more likely and those in the high income range 2.73 times more likely to access care than those earning less than $25,000.

Model 4, which included the set of insurance and health status variables in addition to ethnicity, demographic, and socioeconomic factors in the prediction model, was significantly related to access to care. We found that when insurance and health predictors were added, only employment and high income were significantly associated with access among the previous sets of predictors. Among insurance and health variables, having public insurance and reporting good or fair health, as opposed to poor health, were positively associated with access.

In examining the relationship between perceived barriers and access to care, we omitted ethnicity as a predictor because in the previous models it proved not to be significant. Two models were assessed, the first in which only the set of barriers served as predictors and the second in which insurance and health status variables were also entered (see Table 4.3). Barriers alone did not significantly predict access. Among the individual predictors, the perception of too much paperwork was negatively associated with access; those who stated that too much paperwork was a problem were about half as likely to access care. When insurance and health status variables were added, the model signifi-

Table 4.2 Demographic, Socioeconomic, and Insurance and Health Correlates of Entry into Health Care during the Previous Year

	MODEL 1			MODEL 2			MODEL 3			MODEL 4		
	Odds Ratio	Standard Error	95% Confidence Interval	Odds Ratio	Standard Error	95% Confidence Interval	Odds Ratio	Standard Error	95% Confidence Interval	Odds Ratio	Standard Error	95% Confidence Interval
Ethnicity												
Vietnamese	0.71	0.20	0.46,1.0	1.00	-0.51	0.44,1.13	0.75	0.25	0.45,1.24	0.59	0.21	0.34,1.00
Korean	0.68	0.21	0.42,1.09	0.57[a]	0.20	0.34,0.97	0.54[a]	0.22	0.30,0.98	0.64	0.28	0.35,1.19
Demographic												
Age												
30–44 years				0.68	0.28	0.38,1.23	0.76	0.34	0.40,1.43	0.73	0.34	0.38,1.40
45–64 years				0.96	0.45	0.50,1.84	1.11	0.61	0.54,2.30	0.99	0.57	0.47,2.10
≥65 years				7.99[b]	18.80	1.42,44.84	10.13[a]	40.77	1.14,90.04	5.55	23.71	0.59,52.02
Female				1.37	0.35	0.91,2.06	1.19	0.33	0.77,1.84	1.01	0.30	0.63,1.60
Married				1.09	0.37	0.66,1.81	1.41	0.56	0.79,2.51	1.40	0.57	0.78,2.52
Time in U.S.												
≥6 years in U.S.				1.27	0.40	0.79,2.06	1.28	0.45	0.76,2.16	1.22	0.45	0.71,2.11
Born in U.S.				1.02	0.44	0.56,1.88	0.88	0.44	0.45,1.73	0.84	0.44	0.41,1.71
Socioeconomic												
Employed							0.48[c]	0.17	0.28,0.81	0.52[a]	0.19	0.30,0.90
Education												
High school graduate							0.86	0.36	0.47,1.57	0.79	0.35	0.42,1.49
Some college							0.88	0.48	0.42,1.82	0.80	0.46	0.37,1.70
College graduate							1.41	0.75	0.69,2.89	1.37	0.77	0.65,2.89
Postgraduate							0.83	0.55	0.36,1.90	0.85	0.61	0.35,2.04

(continues)

Table 4.2 (*Continued*)

	MODEL 1			MODEL 2			MODEL 3			MODEL 4		
	Odds Ratio	Standard Error	95% Confidence Interval	Odds Ratio	Standard Error	95% Confidence Interval	Odds Ratio	Standard Error	95% Confidence Interval	Odds Ratio	Standard Error	95% Confidence Interval
Income												
$25,001–$50,000							1.75[a]	0.59	1.05,2.90	1.66	0.59	0.98,2.82
≥$50,001							2.73[c]	1.35	1.39,5.37	2.92[c]	1.52	1.44,5.90
Household size							0.93	0.07	0.81,1.06	0.92	0.07	0.81,1.05
Insurance and health status												
Insurance												
Public										4.34[c]	3.55	1.67,11.30
Private										1.62	0.61	0.93,2.82
Health status												
Excellent										1.63	1.81	0.51,5.18
Good										2.93[a]	2.89	1.00,8.59
Fair										4.06[a]	4.70	1.24,13.28

Source: Data from The Commonwealth Fund Minority Health Survey, 1994.

Note: Referent categories: Chinese, 18–29 years of age, male, unmarried, <6 years in the U.S., unemployed, <high school education, income <$25,001, no insurance, poor health.

[a] $p < 0.05$.

[b] $p < 0.001$.

[c] $p < 0.01$.

Table 4.3   Barriers and Insurance and Health Correlates of Entry into Health Care during the Previous Year

	MODEL 1		MODEL 2	
	Odds Ratio	95% Confidence Interval	Odds Ratio	95% Confidence Interval
Barriers				
No access to specialty care	1.06	0.62,1.81	1.05	0.61,1.81
Cannot get appointment	0.99	0.60,1.64	0.98	0.59,1.63
Pay too much	0.73	0.44,1.22	0.98	0.57,1.68
Language	1.01	0.62,1.65	0.94	0.57,1.56
Nervous/afraid	1.17	0.70,1.96	1.07	0.64,1.81
Wait too long	1.21	0.99,2.81	1.22	0.73,2.04
Transportation	1.67	0.99,2.81	1.75[a]	1.02,3.03
Paperwork	0.53[a]	0.33,0.87	0.51[b]	0.31,0.84
Insurance and health status				
Insurance				
Public			4.80[c]	2.06,11.15
Private			1.92[b]	1.18,3.13
Health status				
Excellent			1.77	0.63,5.02
Good			2.45	0.93,6.49
Fair			3.30[a]	1.13,9.58

Source: Data from The Commonwealth Fund Minority Health Survey, 1994.
Note: Referent categories: no barriers, no insurance, poor health.
[a]$p < 0.05$.
[b]$p < 0.01$.
[c]$p < 0.001$.

cantly predicted access. Transportation and paperwork were significant predictors in opposite directions. Too much paperwork predicted lower access, while the perception of transportation problems was associated with higher access. While this appears to be counterintuitive, it is plausible that seeing a physician may actually heighten the perception of transportation problems because of actual experience. Among the insurance and health status predictors, having public insurance or private insurance were significantly associated with care access. Compared with those in poor health, those who reported fair health were 3.3 times as likely to access care.

Volume of Utilization

Other analyses focus on the issue of volume of utilization and are limited to the subset of respondents who reported visiting a physician at least once during the past year. The actual number of visits was logarithmically transformed to reduce the skewness of the variable. In this section, we employed multiple linear regression as the principal analytic technique. As with access to care, we used the same four prediction models using four sets of factors (ethnicity, sociodemographic, SES, health status, and insurance coverage). We also assessed the relationship of barriers and utilization using two prediction models.

Ethnicity did not significantly predict volume of utilization (data not shown). In model 2, the group of demographic factors was significantly associated with utilization ($F(9,395) = 7.11$, $p < 0.001$, adjusted $R^2_\Delta = 0.12$). Respondents who were older than 44 years and female had more physician visits. When socioeconomic factors were added (model 3), the model significantly predicted utilization ($F(17,375) = 4.34$, $p < 0.001$, adjusted $R^2_\Delta = 0.01$). Again, older and female respondents had more physician visits. Those who were employed had fewer visits. Model 4 included insurance and health status predictors in addition to the previous sets of predictors. A similar pattern of association was found for ethnicity, demographic, and socioeconomic predictors. The group of insurance and health status predictors was significant ($F(22,370) = 4.08$, $p < 0.001$, adjusted $R^2_\Delta = 0.12$), with excellent and good health associated with lower utilization.

As with access to care, we examined the influence of perceived barriers on health care utilization using two models (data not shown). Again, ethnicity was omitted as a predictor because it was not related to utilization. The first model, using only the set of barriers as predictors, did not significantly predict utilization. Among the individual predictors, the perception of lack of access to specialty care was positively associated with utilization, while the perception of high costs was negatively associated. Again, this finding is counterintuitive, but may be reflective of higher utilization increasing awareness of problems. When the set of insurance and health status predictors was included, the model was significant ($F(13,414) = 4.36$, $p < 0.001$, adjusted $R^2_\Delta = 0.08$). Having public insurance was associated with a higher number of physician visits, and excellent and good health were associated with fewer physician visits.

Explaining Health Care Access and Utilization

In these analyses, health status is minimally associated with access and utilization. This raises at least two important points concerning access issues among Asian Americans. First, health status is measured as the respondent's perception of his or her overall health. It is possible that this type of question adequately identifies Asian Americans who are ill and require a physician's care. However, Asian Americans may have different conceptions of health and illness that in turn may affect their overall assessment of their health status. For example, in terms of mental health self-assessment, some analysts speculate that Asian Americans may consider themselves healthy as long as their functioning level allows them to actively perform their work and social roles (Takeuchi and Uehara 1996). It is possible that judgments about physical health are made along similar lines, and Asian Americans may not access health care until their functioning is so impaired that work and social roles cannot be fulfilled.

It is also possible that Asian Americans may see physicians for reasons other than medical care. While survey respondents report seeing a physician at least once in the past twelve months, health status is predictive of access in the counterintuitive direction, in that those reporting good and fair health were more likely to have access to care. This may indicate that there are reasons for seeking out a physician other than poor health. For example, Asian American immigrants, who comprise a majority of the Asians in the United States, may seek referrals from their physicians to gain social and other needed services (Mayeno and Hirota 1994). This may be especially true if health care is delivered in the context of a community clinic in which physicians, nurses, and social workers work at a common site.

Analyses regarding perceived barriers to access and utilization of health care yield a mixed pattern. Some barriers are associated with higher access and utilization, and other barriers are related to lower usage of services. These findings illustrate the difficulty of capturing dynamic, simultaneous psychological processes. That is, although perceived barriers may indeed inhibit the usage of services, the usage of services may, at the same time, increase a person's perceptions of problems.

POLICY IMPLICATIONS

Considerable attention has been given over the past two decades to the delivery of critical preventive care and treatment services in ethnic minority communities. Interest in providing services to "multicultural" populations has intensified during this time period because of the significant demographic transformation the United States has undergone. In 1950, ethnic minorities comprised about 19 percent of the U.S. population. By 1990, this percentage had increased to 23 percent (Lewit and Baker 1994). It is estimated that by the early twenty-first century, approximately one-third of the U.S. population will consist of ethnic minority groups (Jones 1991).

A significant portion of this demographic shift can be attributed to immigration. Over 10 million people have immigrated to the United States in the past twenty years (Portes and Rumbaut 1990). This figure represents one-fourth of the population gain in the United States. In fact, this immigration change parallels a similar change that occurred at the beginning of this century. The major difference between the current immigration pattern and that in the early part of this century is the country of origin. In the early 1900s, immigrants came chiefly from Europe and Canada; more recently, immigrants have come primarily from Asia and Latin America (Muller 1993). For example, as recently as 1950, 68 percent of immigrants were white, while 27 percent were Asian and Latin American. By 1980, these figures had nearly reversed: whites comprised approximately 13 percent of the immigrants living in the United States, and 78 percent were Asian and Latin Americans (Muller 1993). High volumes of immigration have dramatically increased the Asian American population. Between 1980 and 1990, the number of Asian Americans nearly doubled. It is expected to double again by 2010.

Service providers who recognize this demographic shift in communities, particularly in major urban areas, realistically advocate for preventive and medical services that are sensitive to the health needs of diverse populations. A particular concern is tailoring services to people who do not speak English as their first language or who come from different cultures (Takeuchi et al. 1995).

The Means to Access Health Services

As service providers and policymakers turn their attention to access issues, it is equally important to recognize that a substantial number of people in ethnic minority communities may not have the means to access health services even when "special" services are made available. One barrier to receiving health services is the high cost of health care. Health care in the United States costs 40 percent more than in any other developed nation (Schieber and Poullier 1991). Because of these high costs, health care has become virtually unaffordable to a large portion of the American population. While health insurance has evolved to help people meet the cost demands placed on them by medical care, it is estimated that approximately 37 million Americans, or about 14.8 percent of the U.S. population, have neither public nor private health insurance coverage (Mechanic and Aiken 1989).

Although some empirical investigations document the level of insurance coverage in Latino and African American populations, we do not have much information about Asian Americans. In the sparse empirical data that are available, there is some evidence that health insurance coverage in Asian American communities is limited.

In this sample, insurance coverage plays an important part in understanding access and utilization for all three Asian American ethnic groups examined. We find that having health insurance is indeed predictive of access to and utilization of health care. However, almost 40 percent of Korean Americans and about 20 percent of Chinese and Vietnamese Americans report having no insurance coverage. This is a critical finding because past health studies on Asian Americans have neglected insurance coverage in analyses.

Perhaps there are social and cultural factors that enable or prevent Asian Americans from obtaining insurance coverage. For example, the inability to communicate well in English may be a constraining factor. Insurance policies are complicated documents with many legal and bureaucratic terms. Even if insurance guidelines are translated, the insurance terms may not be easily understood to someone whose native language is one other than English. The high percentage of Korean Americans without insurance coverage may reflect the predominance of small business owners in this group. They do not have the option of obtaining insurance through employers, and they may not opt to purchase their own insurance.

The type of insurance may also be critical. In additional analyses performed separately for each ethnic group, we find that having some type of public insurance is predictive of health care access for Chinese and Vietnamese Americans, and we find that private insurance is predictive for Korean Americans. This pattern of results may explain the findings for the effects of employment, which show that unemployed Chinese and Vietnamese tend to access health care more than the employed. Unemployed Chinese and Vietnamese may have better access to Medicaid and Medicare, due to age, citizenship, and disability status; employed Chinese and Vietnamese—like employed Koreans—may work where employer-based health insurance is either unavailable or too costly.

Welfare and Health Care Policy

Placed in the context of the current debates about welfare and health care policy, our findings have several important implications. First, each Asian American ethnic group needs to be considered separately, because any policy is likely to have a differential impact on these groups. Our findings suggest that, among Asian Americans, Korean Americans are more socioeconomically stable, having a relatively higher percentage of individuals who are educated and self-employed. Vietnamese Americans, on the other hand, appear to be younger, less educated, less acculturated, and less economically secure. Chinese Americans appear to be a more diverse group, with a wider range of education and income.

Given these differences among the Asian American groups, it is not surprising that those Chinese and Vietnamese who are unemployed, and who are therefore more likely to have public insurance, are more likely to have access to health care than those who are employed. This raises the possibility that the employed individuals are only marginally employed, and that perhaps makes them ineligible for either public or employer-sponsored insurance coverage. Thus, any further reduction of public benefits may pose a serious constraint to health care access for economically marginal or insecure groups such as the Chinese and Vietnamese.

Given that dramatic changes in the health care system are likely to take place in the next few years, insurance coverage is likely to play an even more salient role than heretofore in the lives of all Americans. This is an issue worthy of increased study, especially for Asian Americans where there is no strong empirical base of knowledge.

References

Asian Week. 1991. Asians in America: 1990 Census Classification by States. San Francisco: *Asian Week*.

Chung, R. C., and Okazaki, S. 1991. Counseling Americans of southeast Asian descent: the impact of the refugee experience. In C. C. Lee and B. L. Richardson, eds., *Multicultural Issues in Counseling: New Approaches to Diversity*. Alexandria, Va.: American Counseling Association.

The Commonwealth Fund. March 20, 1995. National Comparative Survey on Minority Health. New York: The Commonwealth Fund.

Daniels, R. 1988. *Asian America: Chinese and Japanese in the United States since 1850*. Seattle: University of Washington Press.

Daniels, R., and Kitano, H. 1970. *American Racism: Exploration of the Nature of Prejudice*. Englewood Cliffs, N.J.: Prentice-Hall.

Hing, B. O. 1993. *Making and Remaking Asian America Through Immigration Policy 1850-1990*. Stanford, Calif.: Stanford University Press.

Jones, J. M. 1991. A call to advance psychology's role in minority issues. *APA Monitor* 21:23.

Kitano, H. H. L. 1991. *Race Relations*. Englewood Cliffs, N.J.: Prentice-Hall.

Korean Health Survey Task Force. 1989. *Korean Health Survey*. Los Angeles: Korean Health Education, Information and Referral Center.

Lee, S. M. 1998. Asian Americans: diverse and growing. *Population Bulletin* 53(2):1–39.

Lew, R., and Chen, A. October 1989. A community survey of health risk behavior among Chinese Americans. Paper presented at the annual meeting of the American Public Health Association.

Lewit, E. M., and Baker, L. G. 1994. Race and ethnicity: changes for children. *Critical Health Issues for Children* 4:134–144.

Mayeno, L., and Hirota, S. 1994. Access to health care. In N. Zane, D. Takeuchi, and K. Young, eds., *Confronting Critical Health Issues of Asian and Pacific Islander Americans*. Thousand Oaks, Calif.: Sage Publications.

Mechanic, D., and Aiken, L. 1989. Capitation in mental health: potentials and cautions. *New Directions in Mental Health Services* 43:1–16.

Muller, T. 1993. *Immigrants and the American City*. New York: New York University Press.

O'Hare, W. P., and Felt, J. C. 1991. *Asian Americans: America's Fastest Growing Minority Group*. Washington, D.C.: Population Reference Bureau.

Portes, A., and Rumbaut, R. G. 1990. *Immigrant America: A Portrait*. Berkeley: University of California Press.

Rumbaut, R. G., Chavez, L. R., Moser, R. J., Pickwell, S. M., and Wishnik, S. M. 1988. The politics of migrant health care: a comparative study of Mexican immigrants and Indochinese refugees. *Research in the Sociology of Health Care* 7:143–202.

Schieber, G. J., and Poullier, J. P. 1991. International health spending: issues and trends. *Health Affairs* 10:106–116.

Snowden, L., and Cheung, F. 1990. Use of inpatient mental health services by members of ethnic minority groups. *American Psychologist* 45:347–355.

Sue, S., Fujino, D., Hu, L., Takeuchi, D., and Zane, N. 1991. Community mental health services for ethnic minority groups: a test of the cultural responsiveness hypothesis. *Journal of Consulting and Clinical Psychology* 59:533–540.

Takeuchi, D., Chung, R., Lin, K. M., Shen, H., Kuraski, K., Chun C., and Sue, S. 1998. Lifetime and twelve month prevalence rates of major depressive episodes and dysthymia among Chinese Americans in Los Angeles. *American Journal of Psychiatry* 155:1407–1414.

Takeuchi, D., and Uehara, E. 1996. Ethnic minority mental health services: current research and future conceptual directions. In B. L. Levin and J. Petrila, eds., *Mental Health Services: A Public Health Perspective.* New York: Oxford University Press.

Takeuchi, D., Shen, H. K., and Chung, R. C. 1996. Insurance Coverage among Chinese Americans in Los Angeles County. Unpublished paper.

Takeuchi, D. T., Sue, S., and Yeh, M. 1995. Return rates and outcomes from ethnicity-specific mental health programs in Los Angeles. *American Journal of Public Health* 85:638–643.

Uehara, E., Takeuchi, D., and Smukler, M. 1994. Effects of combining disparate groups in the analyses of ethnic differences: variations among Asian American mental health service consumers in level of community functioning. *American Journal of Community Psychology* 22:83–99.

United States Commission on Civil Rights. 1992. *Civil Rights Issues Facing Asian Americans in the 1990s.* Washington, D.C.: U.S. Government Printing Office.

Yu, E., and Cypress, B. K. 1982. Visits to physicians by Asian Pacific Americans. *Medical Care* 20:809–820.

Zane, N., Takeuchi, D., and Young, K. 1994. *Confronting Critical Health Issues of Asian and Pacific Islander Americans.* Thousand Oaks, Calif.: Sage Publications.

5

Health Care for African American and Hispanic Women
Report on Perceived Health Status, Access to Care, and Utilization Patterns

Vickie M. Mays, Ph.D.
Susan D. Cochran, Ph.D., M.S.
J. Greer Sullivan, M.D., M.S.P.H

Over the past decade, health care services in the United States have undergone remarkable changes. Driven largely by the need to control escalating health care costs, innovations in delivering and financing health care have been introduced into the American market. Initiated in the private sector, these innovative approaches (including various types of "managed" care and prospective or capitated funding approaches) are now moving into public sector care (Scanlon, Chernew, and Lave 1997). Although these newer health care strategies do reduce costs, great concern remains about the quality of the care they provide, particularly to vulnerable populations (Lillie-Blanton and Lillie 1996; Blumenthal, Mort, and Edwards 1995). Ethnic minorities, especially those with fewer resources, such as women and the poor, are among the many vulnerable populations that could be affected by these changes. Legislation in a number of states reflects this concern. Bills have been initiated to regulate, or set standards for, our competitive health care market.

One of the fundamental aims of health care reform has been to increase access to primary care for underserved and vulnerable populations (Blumenthal, Mort, and Edwards 1995), such as poor black and Hispanic women. However, it is not clear that access has improved. In a series of recently published studies by The Commonwealth Fund on women's health (Falik and Collins 1996), 14 percent of African Americans and 17 percent of Hispanics were not able to get medical treatment when they needed it (Lillie-Blanton, Bowie, and Ro 1996; Ramirez de Arellano 1996). This difficulty in accessing health services on a regular basis is one of the factors that accounts for high rates of hospitalizations for conditions that could be treated and prevented through primary care visits (Valdez et al. 1993).

Overall in the United States, the number of black and Hispanic women who do not receive medical care when it is needed is increasing (Gaston et al. 1998). This is not inconsequential, given the higher rates of morbidity among these women relative to white women and the high costs of unnecessary hospitalizations both to the patients and to society.

RACIAL DISPARITIES IN WOMEN'S HEALTH

Disparities among the health status of African American, Hispanic, and white women in the United States, and the magnitude of these differences, are of significant concern (Krieger et al. 1993; Lillie-Blanton et al. 1993; Mays, Howard-Caldwell, and Jackson 1996; Zambrana 1987). In the last two decades there has been a greater interest in race and ethnicity as a powerful determinant of health status (Cooper 1986; Harwood 1981; Polednak 1989; Reynolds 1993; U.S. Department of Health and Human Services 1985).

Looking at most indices of health, African Americans and Latinos are worse off than their white counterparts. These differences are not easily explainable by genetic variation. Considering risk factors, such as obesity, hypertension, high cholesterol, and smoking, in findings drawn from the National Health and Nutrition Examination Surveys and National Health Interview Survey, African American women have a greater prevalence of obesity and hypertension than both white and Hispanic women. African American women are more likely than Hispanic women to have high cholesterol, but less likely than white women (Lillie-Blanton et al. 1993). Perhaps, as a consequence, African American women are twice as likely, and Hispanics one-and-a-half times as likely, to rate their own health as fair or poor, as compared to white women (Lillie-Blanton et al. 1993).

More recent investigations into the health of ethnic minorities have begun to examine the effect of not only race/ethnicity and gender but also of social class on health status (Lillie-Blanton et al. 1993; Zambrana 1987). When researchers compare both income and race as factors in the health behaviors of African American, Hispanic, and white women, they find that perceptions of health status are more similar by income than by race/ethnicity, although a larger percentage of the ethnic women, in contrast to white women, rated their health as poor. Perception of health status is inversely related to income; one in four women with incomes under $10,000 report fair/poor health, versus one in 25 with incomes $35,000 or more.

Research repeatedly shows that an individual's social status of origin, an individual's achievement, as well as gender, marital status, ethnic group, and the neighborhood resided in, are all correlates of physical and mental health and the likelihood of premature death (Fang, Madhavan, and Alderman 1996; Geronimus et al. 1996; Macintyre 1986; Miles 1991; Radley 1994; Waldron 1985; Waldron and Jacobs 1988, 1989). Here, women lag behind men on almost every social and economic indicator. In practically every country at every socioeconomic level, women control fewer productive assets than men. They also work longer hours but earn less money, despite the fact that they are responsible for meeting 40 to 100 percent of their family's basic needs (Jacobson 1993; Radley 1994; U.N. Department of International and Economic and Social Affairs 1991). The result is that women are likely to be found in jobs that are labor-intensive, provide little or no health benefits, and experience high levels of occupational risks.

ACCESS TO AND UTILIZATION OF CARE

For poor women and women of color in the United States, race, social class, and gender status are powerful factors that contribute to their poorer health status (Krieger et al. 1993; Lillie-Blanton, Martinez, Taylor, and Robinson 1993). These factors mediate the opportunities that can range from women's restrictive access to employment (which can provide the benefits of health insurance, sick leave, and on-site health clinics), to decision-making about their health—through health care providers' assumptions that women are incapable of making good decisions about their health (Mays 1999). Many of the factors that influence women's use of health care services (such as costs of services, location, or distance and transportation, their willingness and ability to seek services, the infrastructure of services, availability of appointments, waiting time to see health care personnel, and language compatibility) have also been noted as contributing factors in their health care (Timyan et al. 1993). As with demographic risk factors, these access barriers contribute to the poor health outcomes found in women of color in the United States.

Several studies also demonstrate that the poor have significantly less access to health care than others (Aday, Andersen, and Fleming 1980; Aday, Fleming, and Andersen 1984; Anderson 1972; Freeman et al.

1987; Freeman and Corey 1989). Poor but not impoverished women are least likely to visit a physician regardless of ethnic group (Lillie-Blanton et al. 1993). Hispanic women are less likely than both African American and white women to report contact with a physician or to have visited a physician in the last year. Even when income is controlled, both Hispanic and African American women make fewer visits to a physician (Lillie-Blanton et al. 1993).

CHANGING ENVIRONMENT FOR HEALTH COST COVERAGE

For many Latina and African American women, the inability to get medical care stems from a lack of health insurance coverage or a failure to meet eligibility standards for publicly financed health care. Federal and state legislators have investigated ways to extend coverage to these women to ensure that they will receive the necessary health care. This attention rises in part from a recognition that when routine medical care is treated through emergency room visits or hospitalizations for preventable health problems, health care costs rise (Short, Cornelius, and Goldstone 1990). However, with the failure of health care reform, individuals in the United States continue to rely on what have been traditional public and private insurance programs. Even though the unemployment rate is down, jobs with private insurance are hard to get, especially for women (Miles and Parker 1997; Baylis and Nelson 1997).

Miles and Parker (1997) note that health insurance coverage through private, Medicaid, or Medicare sources works differently for men and women in its capacity to act as a safety net for providing necessary health care services. Inequality in health insurance coverage exists because the conditions of men and women are different, particularly for ethnic minority women. Women are more likely to work at jobs in smaller firms, have less union participation, and be employed part-time. These are all situations that lead to fewer benefits. For example, people who work in jobs that do not offer health insurance can make too much money to qualify for Medicaid, although this varies widely from state to state. In one California study of 2 million nonelderly uninsured women, eight out of ten were workers or members of working families (Wyn, Brown, and Ng 1996).

At the same time that innovation and competition are increasing in the health care marketplace, and extending into public insurance programs, the ethnic composition of the American population is changing. The fastest growing population in the United States is the Hispanic population, which by the year 2000 is projected to be the largest racial/ethnic minority group in the United States (Zambrana and Ellis 1995). Hispanics and African Americans have higher-than-average fertility rates. Because ethnic minority women are more likely to be poor and unemployed, or to work in jobs that do not offer private health insurance, ethnic minority populations have traditionally been over-represented in public insurance programs where many of the changes are now occurring (Short, Cornelius, and Goldstone 1990).

To deliver care effectively to ethnic minority populations, in both public and private insurance programs, it is increasingly important to understand more about these populations in terms of their health beliefs, perceptions of barriers to access and utilization of care, and experiences with the health care system. This type of knowledge will facilitate the design of managed care programs to meet and address their needs.

The purpose of this analysis is to examine the differences in perceived health status, access to care, and health care utilization of African American, Hispanic, and white women. It is hoped that the results of this inquiry can serve as a foundation to consider the health policy needs of these women and to provide guidance for managed care providers.

METHODS OF ANALYSIS

Women represented slightly more than one-half of the respondents in The Commonwealth Fund Minority Health Survey (CMHS). For the purposes of this study, only women respondents were selected. Native Americans were excluded because their numbers were too small for meaningful analyses, and the 305 Asian women collected via nonprobability sampling procedures were also excluded because of our inability to assign weights and to determine the true population estimates necessary for multivariate analyses.

Given the nature of the sampling design, we report estimates calculated separately for white, African American, and Hispanic women. This sample was selected using a population-based cluster sampling frame that permitted the use of specialized survey analysis software (SUDAAN; see Shah et al. 1996) to generate both point estimates and their standard errors. Weights were assigned to the sample to adjust for selection probability and for under- or over-representation by ethnicity, gender, educational level, and insurance status. Weights were further adjusted to reflect the actual sample size for each analysis to permit significance testing based on the actual weighted sample size (Aday 1989). Based on this and our interest in focusing on differences between ethnic/racial women's health, we also report when possible on comparisons between African Americans and Latinas.

Women in this sample differed significantly on several key demographic characteristics, including two major factors: age and household income. Specifically, the white women sampled tended to be older, were more likely to be retired, reported greater family incomes, and indicated that no children were present in the household. Because age and household income may confound associations between ethnic/racial background and health and health care utilization, we report both unadjusted and adjusted percentages controlling for these two factors. We conducted further analyses not reported here, controlling for children present in the home or use of prenatal services in the past year, but they did not result in any differences in findings.

To adjust for household income, we used 1993 poverty thresholds (U.S. Census Bureau 1998) as a guide. We first calculated approximate household income (reported income range divided by size of household). Then, because individuals indicated the range of their income and not the precise amount, we created four categories where the median income amount for each income range, divided by the number of individuals per household, was: (1) less than poverty as defined in 1993 (19% of the sample); (2) between 100 percent and 199 percent of poverty (22%); (3) between 200 percent and 299 percent of poverty (20%); and (4) 300 percent or more of poverty (38%).

Adjusted estimates standardize the age and household income distribution for each ethnic group to that of the total sample, thus controlling for age and household income differences across the three groups. We report both chi-square analyses of the unadjusted distributions and after adjustment for stratification by age and poverty status. Findings from the multiethnic sample can be used with some sense of certainty to estimate true population parameters for white, African American, and Hispanic women in the United States. For this reason we report 95 percent confidence intervals (CI) of the estimates to assist in extrapolating current findings.

RESULTS OF ANALYSIS

Perceived Health Status and Healthy Behaviors

Approximately one-fifth of the women in this study perceive their health as fair or poor (Table 5.1). However, African American and Hispanic

Table 5.1   Perceived Health Status and Healthy Habits of White, African American, and Hispanic Women (unadjusted and adjusted for age and poverty status)

Indicator	White %	White 95% Confidence Interval	African American %	African American 95% Confidence Interval	Hispanic %	Hispanic 95% Confidence Interval
Perceived health status rated as fair or poor						
Unadjusted[a]	18.1	14.7,21.5	27.2	22.7,31.7	26.4	21.0,31.8
Adjusted[b]	18.4	15.0,21.8	27.8	23.5,32.1	25.8	20.3,31.3
Dissatisfied with life these days						
Unadjusted	11.9	9.0,14.8	11.0	7.4,14.7	10.1	6.8,13.5
Adjusted	12.3	9.4,15.3	10.1	7.1,13.0	8.3	5.6,11.0
Reports health problem/ disability that impairs activities						
Unadjusted[b]	17.7	14.1,21.2	17.3	13.3,21.2	11.7	8.5,14.8
Adjusted[b]	18.5	15.0,22.1	16.5	13.5,19.5	12.9	9.0,16.8
Smokes cigarettes						
Unadjusted[a]	24.3	20.1,28.5	16.0	12.3,19.7	15.0	11.5,18.6
Adjusted[c]	25.3	21.2,29.5	15.2	11.8,18.5	12.6	9.6,15.7
Eats healthy diet $\geq$ four days a week						
Unadjusted[c]	66.9	62.5,71.4	50.6	46.0,55.2	55.6	50.7,60.2
Adjusted[a]	66.4	61.8,70.9	53.9	49.2,58.7	57.8	53.0,62.5
Exercises $\geq$ one time a week						
Unadjusted	58.2	53.5,62.9	53.8	48.5,59.1	52.1	47.0,57.3
Adjusted	58.8	54.1,63.5	54.8	49.7,59.9	51.5	46.1,56.9

Source: Data from The Commonwealth Fund Minority Health Survey, 1994.
[a] $p < 0.01$.
[b] $p < 0.05$.
[c] $p < 0.001$.

women are significantly more likely, when compared to white women, to rate their health this negatively. This effect is present even after controlling for differences in age and poverty status. In addition, approximately 12 percent of the women in the sample also indicate that they are currently dissatisfied with their lives; no differences were observed among the three ethnic/racial groups. Even though, overall, most women consider themselves healthy, 17 percent of women report having a health problem or a disability that impairs their ability to participate fully in activities. Hispanic women are the least likely to report a health impairment. Contrasting Hispanic and African American women specifically, Hispanic women are significantly less likely to report a disability than African American women (unadjusted chi-square$_{(1)}$ = 4.50, p < 0.05; adjusted chi-square$_{(1)}$ = 4.64, p < 0.05).

Three important aspects of maintaining a healthy lifestyle are refraining from smoking cigarettes, engaging in routine exercise, and eating a healthy diet. Approximately 22 percent of women report that they are current cigarette smokers, with significantly greater numbers of white women reporting that they smoke, compared to African American or Hispanic women, even after controlling for the effects of age and poverty status. Slightly less than two-thirds of the women indicate that they eat a healthy diet four or more days a week; significantly more white women than ethnic minority women report doing so. These ethnic/racial differences hold even after controlling for differences in age and poverty status among the groups. We observe no differences across the ethnic groups in their prevalence of reporting exercising a minimum of one day a week; slightly more than half of all women say they do. Further, we observe no significant differences between African American and Hispanic women in any of the three health behaviors (see Chapter 12).

Health Insurance

Third-party coverage of costs is a major influence on an individual's ability to access medical care when needed. But a quarter of survey respondents (24.3%) report being without health insurance or health coverage at some time during the prior two years (Table 5.2). Risk for noncoverage appears to be far greater for ethnic minority women, even after adjusting for age and poverty status differences among the three ethnic/racial groups. Of particular significance, half of the Hispanic women report being without coverage at some time in the prior two years, in contrast to slightly more than a third of African American women (unadjusted chi-square$_{(1)}$ = 9.72, p < 0.01) and 20 percent of white women (unadjusted chi-square$_{(1)}$ = 26.71, p < 0.001). If the three groups had equivalent age and poverty status distributions, the pattern remains highly similar with 40 percent of Hispanic women reporting lack of coverage, significantly more than the 29 percent of African Amer-

Table 5.2   Health Insurance Status of White, African American, and Hispanic Women (unadjusted percentages and adjusted for age and poverty status)

Indicator	White		African American		Hispanic	
	%	95% Confidence Interval	%	95% Confidence Interval	%	95% Confidence Interval
No health care coverage at some time in past 2 years						
Unadjusted[a]	19.9	15.6,24.3	34.8	28.8,40.9	50.2	44.9,55.5
Adjusted[a]	21.9	17.9,25.9	29.1	24.7,33.6	39.9	35.3,44.5
Current health insurance coverage						
Unadjusted[a]						
None	10.0	6.4,13.6	23.2	28.6,28.9	38.7	32.7,44.6
Medicaid	3.9	1.8,6.0	8.0	4.8,11.2	7.0	4.5,9.6
Private/Medicare— not HMO	68.1	63.4,72.9	48.3	42.7,57.0	37.2	32.2,42.2
Private/Medicare— HMO	18.0	14.5,21.4	20.4	16.7,24.2	17.1	14.1,20.2
Adjusted[a]						
None	11.0	7.4,14.5	18.6	14.5,22.7	29.2	25.0,33.4
Medicaid	4.7	2.5,6.9	6.3	4.1,8.4	5.3	2.8,7.8
Private/Medicare— not HMO	66.4	61.9,71.0	53.8	49.7,57.8	45.3	40.4,50.2
Private/Medicare— HMO	17.9	14.5,21.4	21.4	18.0,24.8	20.3	16.6,23.9
Among those currently insured dissatisfied with health plan or health insurance						
Unadjusted	13.1	10.5,15.7	12.5	9.6,15.3	10.3	7.1,13.5
Adjusted	15.3	11.4,18.5	11.1	8.5,13.6	9.9	6.7,13.0

Source: Data from The Commonwealth Fund Minority Health Survey, 1994.
[a]p < 0.001.

ican women (adjusted chi-square$_{(1)}$ = 10.01, p < 0.01), and 22 percent of white women (adjusted chi-square$_{(1)}$ = 17.77, p < 0.001) who reported lacking coverage.

Current prevalence of health care coverage shows an identical disparity among women according to ethnic/racial background. Overall, 63 percent of women report that they currently have some kind of health insurance coverage, including Medicare, that is not through a health maintenance organization (HMO). An additional 18 percent have HMO coverage, including a Medicare HMO. Approximately 4.7 percent are covered by Medicaid or public aid. Finally, 14 percent indicate that they do not currently have health care coverage. Significantly fewer Hispanic women report coverage, in contrast to both African American (unadjusted chi-square$_{(3)}$ = 10.28, p < 0.01) and white women (unadjusted chi-square$_{(3)}$ = 32.63, p < 0.001) (Table 5.2). Also, significantly fewer African American than white women report having health coverage (unadjusted chi-square$_{(3)}$ = 18.87, p < 0.001). This is true even after controlling for differences in age and poverty status among the women. While current noncoverage is relatively rare among white women (only 10 percent report that they are without any health care coverage), noncoverage is fairly common among Hispanic women (39%) and African American women (23%).

Among those respondents who have health care coverage, levels of dissatisfaction with their plan do not differ across the ethnic groups. Approximately 13 percent of women report being dissatisfied with their health coverage plan.

Accessing Health Care Services

Having a regular doctor or health care provider may facilitate both efficient and effective health care delivery. Over 80 percent of the women surveyed (82.7%) report that they do have a health care provider (Table 5.3). However, the percentage of women responding affirmatively varies by ethnic/racial background. A significantly greater number of white women report having a regular health care provider than either African American or Hispanic women. In turn, more African American women report having a provider than Hispanic women (unadjusted chi-square$_{(1)}$ = 5.93, p < 0.05). This pattern holds even after controlling for age and poverty status differences among the three groups.

One reason for this finding may be that points of access into the health care system vary among the three groups. Approximately 80 percent of white women report that their usual place of getting health care is in a doctor's office, a location more likely to involve a known provider. Some 14 percent of white women normally receive care at a clinic or outpatient department, and only 6 percent indicate that an emergency room is their usual place. In contrast, approximately two-

Table 5.3 Points of Access to Health Care Services among White, African American, and Hispanic Women (unadjusted percentages and adjusted for age and poverty status)

Point of Access	White %	White 95% Confidence Interval	African American %	African American 95% Confidence Interval	Hispanic %	Hispanic 95% Confidence Interval
Has a regular doctor or health care provider						
Unadjusted[a]	85.7	82.2,89.2	75.6	70.8,80.4	65.4	60.2,70.6
Adjusted[a]	85.4	81.9,88.9	77.3	73.3,81.4	69.6	65.0,74.3
Usual place of getting care Unadjusted[a]						
Doctor's office or group practice	79.7	75.7,86.7	66.3	61.2,71.4	64.0	58.7,69.3
Clinic, outpatient department, health center	14.1	10.4,17.7	19.3	14.2,24.3	27.2	22.7,31.7
Emergency room	6.2	3.8,8.6	14.5	10.8,18.1	8.8	5.6,12.0
Adjusted[b]						
Doctor's office or group practice	78.7	74.5,82.8	67.1	62.4,71.8	68.9	63.8,74.0
Clinic, outpatient department, health center	15.1	11.3,18.8	18.3	13.8,22.8	24.4	19.9,29.0
Emergency room	6.3	3.8,8.7	14.6	11.2,18.0	6.7	4.2,9.1

Source: Data from The Commonwealth Fund Minority Health Survey, 1994.
[a]$p < 0.001$.
[b]$p < 0.01$.

thirds of African American and Hispanic women report that their usual place of care is a doctor's office. Significantly, more African American women (14.5%) than either white (6.2%, unadjusted chi-square$_{(3)}$ = 16.38, $p < 0.001$) or Hispanic (8.8%, unadjusted chi-square$_{(3)}$ = 8.21, $p < 0.05$) women report that an emergency room is their usual point of health care access. More than a quarter of Hispanic women report they normally receive care in a clinic or outpatient department.

Several barriers can impede access to health care. These include difficulties in getting convenient appointments, excessive waiting times at health care sites, not knowing where to go for care or having transportation difficulties getting there, language barriers, cost, and a service provider's outright refusal to provide services. Approximately 11 percent of all of the women in the study (11.3%) report that access difficulties had kept them from getting health care when needed in the past year. Significantly fewer numbers of African American, as opposed to white (unadjusted chi-square$_{(1)}$ = 4.92, p < 0.05) or Hispanic (unadjusted chi-square$_{(1)}$ = 7.29, p < 0.01) women report that access difficulties kept them from getting care—perhaps in part due to their greater use of emergency rooms (Table 5.4). In addition, 18 percent of women report that they put off getting care because of access difficulties. Outright refusal of care by service providers was not commonly reported; only 2.5 percent of women indicate that this had happened in the prior year, with prevalence not differing significantly among the three ethnic/racial groups.

Table 5.4 Indicators of Health Access Difficulties among White, African American, and Hispanic Women (unadjusted percentages and adjusted for age and poverty status)

Indicator	White		African American		Hispanic	
	%	95% Confidence Interval	%	95% Confidence Interval	%	95% Confidence Interval
Did not get care in past year due to access difficulties[a]						
Unadjusted[b]	11.8	8.3,15.2	6.7	4.0,9.4	14.0	10.4,17.5
Adjusted[c]	12.8	9.5,16.2	5.8	3.5,8.1	12.3	8.9,15.7
Put off getting care in past year due to access difficulties[a]						
Unadjusted[b]	18.1	14.1,24.9	16.3	12.2,20.4	22.0	17.7,26.3
Adjusted[c]	19.2	15.4,22.9	14.2	10.7,17.8	19.8	15.8,23.8
Refused care in past 12 months						
Unadjusted[b]	2.2	0.2,4.3	4.0	1.6,6.3	2.8	1.1,4.5
Adjusted[c]	2.5	0.4,4.7	3.6	1.5,5.7	1.8	0.7,3.0

Source: Data from The Commonwealth Fund Minority Health Survey, 1994.

[a]Access difficulties included unavailability of appointment, inconvenient appointment hours, wait at site, paperwork or bureaucracy, language barriers, not knowing who to see or where to go, cost, lack of insurance coverage, and transportation difficulties.

[b]p < 0.05.

[c]p < 0.01.

Utilization of Health Care Services

The great majority of women in the study (91.7%) report that they saw a health care provider at least once during the course of the prior year. However, Hispanic women, in contrast to both white (unadjusted chi-square$_{(1)}$ = 14.63, p < 0.001) and African American women (unadjusted chi-square$_{(1)}$ = 13.59, p < 0.001) are significantly less likely to report having seen someone (Table 5.5). Approximately three-quarters of women report that they received some form of preventive care, such as blood pressure checks, Pap smears, or cholesterol level readings. However, once again Hispanic women report significantly less frequently having received preventive care than either white (unadjusted chi-square$_{(1)}$ = 16.57, p < 0.001) or African American women (unadjusted chi-square$_{(1)}$ = 14.03, p < 0.001). Hispanic women are also less likely to report that they had been hospitalized in the previous year than either African American (unadjusted chi-square$_{(1)}$ = 5.32, p < 0.05) or white women (unadjusted chi-square$_{(1)}$ = 7.68, p < 0.01). These differences remain even after controlling for age and poverty status.

Because African American women are more likely than white or Hispanic women to have an emergency room as their usual point of access to health care, a greater percentage of African American women than Hispanic women also report having used an emergency room in the prior year (unadjusted chi-square$_{(1)}$ = 5.24, p < 0.05). When age and poverty status differences among the three groups are statistically controlled, African American women are still more likely than Hispanic women to report using an emergency room (adjusted chi-square$_{(1)}$ = 6.55, p < 0.05).

We also studied other indicators of the breadth of health care utilization (Table 5.5). Although the percentages of women reporting the receipt of prenatal care did not differ across the three ethnic/racial groups, greater percentages of white women report obtaining a second medical opinion, seeing a mental health care provider, and receiving treatment from a chiropractor.

Levels of Satisfaction and Experiences with Discrimination

Women in the study were asked several questions related to satisfaction and comfort with health care services. Overall, 76 percent of women report being very satisfied with their regular provider. For this and other responses to satisfaction questions concerning women's regular provider,

Table 5.5   Indicators of Health Care Utilization in Past Year among White, African American, and Hispanic Women (unadjusted percentages and adjusted for age and poverty status)

Indicator	White %	White 95% Confidence Interval	African American %	African American 95% Confidence Interval	Hispanic %	Hispanic 95% Confidence Interval
Saw a health care provider						
Unadjusted[a]	92.6	90.3,95.0	92.2	89.4,94.9	81.6	77.0,86.3
Adjusted[a]	92.8	90.5,95.1	93.2	90.7,95.7	83.8	79.6,88.1
Received preventive care						
Unadjusted[a]	74.8	70.7,79.0	73.3	68.5,78.0	59.1	54.5,63.7
Adjusted[a]	74.4	70.2,78.5	75.0	71.1,79.0	59.8	54.7,64.9
Used an emergency room						
Unadjusted	20.1	16.0,24.1	25.6	21.6,29.6	18.7	15.0,22.4
Adjusted[b]	21.0	17.1,24.8	24.5	20.5,28.4	18.6	14.9,22.3
Was hospitalized						
Unadjusted[b]	17.7	13.9,21.5	15.5	12.0,19.0	10.6	7.7,13.5
Adjusted	17.9	14.1,21.7	16.1	12.5,19.7	10.2	7.3,13.1
Received prenatal care						
Unadjusted	6.4	3.7,9.1	8.6	5.9,11.4	8.0	5.4,10.7
Adjusted	7.1	4.2,10.1	6.9	4.8,9.1	5.7	4.0,7.4
Received a second medical opinion						
Unadjusted[b]	20.0	16.2,23.8	14.4	11.6,17.1	13.3	9.2,17.4
Adjusted[b]	20.3	16.5,24.1	13.7	11.0,16.4	12.6	9.1,16.1
Saw mental health care provider						
Unadjusted	8.1	5.6,10.6	4.6	2.5,6.6	5.3	3.1,7.5
Adjusted[b]	8.6	5.9,11.2	4.1	2.3,5.9	4.6	2.9,6.2
Treated by a chiropractor						
Unadjusted[a]	14.4	11.1,17.6	3.8	2.2,5.4	8.0	5.2,10.9
Adjusted[a]	14.3	11.2,17.4	4.2	2.5,5.8	8.9	5.6,12.2

Source: Data from The Commonwealth Fund Minority Health Survey, 1994.

[a]$p < 0.001$.

[b]$p < 0.05$.

there are no statistical ethnic/racial differences among the three groups of women sampled. Regular providers were viewed by 70 percent of women as doing an excellent job of treating them with respect. Sixty-four percent of women report that their provider does an excellent job of making sure they understand instructions. Additionally, 62 percent report that their regular provider does an excellent job of listening to their concerns, and 58 percent feel that their provider does an excellent job at providing good health care. Women are less sanguine about their provider's availability; only 51 percent feel that their provider does an excellent job of being accessible by telephone or in person.

Despite the lack of ethnic/racial differences in women's satisfaction with their regular provider, women in the study do differ in their overall satisfaction with the quality of their health care services (Table 5.6). White women are more likely to report being very satisfied with the quality of their health care services in contrast to African American (unadjusted chi-square$_{(1)}$ = 11.56, p < 0.001) and also to Hispanic women (unadjusted chi-square$_{(1)}$ = 9.94, p < 0.001), who do not differ significantly from each other. Although this overall difference does not quite achieve overall statistical significance (p = 0.06) when the possible confounding effects of age and poverty status are controlled for, a higher percentage of white women report being very satisfied with the quality of their health care services when contrasted with African American women (adjusted chi-square$_{(1)}$ = 5.61, p < 0.05).

Women were also asked about levels of satisfaction with four other aspects of their medical care. We observed no ethnic/racial differences in terms of women's satisfaction with the convenience of hours and location of their health care setting (with the overall percent reporting that they are very satisfied being 66%), and in terms of sensitivity of the office staff to cost concerns (with the overall percent reporting that they were very satisfied being 47%). However, white women most frequently report being very satisfied with the skills of the medical staff and the helpfulness of the office staff. This satisfaction level is in contrast, particularly, to Hispanic women, who appear to be the most dissatisfied ethnic/racial group concerning aspects of their health care services. Contrasting specifically Hispanic and African American women, we observed no differences in satisfaction in the perceived skill of the medical staff or in the quality of health care, but Hispanic women are also more likely than African American women to report being less satisfied with the helpfulness of office staff (unadjusted chi-square$_{(1)}$ = 9.58, p < 0.01: adjusted chi-square$_{(1)}$ = 6.83, p < 0.01).

Table 5.6 Satisfaction with Health Care Services and Experiences with Discrimination among White, African American, and Hispanic Women

Indicator	White %	White 95% Confidence Interval	African American %	African American 95% Confidence Interval	Hispanic %	Hispanic 95% Confidence Interval
Overall, very satisfied with:						
Skill of medical staff						
Unadjusted[a]	73.0	68.7,77.2	63.1	58.2,68.0	56.0	49.7,62.2
Adjusted[b]	72.6	68.4,76.8	65.5	60.8,70.2	57.7	52.2,63.2
Helpfulness of office staff						
Unadjusted[a]	68.5	64.1,72.9	61.7	57.1,62.2	50.3	45.5,55.1
Adjusted[b]	67.6	63.3,71.9	64.6	60.6,68.7	52.5	47.6,57.3
Quality of health care services						
Unadjusted[a]	61.5	57.0,66.1	48.8	43.6,56.9	49.3	44.1,54.5
Adjusted	60.4	55.7,65.0	50.5	45.7,55.3	53.1	47.9,58.3
Has ever changed doctors because dissatisfied						
Unadjusted[b]	44.2	39.6,48.9	33.6	29.5,37.8	32.7	28.2,37.2
Adjusted[a]	45.2	40.6,49.8	33.2	29.3,37.2	32.5	28.3,36.6
Believes there was a time she would have received better care if of a different race						
Unadjusted[a]	2.8	1.0,4.6	16.0	12.7,19.4	13.0	8.9,17.2
Adjusted[a]	3.2	1.2,5.2	14.9	11.8,17.9	10.2	6.9,13.5
Was treated badly or felt uncomfortable when getting health care in past year						
Unadjusted	8.8	6.1,11.5	6.6	4.5,8.8	8.5	6.1,11.0
Adjusted	9.4	6.5,12.2	5.5	3.6,7.4	8.3	5.5,11.1

Source: Data from The Commonwealth Fund Minority Health Survey, 1994.
[a]$p < 0.001$.
[b]$p < 0.01$.

White women, more frequently than either African American (unadjusted chi-square$_{(1)}$ = 7.76, p < 0.01) or Hispanic women (unadjusted chi-square$_{(1)}$ = 10.14, p < 0.001), report that they had changed doctors at some time in the past because they were dissatisfied with their care (Table 5.6). But a sizable minority of African American women, followed by Hispanic/Latina women, believe that at some time in the past they would have received better care if they had been of a different race. This effect is quite robust and holds even after the effects of age and poverty status differences are statistically controlled. But when women are asked specifically about experiences of being treated badly in the prior year, we find no statistically significant differences by ethnic minority.

DIFFERENCES REMAIN BETWEEN WHITES AND MINORITY GROUPS

We find, like other researchers (Lillie-Blanton et al. 1993; Zambrana and Ellis 1995), that African American and Hispanic/Latina women are worse off than white women in their level of health care coverage, in their utilization of health care services, and in the perceived quality of their health care. This is true even after controlling for the effects of poverty. Further, our results suggest that patterns of access to health care for African American and Hispanic women are less likely to result in optimum health care than other patterns of access. Both African American and Hispanic women are less likely than white women to have a regular health care provider. Also, African American women are more likely than white or Hispanic/Latina women to use emergency rooms as their usual place of care, which is an environment unlikely to provide preventive health services well (although in the current study we observe no differences between African American and white women in their receipt of preventive care the prior year) or continuity of care.

Hispanic Women Have Less Coverage and Care

The Hispanic/Latina women in our study often have the least health care coverage, resources, and utilization of services of all the ethnic groups. Of pressing concern is our finding that approximately half of the Hispanic/Latina women report that they have not had any health care coverage at some point during the past two years. Also, in contrast to the African American and white women respondents, the Hispanics are most likely to report that they currently have no health insurance coverage.

Unfortunately, the pattern of Hispanics/Latinos accounting for a large proportion of the uninsured population is one that is increasing rather then decreasing (Weissman and Epstein 1994). It is therefore not surprising that in this study the Hispanic/Latina women are the most likely group not to get care, to put if off because of difficulties in accessing health services, or not to have received preventive services or to have seen a health care provider within the last year. These findings increase our concern for the health of Hispanic women, in light of the fact that heart disease, diabetes, and breast and lung cancer are the leading causes of death in this population (Zambrana and Ellis 1995). These are all diseases whose outcomes benefit from early screening, preventive services, and monitoring.

The Hispanic women in our study are also the least likely to believe that their health problems impair their activities. What our findings cannot tell us, however, is whether the health problems of the Hispanic/Latina women respondents are mild, and present no handicap to the business of meeting their daily activities, or whether these women's definitions and/or cultural norms of illness and health (as an impediment in meeting their obligations) account for their responses. Other studies indicate that Hispanics seek health care only when they view their illness as serious (Andersen et al. 1981 and 1986). Merely documenting that Hispanic/Latina women do not perceive that their health problems hamper them from meeting daily obligations does not give us an adequate insight into the true nature of their health problems. It is not clear, for example, whether it is culturally unacceptable (in the press of family obligations) to fail to meet those obligations except in the face of serious illness, or whether the intolerance of ill health differs from other cultural groups.

The Hispanic women in our study, when they do access health care, are the least satisfied with the health care services they receive. While both African American and Latinas perceive less satisfaction than others with the quality of health care and skills of their medical professionals, only approximately half of the Latinas feel that the office staff is helpful. As managed care providers seek to provide quality health care, and to design measures of patient satisfaction that will review their service delivery performance, this study indicates that there may be differences in cultural expectations of how service delivery should be structured.

In contrast to minority women, white women appear to make greater and perhaps better use of health care resources, including getting second medical opinions, mental health care services, and chiropractic care, and in changing doctors when they are dissatisfied with their care. They also perceive, in contrast to African American women or Hispanic/Latina women, both their health and the quality of their health services as being better. The white women in our study were more likely to eat a healthy diet, but they were also more likely to be smokers. White women, however, did not significantly differ from African American or Hispanic/Latina women in their amount of exercise, or their perception of being treated badly or feeling uncomfortable when getting health care.

The Social Nature of Health Disparities

Results of the CMHS indicate that a small but nonetheless important percentage of women have not seen a health care provider in the last year, do not receive preventive health care services, do smoke, and do not eat a healthy diet or exercise at least once a week. The social nature of health disparities requires a broader focus on more issues than the physical aspects of disease. The medical care delivery sector alone is not an adequate source for the improvement of women's health (U.S. Department of Health and Human Services 1994), particularly the health disparities experienced by African American and Hispanic/Latina women. Although changes in the delivery of health care services by managed care and capitated health plans will increase accessibility, preventive services, and the quality of those services (U.S. Department of Health and Human Services 1994), it is not clear whether African American and Hispanic women would benefit if these were the sole changes to the delivery of their health care.

On the other hand, relying on the public health system to monitor the health status of women, to assure quality accessibility and accountability in medical care and planning for women, is not without its own problems. Public health activities accounted for less than 1 percent of the aggregate amount spent in budget year 1992 on health care in the United States (U.S. Department of Health and Human Services 1994). Rather, a better collaborative relationship between the medical care delivery service and public health systems will be necessary if the country is to meet the Healthy People 2000 goals outlined for the health of women (U.S. Department of Health and Human Services 1991).

In this status report on perceptions of access to health care, health status, and utilization patterns of African American and Latina women, based on a national probability sample, we have found some striking differences between these two groups. Despite the fact that both African

American and Latina women report poorer health relative to that reported by whites, Hispanics are far more likely to lack health insurance. One of every three Latina women interviewed lacked health insurance in the past year, compared to one of every five African American women. These alarming results are similar to facts revealed in the 1990 Census, in which 40 percent of Latinos were uninsured, compared to one-fourth of African Americans and only one-seventh of whites (Valdez et al. 1993).

BETTER HEALTH POLICIES FOR ALL WOMEN

More attention is now being focused on strategies and policies aimed at reducing the burden of illness and rectifying the disparities in the health of poor and ethnic minority women. It is important for these efforts to focus on two distinctly different but interrelated areas. First, as women have long been neglected as the subjects of biomedical research, much of the data that guides clinical practice for the treatment and prevention of disease is based on studies of men (Mastroianni, Faden, and Federman 1994). For epidemiologic and biomedical research to contribute to a clearer understanding of disease etiology and transmission, and to offer better choices in pharmacologic, surgical, and other medical interventions, it will be important to prioritize more female-specific (Leslie 1992) and race-specific research (Mays 1999). However, we must also concentrate equally on efforts to gain a clearer understanding about how culture, ethnicity, social status, socioeconomic resources, and individual priorities *interact* with women's health to positively affect their health behaviors and health status (Kreiger 1987, 1989, 1990a,b; Bassett and Krieger 1986; Krieger et al. 1993; Lillie-Blanton et al. 1993; Zambrana 1987).

The decisions that women make about when to seek help, or whether to seek traditional or informal sources of care for their health problems, are decisions made within the context of other priorities, availability of resources, and role demands in women's lives (Leslie 1992; Mays, Beckman, Ornacheck, and Harper 1994; Mays, Howard-Caldwell, and Jackson 1996). Previous studies demonstrate the significance of families, social networks, and peer groups in influencing the engagement in or resistance to such health behaviors as smoking, diet, and exercise (Mays 1999).

Anticipatory responses of possible discrimination and mistreatment based on race and/or gender also influence an individual's search for help for health concerns (see Chapter 11). African American and Hispanic women in this study feel that if their race had been different they would have received better health services. What our results help to illustrate is that the health status of women is not just a matter of individual behaviors. Women's health behaviors and health status may be influenced or constrained by other factors. While researchers are beginning to document that the health problems of women are an interaction of family, resource availability, cultural and social status norms of illness and health, and biological factors, policymakers should review how interventions to enhance women's health should take contextual factors into account (Leslie 1992; Cochran and Mays 1994; Zambrana 1987). As managed care companies extend into populations of ethnic minority women, they need to realize that they cannot be effective without being sensitive to the issues of poverty, culture, and intragroup diversity that characterize these populations.

Women's Cultural Patterns about Health Practices

Studies of women's health must begin to move beyond mere documentation of the problems to investigating better answers to the questions of why and how poor and ethnic women experience the worst health of all women. To do this, we need to include contextual questions that assess social inequalities—such as how racism, discrimination, and oppression influence women's health (Cochran and Mays 1994; Mays, Coleman, and Jackson 1996). These contextual questions will require greater attention to the demand side of women's health utilization by increasing our knowledge of women's cultural patterns concerning their health practices (Timyan, Brechin, Measham, and Ogunleye 1993). It will be necessary to take into account women's relationships with their families, their systems of social support, their use of alternative sources of care for health problems, their priorities, and their definitions of ill health. This can only be accomplished by listening and talking with women before designing and implementing research endeavors, health programs, or health policies that affect women or their families (Brems and Griffith 1993; Baylis and Nelson 1997).

What we have failed to accomplish here is to explore the unique health needs and health habits of the intra-ethnic groups of the women in this study. While data were collected that identifies Caribbean-born African Americans and subgroups of the Hispanic/Latina populations, sample size and data collection methods do not allow for comparisons.

Yet, to make quantitative advancements in understanding the health of ethnic women, we need to examine ethnic subgroup differences— because the incidence and prevalence of disease as well as health behaviors, cultural norms, access and utilization can be expected to differ by subpopulations.

For example, our study has found that Hispanics are the least likely to have health insurance. But any design of health policy on this issue would be best guided by data broken down by geographic region, ethnic subpopulations, and age. Women's health insurance coverage differs substantially among Hispanic subpopulations; Puerto Ricans are most likely to be insured and Mexican-origin women the least likely (Torre et al. 1996). Several factors contribute to these differences. Puerto Ricans are more likely to be U.S. citizens and to reside in the Northeast, where states have favorable benefits and eligibility requirements for Medicaid (Valdez et al. 1993). Mexican-origin women, on the other hand, face stringent immigration laws, and they tend to reside in the Southwest, where Medicaid eligibility is among the most restrictive, with fewer benefits (Valdez et al. 1993).

The labor force participation of Hispanics differs from that of whites and African Americans just enough to make a difference in the type of health care coverage that is based in employer-sponsored benefits. Latinos are most likely to be employed in agriculture, sales, and personal service industries, and to work for employers with small businesses; these are conditions that traditionally offer few to no health benefits (Valdez et al. 1993). Thus, although our study presents results for Hispanics as a group, the reader is cautioned that identifying a particular Hispanic subpopulation, and noting where that group geographically resides, are important considerations when formulating health policies that will be adequate and effective for that subgroup.

Policies Must Be Multifaceted to Address Ethnic Differences

From a policy standpoint, the data in this study question the wisdom of developing policies and managed care strategies that attempt to address the broad group of "racial/ethnic minorities." While many managed care settings will contain a mixed-ethnic population of both African Americans and Hispanics, planners must accept that not all policies will serve each group equally well. *Significant* differences exist between these two ethnic groups as well as within them in terms of labor force participation, family formation, immigration status, and state eligibility requirements for publicly financed coverage. Proposals for reforming either the design or financing of health care should be based on an examination of whether outcomes will be equitable, given the many differences among and within the ethnic groups' participation in the larger societal structure. Designers of managed care programs for these populations should learn about the differences, particularly between African American and Hispanic women, in their perceived health status.

For health care reform to be effective for all ethnic groups, the unique structural and cultural experiences of each group (for whom we are responsible for delivering medical services) must be a part of the discussion for solutions. Sensitivity to how poverty and culture influence perceived health status and interact with affordability, acceptability, and accessibility of services, is critical if managed care groups are to maintain optimal and cost-efficient health care services to ethnic minority women.

To ensure adequate and effective health care services for ethnic minority women, reform must address cultural competence among providers and systems as well as financing mechanisms and medical care delivery system structures. Systems that recognize the cultural realities of women's lives will be more effective in their treatment and prevention of the morbidity and mortality that is disproportionately high for these populations.

By including standards of cultural competence in the delivery of health care for women of all ethnicities, health care treatment and prevention efforts based on reality will emerge. Providers will understand that treating hypertension, obesity, or diabetes occurs within the context of how that woman's cultural, social class, work and community life, age, household composition, immigration status, and a host of other factors affect the way she takes care of herself.

References

Aday, L. A. 1989. *Designing and conducting health surveys.* San Francisco: Jossey-Bass.

Aday, L. A., Andersen, R, and Fleming, G. V. 1980. *Health Care in the U.S.: Equitable for Whom?* Newbury Park, Calif.: Sage Publications.

Aday, L. A., Fleming, G. V., and Andersen, R. M.. 1984. *Access to Medical Care in the U.S.: Who Has It, Who Doesn't.* Chicago: Pluribus Press.

Andersen, R., Lewis, S., Giachello, A. L., Aday, L. A., and Chiu, G. 1981. Access to medical care among Hispanic population of the Southwestern United States. *Journal of Health and Social Behavior* 22:78–89.

Andersen, R. M., Giachello, A. L., and Aday, L. A. 1986. Access of Hispanics to health care and cuts in services: a state-of-the-art overview. *Public Health Reports* 101(3):238–252.

Anderson, O. W. 1972. *Health Care: Can There Be Equity?* New York: John Wiley.

Bassett, M. T., and Krieger, N. 1986. Social class and black-white differences in breast cancer survival. *American Journal of Public Health* 76(12): 1400–1403.

Baylis, F., and Nelson, H. L. 1997. Access to health care for women. *New England Journal of Medicine* 336(25):1841.

Blumenthal, D., Mort, E., and Edwards, J. 1995. The efficacy of primary care for vulnerable population groups. *Health Services Research* 30(1):253-273.

Brems, S., and Griffith, M. 1993. Health women's way: learning to listen. In M. Koblinsky, J. Timyan, and J. Gay, eds., *The Health of Women: A Global Perspective*. Boulder, Colo.: Westview Press.

Cochran, S. D., and Mays, V. M. 1994. Depressive distress among homosexually active African American men and women. *American Journal of Psychiatry* 4:524-529.

The Commonwealth Fund. March 20, 1995. National Comparative Survey on Minority Health. New York: The Commonwealth Fund.

Cooper, R. 1986. Race, disease and health. In T. Rathwell and D. Phillips, eds., *Health, Race and Ethnicity*. London: Croom Helm.

Falik, M. M., and Collins, K. S. 1996. *Women's Health: The Commonwealth Fund Survey*. Baltimore: Johns Hopkins University Press.

Fang, J., Madhavan, S., and Alderman, M. H. 1996. The association between birthplace and mortality from cardiovascular causes among black and white residents of New York City. *New England Journal of Medicine* 335(21): 1545-1551.

Freeman, H. E., Blendon, R. J., Aiken, L. H., Sudman, S., Mullinix, C. F., and Corey, C. R. 1987. Americans report on their access to health care. *Health Affairs* 6(1):6–18.

Freeman, H. E., and Corey, C. R. 1989. *Health Insurance and Access to Medical Services: A Secondary Analysis of Three Years of NCHS Health Interview Surveys*. Santa Monica, Calif.: A RAND Note, N-3584-HFCA.

Gaston, M. H., Barrett, S. E., Johnson, T. L., and Epstein, L. G. 1998. Health care needs of medically underserved women of color: the role of the Bureau of Primary Health Care. *Health and Social Work* 23(2):86–95.

Geronimus, A. T., Bound, J., Waidmann, T. A., Hillemeir, M. M., and Burns, P. B. 1996. Excess mortality among blacks and whites in the United States. *New England Journal of Medicine* 335(21):1552–1558.

Harwood, A. 1981. *Ethnicity and Medical Care*. Cambridge: Harvard University Press.

Jacobson, J. L. 1993. Women's health: the price of poverty. In M. Koblinsky,

J. Timyan, and J Gay, eds., *The Health of Women: A Global Perspective.* Boulder, Colo.: Westview Press.

Krieger, N. 1987. Shades of differences: theoretical underpinnings of the medical controversy on black/white differences in the United States, 1830–1870. *International Journal of Health Services* 17:256–278.

Krieger, N. 1989. Exposure, susceptibility, and breast cancer risk: hypothesis regarding exogenous carcinogens, breast tissue development, and social gradients, including black/white differences, in breast cancer incidence. *Breast Cancer Research and Treatment* 13:205–223.

Krieger, N. 1990a. Social class and the black/white crossover in the age-specific incidence of breast cancer: a study linking census-derived data to population-based registry records. *American Journal of Epidemiology* 131:804-814.

Krieger, N. 1990b. Racial and gender discrimination: risk factors for high blood pressure? *Social Science and Medicine* 30:1273–1281.

Krieger, N., Rowley, D. L., Herman, A. A., Avery, B., and Phillips, M. T. 1993. Racism, sexism, and social class: implications for studies of health, disease, and well-being. *American Journal of Preventive Medicine* 9(Suppl.):82–122.

Leigh, W. A. 1995. The health of African American women. In D. L. Adams, ed., *Health Issues of Women of Color: A Cultural Diversity Perspective.* Thousand Oaks, Calif.: Sage Publications.

Leslie, J. 1992. *Women's Lives and Women's Health: Using Social Science Research to Promote Better Health for Women.* New York / Washington, D.C.: Population Council, International Center for Research on Women.

Lillie-Blanton, M., Bowie, J., and Ro, M. 1996. African American women: social factors and the use of preventive health services. In M. M. Falik and K. S. Collins, eds., *Women's Health: The Commonwealth Fund Survey.* Baltimore: Johns Hopkins University Press.

Lillie-Blanton, M., and Lillie, C. 1996. Re-examining federal and state roles in assuring equitable access to health care. In M. D. Lillie-Blanton, W. Leigh, and A. I. Alfaro-Correa, eds., *Achieving Equitable Access: Studies of Health Care Issues Affecting Hispanics and African Americans.* Landham, Md.: Joint Center for Political and Economic Studies.

Lillie-Blanton, M., Martinez, R. M., Taylor, A. K., and Robinson, B. G. 1993. Latina and African American women: continuing health disparities. *International Journal of Health Services* 23(3):555–584.

Macintyre, S. 1986. The patterning of health by social position in contemporary Britain: directions for sociological research. *Social Science and Medicine* 23(4):393–415.

Mastroianni, A. C., Faden, R., and Federman, D. 1994. *Women and Health Research: Ethical and Legal Issues of Including Women in Clinical Studies. Volume 1.* Washington, D.C.: National Academy Press.

Mays, V. M. 1999. Psychological differences between men and women: implications for a research agenda on women's physical and mental health. *Agenda for Research on Women's Health for the 21st Century. A Report of the Task Force on the NIH Women's Health Agenda for the 21st Century.* Vol. 5, *Sex and Gender Perspectives for Women's Health Research.* Bethesda, Md.: USDHHS, PHS, NIH; NIH Publication 99-4389:54–64.

Mays, V. M., Beckman, L. J., Oranchak, E., and Harper, B. 1994. Perceived support for helpseeking of black heterosexual and homosexually active women alcoholics. *Psychology of Addictive Behaviors* 8(4):235–242.

Mays, V. M., Coleman, L. M., and Jackson, J. S. 1996. Race-based perceived discrimination, employment status, and job-stress in a national sample of black women: implications for health outcomes. *Journal of Occupational Health Psychology* 1(3):319–329.

Mays, V. M., Howard-Caldwell, C. S., and Jackson, J. S. 1996. Mental health symptoms and service utilization patterns of African-American women in the United States. In H. W. Neighbors and J. S. Jackson, eds., *Mental Health in Black America.* Newbury Park, Calif.: Sage Publications.

Miles, A. 1991. *Women, Health and Medicine.* Buckingham: Open University Press.

Miles, S., and Parker, K. 1997. Men, women and health insurance. *New England Journal of Medicine* 336(3):218–221.

Polednak, A. P. 1989. *Racial and Ethnic Differences in Disease.* New York: Oxford University Press.

Radley, A. 1994. *Making Sense of Illness: The Social Psychology of Health and Disease.* London / Thousand Oaks, Calif.: Sage Publications.

Ramirez de Arellano, A. B. 1996. Latino women: health status and access to health care. In M. Falik and K. S. Collins, eds., *Women's Health: The Commonwealth Fund Survey.* Baltimore: Johns Hopkins University Press.

Reynolds, G. 1993. Foreword to special issue on mortality/morbidity gap: is it race or racism? *Annals of Epidemiology* 3(2):119.

Scanlon, D. P., Chernew, M., and Lave, J. R. 1997. Consumer health plan choice: current knowledge and future directions. *Annual Review of Public Health* 18:507–528.

Shah, B. V., Barnwell, B. G., and Bieler, G. S. 1996. *SUDAAN User's Manual, Version 6.40, Second Edition.* Research Triangle Park, N.C.: Research Triangle Institute.

Short, P. F., Cornelius, L. J., and Goldstone, D. E. 1990. Health status of minorities in the United States. *Journal of Health Care for the Poor and Underserved* 1(1):9–24.

Timyan, J., Brechin, S. J. G., Measham, D. M., and Ogunleye, B. 1993. Access to care: more than a problem of distance. In M. Koblinsky, J. Timyan, and J. Gay, eds., *The Health of Women: A Global Perspective.* Boulder, Colo.: Westview Press.

Torre, A. de la, Friis, R, Hunter, H. R., and Garcia, L. 1996. The health insur-

ance status of U.S. Latino women: a profile from the 1982–1984 *HHANES.*
American Journal of Public Health 86(4):533–537.

United Nations Department of International and Economic and Social Affairs.
1991. *The World's Women: Trends and Statistics 1970–1990.* New York:
United Nations.

U.S. Census Bureau. 1998. *Poverty Thresholds 1993.* Available at: http://www
.census.gov/hhes/poverty/threshld/thresh93.html.

U.S. Department of Health and Human Services. 1985. *Health Status of Minorities and Low-income Groups.* Public Health Service. Washington, D.C.:
U.S. Government Printing Office.

U.S. Department of Health and Human Services. 1991. *Healthy People 2000:
National Health Promotion and Disease Prevention Objectives.* Public
Health Service. Washington, D.C.: U.S. Government Printing Office.

U.S. Department of Health and Human Services. 1994. *For a Healthy Nation:
Returns on Investment in Public Health.* Public Health Service. Washington,
D.C.: U.S. Government Printing Office.

Valdez, R. B., Morgenstern, H., Brown, E. R., Wyn, R., Wang, C., and Cumber-
land, W. 1993. Insuring Latinos against the cost of illness. *Journal of the
American Medical Association* 269:889–894.

Waldron, I. 1985. Sex differences in illness incidence, prognosis and mortality:
issues and evidence. *Social Science and Medicine* 17(16):1107–1123.

Waldron, I., and Jacobs, J. A. 1988. Effects of labor force participation on
women's health: new evidence from a longitudinal study. *Journal of Occupational Medicine* 30(12):977-983.

Waldron, I., and Jacobs, J. A. 1989. Effects of multiple roles on women's
health—evidence from a national longitudinal study. *Women and Health*
15(1):3-19.

Weissman, J. S., and Epstein, A. M. 1994. *Falling Through the Safety Net: Insurance Status and Access to Health Care.* Baltimore, Md.: Johns Hopkins University Press.

Wyn, R., Brown, E. R., and Ng, L. 1996. Health Insurance Coverage of Women
in California. Policy Brief (#PB96-1). Los Angeles, Calif.: UCLA Center for
Health Policy Research.

Zambrama, R. E. 1987. A research agenda on issues affecting poor and minority
women: a model for understanding their health needs. *Women's Health*
12(3/4):137–160.

Zambrana, R. E., and Ellis, B. K. 1995. Contemporary research issues in
Hispanic/Latina women's health. In D. Adams, ed., *Health Issues for
Women of Color.* Thousand Oaks, Calif.: Sage Publications.

6

Financial Barriers for Working-Age Minority Populations
Poverty and Beyond

Llewellyn J. Cornelius, Ph.D.
Karen Scott Collins, M.D., M.P.H.

The ability to pay for medical services has been and continues to be a significant barrier to obtaining medical services (Andersen et al. 1987; Cornelius 1993). Before the development of private health insurance plans, obtaining medical care depended on one's ability to pay for care out-of-pocket, or the good will of charitable institutions (Starr 1982; Anderson 1990). The development of private insurance plans and public insurance options (most notably Medicare and Medicaid in 1965) vastly increased the proportion of Americans who had some form of health insurance. By 1953, some 41 percent of low-income families (<$3,000 in 1953) and 80 percent of upper-income families in America (>$4,999 in 1953) had health insurance (Andersen and Anderson 1967). In 1963, 51 percent of low-income families (<$4,000 in 1963) and 89 percent of upper-income families in America (>$7,000 in 1963) had health insurance (Andersen and Anderson 1967). By 1989, 65 percent of low-income families (<$14,000) and 95 percent of upper-income families (>$50,000) had health insurance (National Center for Health Statistics 1995).

INSURANCE SYSTEMS INCREASE COVERAGE

Having a means to pay for health care and having a regular place to go for health care are typically seen as prerequisites for visiting a health care provider on either an ambulatory or an inpatient basis. For this reason, access to medical care can be defined as visiting a health care provider. As the percentage of insured Americans grew, there was also an increase in the percentage of people who visited a physician. By 1970, 70 percent of whites and 58 percent of non-whites in the United States made at least one ambulatory visit to a physician during the year (Andersen, Lion, and Anderson 1975). Whites also reported an average of 4.1 ambulatory visits to a physician during 1970, compared with 3.6 visits for non-whites (Andersen, Lion, and Anderson 1975). By 1982, 80 percent of Hispanic Americans and 82 percent of whites and African Americans saw a physician at least once a year. At the same time African Americans and Hispanic Americans averaged 6.7 visits to a physician, compared with 5.9 visits for whites (Aday, Fleming, and Andersen 1984).

These improvements in access to care did not come without problems, some of which reflect the design and administration of U.S. private and public health insurance programs. A case in point is the Medicaid program. In the years since its enactment, Medicaid has become a critical component of the U.S. health care system and the primary national program that finances health care for the poor and medically needy. It currently constitutes one of the largest single components of state budgets, with expenditures totaling $125 billion (57% federal and 43% state) for medical services to more than 25 million individuals in the 1993 federal fiscal year (Liska et al. 1995).

The Arrival of Medicaid

The Medicaid program was enacted in 1965 to encourage states to increase the provision of medical care to the poor. However, it was built on then-existing federally supported welfare programs for families with dependent children, and this provision limited eligibility to the population covered by those programs. In addition to covering a subset of the poor, Medicaid extended eligibility to the aged, blind, and disabled. Medicaid also covered individuals whose income was too high to make them eligible for a cash payment, but who had high medical expenses relative to income and met the nonfinancial eligibility (called *categorical*) criteria for welfare. These people were the "medically needy." There have been some other eligibility expansions throughout the history of the program, notably recent mandates to cover low-income pregnant women and women and children with incomes above the poverty line. For the most part, however, the program remains limited to certain categories of the poor (Iglehart 1993).

As of 1995, Medicaid provided health care coverage to more than 35.1 million Americans; nearly half (17.5 million) of these beneficiaries were children (Liska et al. 1997). Medicaid also provided coverage for services provided to 3.9 million elderly, 5.8 million blind and disabled persons, and 8 million low-income adults, including pregnant women (Liska et al. 1997). For the groups targeted by the Medicaid program, the availability of Medicaid has led to increases of the chances of being seeing by a physician, improvement in prenatal care, and improvements in health status (Davis 1979).

Despite Medicaid's commitment to providing care for the indigent, most critics contend that the program is seriously flawed. First, Medicaid expenditures have more than doubled since 1989 (Iglehart 1993), and Medicaid has become a prime target for cost containment, cutbacks in programs for the poor, attempts to increase general state taxes, and attempts to reduce other state programs (Coughlin et al. 1994). Second, although Medicaid was designed to provide access to care for the poor, most estimates are that it covers less than 50 percent of the non-institutionalized poor. Third, less than half of participating Medicaid physicians accept all patients (Perloff, Kletke, and Fossett 1995). Fourth, the majority (59%) of health care expenditures for Medicaid are for the disabled, the blind, and the aged, who constitute only 27 percent of Medicaid enrollees (Liska et al. 1995). Finally, because states administer the program, the federal government collects only limited data and finds it difficult to estimate nationally the proportion of the near poor, the aged, the disabled, minorities, and other groups who benefit from Medicaid.

Like Medicaid, private health insurance in the United States is at best a partial solution to the more global problem of a lack of universal health insurance. The provision of some form of universal health insurance has been achieved by other countries, such as Canada, England, and Denmark (Raffel 1984), but it has been an elusive goal in the United States. Opposition to universal coverage in this country began at the turn of the century. However, since the Depression, several private insurance options have made health care affordable for most Americans. Starting with "fee-for-service" plans at Baylor University in 1929 and the development of health maintenance organizations (HMOs) in the 1940s, such as Kaiser Permanente and the Health Insurance Plan of New York (Starr 1982; Anderson 1990), private insurance has become the pillar of the U.S. health insurance system.

Growth of Managed Care

Until the 1980s, HMOs—managed care organizations (MCOs), coordinated care approaches, or capitated payments systems—covered only a small portion of the U.S. population. As of 1982, only 9 million Americans were enrolled in an MCO (Goldsmith 1997). Recently, however, the spiraling cost of health expenditures have fueled an exponential growth of MCOs as a cost containment strategy for both public and private insurance patients. In 1996, 52.5 million Americans were enrolled in an MCO (National Center for Health Statistics 1997). As of 1996, slightly over 13.3 million Medicaid patients across 23 states were enrolled in an MCO (Long and Liska 1998).

Along with the evolution of MCOs, other cost containment strategies have evolved. These include the frequent elimination of health insurance as a fringe benefit (as an employer cost-savings strategy); the restriction of the scope of health coverage; and an increase in out-of-pocket costs for those individuals and families who have health insurance.

Policies that address the financing of medical care have contributed to an improvement in access to care for all Americans. However, gaps in the financing of care produce problems in access to care for the underserved. Current health care financing arrangements tend to underserve African and Latino Americans, the poor (especially poor men), the unemployed, the employed who work in industries without health coverage, and low-wage workers (Short, Monheit, and Beauregard 1989; Short, Cornelius, and Goldstone 1990).

Socioeconomic and sociodemographic trends, which disproportionately affect African and Latino Americans, have influenced these gaps in insurance coverage. First, a considerable portion of the increase in uninsured Latinos stems from the increase in the Latino population during the 1980s (Short, Cornelius, and Goldstone 1990). Second, during the 1960s and 1970s, Anglo Americans fared better than Latino Americans and African Americans in the areas of education and employment (Jaynes and Williams 1989; National Association of Hispanic Publications 1996). Human capital theorists have often linked the achievement of advanced degrees to higher lifetime earnings (Ehrenberg and Smith 1982). During the same two decades the disparity in earnings between Latino, African, and Anglo Americans increased (Jaynes and Williams 1989; National Association of Hispanic Publications 1996). This trend in earnings carried into the 1980s, a decade that revealed a gap in factors related to economic progress and the ability to obtain health insurance coverage.

The first purpose of this analysis is to use recent data to examine how working-age (18–64) African and Latino Americans fare on correlates of the financing of care (insurance, income, and insurance premiums). The second purpose is to examine whether differences in these financing mechanisms translate into differences in health care access and utilization (probability of a physician visit and the number of ambulatory visits to a physician). We use 1994 data from The Commonwealth Fund Minority Health Survey (CMHS) to address these issues.

METHODS OF ANALYSIS

This study focused on a subpopulation of persons between the ages of 18 and 64. We use the terms "Hispanics," "Latinos," and "Latino Americans" interchangeably in this chapter to describe the experiences of individuals identified as Hispanics in the survey. We use the terms "African American" and "blacks" interchangeably to describe the experiences of survey respondents who identified themselves as non-Hispanic blacks or non-Hispanic African Americans.

Insurance

Insurance data presented in this chapter are based on self-reported data from survey respondents. Questions were asked to determine whether the respondent was covered by health insurance on the date of the interview through work or union; through someone else's work or union; through direct purchase by the respondent or another member of the family; or through some other group insurance, Medicare, or Medicaid. The category "private insurance only" represents people who had health insurance either through work or a union, or health insurance purchased directly by the respondent or a family member, or some other group insurance, but who did not have Medicare, Medicaid, or some other public insurance. The category "any public insurance" represents people who had either Medicaid or Medicare on the interview date, regardless of whether they also had some form of private insurance. The category "uninsured" represents people who did not fall into any of the above insurance categories.

Usual Source of Care

Respondents were asked to indicate the location where they usually go when they are sick or need health care. The choices provided were: doctor's office, HMO or physician group practice, hospital emergency room, hospital outpatient department, community health center, public clinic, military hospital, or other. For this analysis the categories community health center, public clinic, and military hospital were combined with the "other" category. Respondents who indicated an HMO as their usual source of care did so independently of whether they were insured by an HMO.

Discrimination Levels

Questions regarding any discrimination experienced by the respondent were based on self-reports of mistreatment or discrimination. The variable "any discrimination" represents people who reported having health care experiences in the previous twelve months during which they were mistreated. It also includes people who felt they would have received better care had they belonged to a different race or ethnic group, or people who felt they were treated badly because of race/ethnicity, sex, age, health or disability, income level, or any other reason.

Measures of Access to Care

The probability of a physician visit is a variable that we computed based on a variable, which asked how many times the respondent visited a doctor or medical facility in the last twelve months. Respondents who made at least one visit to a doctor's office or medical facility were coded as 1 (yes—the person saw a physician). All others were coded as 0 (no—the respondent did not see a doctor).

The number of physician visits is a variable that we computed based on the number of times the respondent visited a doctor or medical facility in the last twelve months. Persons with no visits were excluded from analyses of physician visits.

Tests of Significance

Tests of significance were conducted using SUDAAN (Shah et al. 1992) to determine the statistical significance of findings. Two tests of statistical significance detected whether the data reported in these analyses are statistically significant. The first statistic used was the standard error of a percent. A major purpose of the CMHS was to allow for the construction of population estimates based on sample data. Like all probability samples, there is a margin of error in this survey between the response given by a sampled respondent and what the actual response to a question would be if a census were taken. The standard error represents the difference between the reported results and what the results would have been if a census of the total population were taken (Loether and Mc-Tavish 1980). Percents displayed in tables and figures with a relative standard error of more than 30 percent are noted. This indicates that the actual response by the population for a given question may be at least 30 percent higher or lower than what is listed in the table.

The second statistic used to perform tests of statistical significance in this study is the Student T test. This test was used to determine the statistical significance of two percents or means being compared in the analysis and to test the significance of the coefficients reported in the regression analyses. Unless otherwise noted, only statistically significant differences ($p < 0.05$) are discussed in the text.

RESULTS OF ANALYSIS

Insurance Coverage Varies by Ethnicity and Work Status

One out of every five (18.6%) working-age adults was uninsured in 1994. Slightly over 9 percent (9.4%) had either Medicaid, Medicare, or some other public insurance, while 71.9 percent had private insurance. The uninsured were less likely than people with public insurance or private insurance to see a physician in 1994 (76.3% vs. 92.0% and 87.9%, respectively) ($p < 0.01$). (See Chapter 7 for a more thorough discussion of the uninsured and their challenges in seeking medical care.)

African Americans and Latino Americans, the poor, and non-full-time workers were disproportionately represented among the uninsured. Nearly one-third (32.3%) of Latino Americans were uninsured, compared with 25.5 percent of African Americans and 14.4 percent of whites ($p < 0.001$). Poor Americans, with incomes less than $15,000, were more than seven times as likely as upper-income Americans, those with incomes over $50,001 (39.8% vs. 5.5%), to lack health insurance ($p < 0.001$).

Finally, part-time workers and individuals not in the labor force were more likely than full-time workers to be uninsured ($p < 0.01$). Full-time workers generally had private insurance (81.4%), whereas only 4.1 percent of full-time workers had public insurance and 14.4 percent had no insurance. Among part-time workers, 56.9 percent had private insurance, 11.8 percent had public insurance, and 31.3 percent were uninsured.

Assessing Disparities in Premiums

One out of every eight (13.4%) working-age Americans spent more than $200 per month in insurance premiums in 1994. Middle- and upper-income Americans, as well as whites, are disproportionately represented in this group. Nearly 15 percent of whites (14.4%) spent more than $200 per month in premiums, compared with 9.4 percent of Latino Americans and 7.7 percent of African Americans ($p < 0.01$). In addition, over 14 percent of the middle- and upper-income Americans (14.2% and 18.2%, respectively) spent more than $200 per month in insurance premiums, compared to 8.2 percent of the lowest-income group ($p < 0.05$).

The disparities by income and employment status on insurance and monthly premiums appear even larger when one examines ethnic and racial differences within these categories. Half of poor Latinos (49.9%) lacked health insurance coverage, while 13.6 percent of the upper-income Latino Americans were without coverage in 1994 ($p < 0.001$) (Table 6.1). Likewise, over 40 percent (43.2%) of poor African American respondents had no health insurance, compared with 11 percent of higher-income African Americans ($p < 0.001$) (Table 6.1). African Americans and Latino Americans who were not in the labor force were twice as likely (39% and 47%, respectively) as full-time workers (18.1% and 25%, respectively) to lack insurance coverage in 1994 (Table 6.1). Finally, whites employed full-time were disproportionately more likely (13.2%) than African Americans employed full-time (6.8%) to pay more than $200 per month in insurance premiums ($p < 0.05$) (Table 6.2).

These differences in premiums by income and race may be because of the affordability of health insurance or because the individual may be in a job that does not provide adequate insurance coverage. Data from the 1987 National Medical Expenditure Survey indicate that average insurance premiums increased with wages (Cooper and Johnson 1993). Cooper and Johnson also found that the availability of insurance varied by whether the person was a member of a labor union, whether the person was a member of a transitory workforce, or whether the person was employed all year (Cooper and Johnson 1993). This makes sense, in that the poor may not be able to afford high insurance premiums. At the

Table 6.1   Percentage Distribution of Insurance Coverage by Race/Ethnicity and Income, Employment Status, Ages 18–64

	Insurance Status		
	Private Only	Any Public Insurance	Uninsured
Income <$15,000			
Whites	38.2	25.1	36.7
African Americans	25.7	31.1	43.2
Latino Americans	27.2	22.9	49.9
Income $15,001–$25,000			
Whites	73.3	8.1	18.7
African Americans	60.9	9.7[a]	29.4
Latino Americans	46.4	8.3	45.3
Income $25,000–$50,000			
Whites	86.5	4.2	9.3
African Americans	74.1	11.8	14.1
Latino Americans	73.1	4.2	22.8
Income ≥$50,001			
Whites	94.2	2.0	3.8
African Americans	77.4	11.5[a]	11.0[a]
Latino Americans	82.2	4.2	13.6
Full-time work			
Whites	85.3	3.6	11.2
African Americans	73.7	8.2	18.1
Latino Americans	70.7	4.3	25.0
Part-time work			
Whites	65.2	9.1[a]	25.7
African Americans	37.8	17.9[a]	44.3
Latino Americans	39.6	5.5[a]	54.9
Not in labor force			
Whites	49.3	27.1	23.6
African Americans	30.9	30.1	39.0
Latino Americans	31.3	21.7	47.0
Unemployed			
Whites	69.0	15.3	15.7
African Americans	31.3	38.5	30.3
Latino Americans	45.5	24.5[a]	30.3

Source: Data from The Commonwealth Fund Minority Health Survey, 1994.
[a]Standard error >30 percent.

Table 6.2   Percentage Distribution of Monthly Insurance Premiums by Income and Employment Status, Controlling for Race/Ethnicity

	Cost of Monthly Insurance Premiums				
	None	$1–$49	$50–$99	$100–$199	≥$200
Income <$15,001					
Whites	48.7	21.9	11.8	9.4	8.3
African Americans	44.3	29.4	12.1	8.0[a]	6.2[a]
Latino Americans	48.8	20.5	17.6[a]	10.7[a]	2.5[a]
Income $15,001–$25,000					
Whites	30.0	24.5	15.8	21.5	8.1
African Americans	20.6	38.9	21.3	14.4[a]	4.8[a]
Latino Americans	26.2	30.4	13.3	19.1	11.0[a]
Income $25,001–$50,000					
Whites	33.8	20.4	13.5	16.9	15.3
African Americans	29.6	30.0	19.9	11.8	8.8
Latino Americans	25.9	27.5	17.7	20.4	8.5
Income ≥$50,001					
Whites	20.5	26.8	14.7	18.8	19.3
African Americans	26.9	32.4	17.9	15.8	7.0[a]
Latino Americans	31.1	21.9	16.4	15.6	15.1
Employed full-time					
Whites	27.5	27.7	14.7	17.0	13.2
African Americans	23.8	34.1	21.7	13.5	6.8
Latino Americans	26.3	26.8	18.8	18.3	9.8
Employed part-time					
Whites	40.9	9.0[a]	11.6[a]	21.5	17.0[a]
African Americans	33.3	34.0	12.7[a]	11.9[a]	8.1[a]
Latino Americans	22.6	36.0[a]	15.3[a]	17.2[a]	8.9[a]
Not in labor force					
Whites	48.3	12.1	9.1[a]	12.6	17.8
African Americans	52.5	19.5[a]	10.6[a]	6.6[a]	10.7[a]
Latino Americans	42.8	14.7[a]	13.8[a]	20.4	8.3[a]
Unemployed					
Whites	36.8	11.5[a]	14.9	19.0	17.9
African Americans	48.0	29.7	7.6[a]	9.5[a]	5.1[a]
Latino Americans	34.4	22.1	10.5[a]	12.5[a]	20.6[a]

Source: Data from The Commonwealth Fund Minority Health Survey, 1994.

Note: Premiums for persons with private insurance.

[a]Standard error ≥ 30 percent.

same time it suggests that factors outside of full-time employment (e.g., being a member of a union) influence an employee's share of the health insurance premium.

MULTIVARIATE FINDINGS

Probability of at Least One Visit to a Physician in the Past Year

We analyzed the relative odds of respondents' seeing a physician in 1994 by insurance status (Table 6.3). Using logistic regression, we developed three multivariate models, one for each of the insurance categories. In the context of other factors, socioeconomic factors play only a modest role in the decision to see a physician for those with private insurance, public insurance, or no insurance. Even so, race/ethnicity continues to play a role in the uninsured's access to care.

Among the privately insured, high school graduates were less likely to see a provider than were college graduates. For the publicly insured, those with incomes of $25,000 to $50,000 were more likely to see a provider than were those with incomes over $50,000 (log odds = 6.61). This middle-income category may represent better access to care through Medicaid among the disabled and medically needy, as well as greater utilization of services through Medicare. People with private insurance who regularly use a physician's office were more likely than people using other sources of care to see a physician during 1994 (log odds = 2.93, $p < 0.001$). Regardless of insurance status, females were more likely than males to see a physician ($p < 0.001$). Young adults with private insurance and middle-aged adults with public insurance were more likely than other adults with private or public insurance to see a physician.

The uninsured living in urban or rural areas were more likely to see a physician than were the uninsured in suburban areas (log odds = 2.03 and 2.73, $p < 0.05$). These findings may reflect the availability of uncompensated care (charity care) to these patients at urban and rural public hospitals, as well as in teaching hospitals.

In addition to age, income, and gender, for 1994 survey participants who had public insurance, the added variables of place of birth, perceptions of discrimination, and perceived health status were correlated with having seen a physician in the previous year. Individuals who had public insurance, were either born outside of the United States, were in good or excellent health, or felt that they had been discriminated against on the basis of race/ethnicity, sex, age, health, disability, or income level, were less likely than other individuals with public insurance to see a physician ($p < 0.01$).

Table 6.3   Predictors of a Physician Visit, Ages 18–64 (adjusted odds ratios)

	Private Insurance Only	Any Public Insurance	Uninsured
Birthplace outside U.S.	0.92	0.10[a]	0.72
Race/ethnicity			
African Americans	1.14[a]	1.03	1.61
Latino Americans	0.99[b]	0.29	0.20[a]
Insurance premiums (monthly)			
$1–$49	1.09	—	—
$50–$99	1.60	—	—
$100–$199	1.21	—	—
≥$200	1.27	—	—
Income			
<$15,000	0.71	2.86	0.36
$15,000–$25,000	0.69	5.74	1.71
$25,001–$50,000	1.09	6.61[b]	1.02
Employment status			
Part-time	0.86	1.09	1.66
Not in labor force	0.84	0.31	1.31
Unemployed	0.98	1.07	1.77
Education level			
<High school	0.54	0.38	2.01
High school graduate	0.59[b]	1.87	1.29
Usual source of care			
Doctor's office	2.93[c]	0.61	2.11[b]
HMO	1.36	0.05	6.40[b]
Hospital OPD	1.85	0.30	3.20[a]
Hospital ER	0.74	3.03	5.17[a]
Perceived health			
Fair/poor	1.65	9.71[b]	4.01
Any discrimination	1.10	0.14[c]	1.31
Gender			
Female	2.35[c]	6.77[a]	3.24[c]
Age			
18–24	3.60[b]	1.84	2.44
25–50	1.20	4.89[b]	1.72
Region			
Northeast	0.66	0.51	0.76
Midwest	0.84	4.75	1.33
South	0.60	1.47	0.67
Urban			
Urban	0.98	0.47	2.03[b]
Rural	0.96	0.28	2.73[b]

(*continues*)

Table 6.3 (*Continued*)

	Private Insurance Only	Any Public Insurance	Uninsured
Chi-square	127.78[c]	57.34[a]	151.10[c]
Degrees of freedom	28	24	24
N	2023	324	344

Source: Data from The Commonwealth Fund Minority Health Survey, 1994.

Note: Referent categories: born in the U.S., white, no monthly premiums, no out-of-pocket costs, income >$50,000, employed full-time, college educated, other sources of care, good/excellent health, no reported discrimination, male, age 51–64, Western, suburban resident. Each column represents a separate multiple logistic model; within each model, odds ratios are adjusted for all independent variables.

A dash = not applicable.

[a]$p < 0.01$.

[b]$p < 0.05$.

[c]$p < 0.001$.

Factors Contributing to Ongoing Physician Visits

The number of physician visits was modeled as a continuous dependent variable in three multiple regression models corresponding to the three insurance statuses. Individuals who had not accessed medical care in the previous twelve months were not included. As contrasted with having seen a physician, the volume of ambulatory physician visits was correlated with fewer factors (data not shown). Income, age, place of residence (rural, urban, or suburban), and employment status were not correlated with the volume of physician visits. However, race/ethnicity, gender, usual source of care, and perceptions of discrimination were correlated with the volume of physician visits. In addition, perceptions of discrimination were correlated with the number of physician visits for those people with public insurance.

The findings show that respondents with public insurance who perceived they were discriminated against were less likely to see a physician (see Table 6.3), but reported more visits after initiating their first visit (data not shown). This suggests that perceptions of discrimination may serve a role in hindering someone from obtaining any care. The stigma felt by the victims of discrimination may lead to a person's delaying the initiation of medical care. Once in the system, a greater number of exposures to the system may result in greater risk of experiencing discrimination.

African Americans with private insurance made more ambulatory visits to a physician in 1994 than others with private insurance (beta = 0.0280, p < 0.05). Females with private insurance made more ambulatory visits to a physician than men with private insurance (beta = 0.888, p < 0.05). People with private insurance whose usual source of care was a physician's office made more ambulatory physician visits than people with private insurance using other sources of care (beta = 0.0484, p < 0.05). Working-age adults with no insurance who lived in the South made fewer visits than the uninsured in other regions. Finally, although respondents who were privately insured who lived in the Northeast made fewer visits than others (p < 0.05), those with public insurance (p = 0.05) who lived in the Northeast made more visits than the other groups studied.

TRENDS AND POLICY IMPLICATIONS

Our results show that financing issues continue to persist, especially by race/ethnicity. Our study reveals that close to one out of every five adults interviewed was uninsured. This represents a 50 percent increase (from 12.5% to 18.6%) in the percentage of uninsured Americans under 65 between 1980 and 1994 (National Center for Health Statistics 1995). These trends in the financing of health care highlight a paradox. During the time America has enrolled more and more individuals with private and public insurance programs in MCOs, the percentage of uninsured Americans has dramatically increased. These Americans are typically uninsured because private insurance is unaffordable or because they are ineligible for public insurance programs.

Race and Ethnicity Effects on Insurance Coverage

Uninsured survey respondents were less likely than those with insurance to see a physician, and they also reported fewer visits to a physician than those with public or private insurance. In 1994, African Americans and Latino Americans were still more likely to be uninsured than whites (25.5% and 32.3%, vs. 14.3%, respectively). These gaps were even larger when the African Americans and Latino Americans were poor and unemployed. Even in the context of disparities by income and employment status, race/ethnicity was correlated with the likelihood of seeing a physician. Uninsured Latino Americans were less likely than other groups to see a physician.

Regarding race and ethnicity, the findings are even more distressing, in light of the consequences of an individual's being without insurance. Hadley, Steinberg, and Feder (1991) have shown that the mortality rates for people without health insurance is three times that of people with insurance. In addition, Franks et al. have reported that a long-term lack of insurance coverage increases the rate of premature death among Americans (Franks, Clancy, and Gold 1993). Survival after the onset of chronic illness is also worse for low-income Americans (Epstein, Weissman, and Gatonis 1992; Hallstrom et al. 1993).

Given the growth of the uninsured population and the persistent gaps in insurance coverage by race/ethnicity, it is clear that disparities in coverage for African Americans and Latino Americans will not be resolved without a fundamental decision that health coverage is a right for all Americans, not just a privilege for people who can afford it. In addition, this problem will only be resolved through the development of a more universal, inclusive policy that benefits all Americans, not just African Americans and Latino Americans. This will require that all Americans, especially the disadvantaged, advocate for the provision of some minimum level of health coverage.

From a public policy point of view, this idea may work only if health insurance is not tied to employment, nor to a needs-based social welfare program such as Medicaid. Keeping health insurance tied to employment will not work over time because employers can simply reduce or eliminate health insurance as a fringe benefit. Currently, a large proportion of uninsured Latino Americans are in jobs without insurance coverage (Short, Cornelius, and Goldstone 1990). Keeping health insurance tied to needs-based social welfare programs will not work because of the stigma attached to income-based social welfare programs, which serve disproportionately larger groups of African Americans and Latino Americans than other groups. In addition, this approach will not work because needs-based programs do not serve all of the people who may need help with health insurance.

Changes in Policy Approaches

Two important changes would foster making health insurance a right for all Americans: (1) the promotion of a broad-based conviction by all Americans that health insurance coverage is a fundamental right to be guaranteed by virtue of being a U.S. citizen (which by default would make the provision of health coverage a critical governmental responsibility); and (2) the serious consideration of a more broad-based tax to pay for health insurance for all Americans, such as a value-added tax (VAT) on all nonessential goods and services, excluding necessities such as food, clothing, housing, and medical care.

The first change would require advocacy and coalition-building across racial/ethnic, gender, and income lines to push for universal health coverage. The second change would require more consensus around the belief and acceptance that health insurance is a social cost that all citizens must bear, and that some tax mechanism would enable us to pay for the cost. The VAT is just one example of a policy that would spread the social cost around among all Americans.

A VAT is based on what society consumes (Rifkin 1995). In this case, society does not levy a tax on what it costs to produce a product, but rather levies a tax on the difference between what it costs a firm to produce a product and the final product itself. By excluding essential goods and services from the tax, one eliminates most of the regressive nature of the tax (Rifkin 1995). Although the VAT has not been tried in the United States, it is currently in use in more than 59 countries, including most of Europe (Rifkin 1995).

Other examples of taxes that could be used for such an effort include a gasoline tax or a tax on tobacco or alcohol use. The problem with these approaches is that they would be targeted to a subset of Americans who may feel they are unfairly penalized. A second problem is that they would require an additional levy on taxes already being collected from the same source.

Our findings suggest that the underlying health care financing problem for minorities is that current policies, despite the growth in MCOs, still allow significant numbers of people to remain uninsured. Current health care financing policy arrangements are merely patchwork solutions based on a history of patchwork solutions. For example, even under managed care, if one's job does not provide health insurance, or if one is not covered by public insurance, there are few affordable alternatives. Thus, the health insurance problem for minorities is neither employment nor income enhancement, but a lack of access to universal health coverage. Without a bold policy leap to offering universal health coverage, our country will begin the next century with the same sets of policy problems that we currently face.

References

Aday, L. A., Fleming, G. V., and Andersen, R. M. 1984. *Access to Medical Care in the U.S.: Who Has It, Who Doesn't.* Chicago: Pluribus Press.

Andersen, R. M., and Anderson, O. W. 1967. *A Decade of Health Services.* Chicago: University of Chicago Press.

Andersen, R. M, Lion, J., and Anderson, O. W. 1975. *Two Decades of Health*

Services: Social Survey Trends in Use and Expenditures. Cambridge, Mass.: Balinger.

Andersen, R. M., Aday, L. A., Lyttle, C. S., Cornelius, L. J., and Chen, M. S. 1987. *Ambulatory Care and Insurance Coverage in an Era of Constraint.* Chicago: Pluribus Press.

Anderson, O. W. 1990. *Health Services as a Growth Enterprise in the United States Since 1875.* Ann Arbor, Mich.: Health Administration Press.

The Commonwealth Fund. March 20, 1995. *National Comparative Survey on Minority Health.* New York: The Commonwealth Fund.

Cooper, P., and Johnson, A. E. 1993. Employment related health insurance in 1987. *National Medical Expenditure Survey Research Findings 17.* AHCPR Pub. No. 93-0044. Rockville, Md.: U.S. Department of Health and Human Services, Agency for Health Care Policy and Research.

Cornelius, L. J. 1993. Ethnic minorities and access to medical care: where do they stand? *Journal of the Association of Academic Minority Physicians* 4(1):16–25.

Coughlin, T. A., Ku, L., Holahan, J., Hesiam, D., and Winterbottom, C. 1994. State responses to the Medicaid spending crisis: 1988 to 1992. *Journal of Health Politics, Policy and Law* 19:837–864.

Davis, K. 1979. Achievements and problems of Medicaid. In A. D. Speigel, ed., *The Medicaid Experience.* Germantown, Md.: Aspen Systems.

Ehrenberg, R. G., and Smith, R. S. 1982. *Modern Labor Economics: Theory and Public Policy.* Glenview, Ill.: Scott, Foresman.

Epstein, A., Weissman, J., and Gatonis, C. 1992. Rates of avoidable hospitalization by insurance status in Massachusetts and Maryland. *Journal of the American Medical Association* 68:2388–2394.

Franks, P., Clancy, C. M., and Gold, M. R. 1993. Health insurance and mortality: evidence from a national cohort. *Journal of the American Medical Association* 270:737–741.

Goldsmith, J. 1997. Harnessing information resources and technology for improving community health: visions of the future. In *Proceedings of the 46th Anniversary Symposium of the National Committee on Vital and Health Statistics.* Hyattsville, Md.: U.S. Department of Health and Human Services, Centers for Disease Control and Prevention, National Center for Health Statistics.

Hadley, J., Steinberg, E. P., and Feder, J. 1991. Comparison of uninsured and privately insured hospital patients: condition on admission, resource use, and outcome. *Journal of the American Medical Association* 265:374–379.

Hallstrom, A., Boutin, P., Cobb, L., and Johnson, E. 1993. Socioeconomic status and prediction of ventricular fibrillation survival. *American Journal of Public Health* 83(2):245–248.

Iglehart, J. K. 1993. The American health care system: Medicaid. *New England Journal of Medicine* 328:896–900.

Jaynes, G. D., and Williams, R. M. Jr. 1989. *A Common Destiny: Blacks and American Society.* Washington, D.C.: National Academy Press.

Liska, D., Bruen, B., Salganicoff, A., Long, P., and Kessler, B. 1997. *Medicaid Expenditures and Beneficiaries: National and State Profiles and Trends, 1990–1995.* 3d ed. Washington, D.C.: Kaiser Commission on the Future of Medicaid.

Liska, D., Obermaier, K., Lyons, B., and Long, P. 1995. *Medicaid Expenditures and Beneficiaries: National and State Profiles and Trends, 1984–1993.* Washington, D.C.: Kaiser Commission on the Future of Medicaid.

Loether, H. J., and McTavish, D. G. 1980. *Descriptive and Inferential Statistics: An Introduction.* 2d ed. Boston, Mass.: Allyn and Bacon.

Long, P., and Liska, D. 1998. *State Facts: Health Needs and Medical Financing.* Washington, D.C.: Kaiser Commission on Medicaid and the Uninsured.

National Association of Hispanic Publications. 1996. *Hispanic-Latinos: Diverse People in a Multicultural Society.* Washington, D.C.: National Association of Hispanic Publications.

National Center for Health Statistics. 1995. *Health, United States, 1994.* Hyattsville, Md.: U.S. Department of Health and Human Services, Public Health Service.

National Center for Health Statistics. 1996. *Health, United States, 1995.* Hyattsville, Md.: U.S. Department of Health and Human Services, Public Health Service.

National Center for Health Statistics. 1997. *Health United States, 1996–1997, and Injury Chartbook.* Hyattsville, Md.: National Center for Health Statistics.

Perloff, J. D., Kletke, P., and Fossett, J. W. 1995. Which physicians limit their Medicaid participation and why. *Health Services Research* 30:7–26.

Raffel, M. W. 1984. Comparative Health Systems. University Park: Pennsylvania State University Press.

Rifkin, J. 1995. *The End of Work: The Decline of the Global Labor Force and the Dawn of the Post Market Era.* New York: G. P. Putnam's Sons.

Shah, B. V., Barnwell, B. G., Hunt, P. N., and LaVange, L. M. 1992. *SUDAAN Users Manual: Professional Software for Survey Data Analysis for Multistage Designs.* Research Triangle Park, N.C.: Research Triangle Institute.

Short, P. F., Cornelius, L. J., and Goldstone, D. E. 1990. Health insurance of minorities in the United States. *Journal of Health Care For the Poor and Underserved* 1(1):9–24 discussion, 28–30.

Short, P., Monheit, A., and Beauregard, K. 1989. *A Profile for Uninsured Americans.* Rockville, Md.: U.S. Department of Health and Human Services, Agency for Health Care Policy and Research.

Starr, P. 1982. *The Social Transformation of American Medicine.* New York: Basic Books.

7

Uninsurance and Its Impact on Access to Health Care

What Are the Challenges for Policy?

Martha A. Hargraves, Ph.D., M.P.H.

THE HISTORICAL SETTING AND WELFARE REFORM

Several of the preceding chapters have validated the importance placed on access to health care by race/ethnicity, income, and insurance status. The incremental nature of policy changes in the United States since the Depression has removed some, but not all, of the barriers to health and medical care through a number of reforms. The Depression revealed the dire circumstances of most Americans, who could not afford health care. During the 1930s, the majority of Americans became eligible for newly introduced private insurance through the workplace. However, the elderly, the poor, and many employed persons were left out. Later, in the 1960s, expansion of public insurance to cover the elderly and the indigent helped to close the health insurance gap in the United States (Aday and Anderson 1981; Starr 1982).

Even so, some Americans remain uninsured. As policymakers have tried to cover individuals who need health and medical care, fragmentation has increased. In the early 1990s, the comprehensive approach advocated through health care reform was defeated, with preference going to a managed, market-driven health care system.

As a result of this incremental approach, a large and growing portion of the American population remains uninsured. In 1994 the uninsured population represented 17.3 percent of the nonelderly population, or 39.4 million individuals. In 1995, an estimated 15.4 percent of all ages including the elderly, or 40.6 million people, were without health insurance. In one year's time, this estimate increased by 1.1 million

Americans in 1996, a figure that, while not statistically significant owing to sampling, suggests an alarming trend upward. The trend continued in 1997, when 43.4 million people, or 16.1 percent of the total U.S. population, were without health insurance. Racial and ethnic minorities, and the poor or near poor, were more likely than others not to have insurance. In 1997, for example, Hispanics had the highest risk of being uninsured, with a rate of 34.2 percent, compared to 12.0 percent for non-Hispanic whites and 21.5 percent for African Americans (Bennefield 1995–1998).

Income and Employment

Historically, several populations have been at risk of being uninsured, namely poor and low-income Americans, African and Latino Americans, people who work either part-time or in small firms, low-wage workers, and individuals not in the labor force (Seccombe, Clarke, and Coward 1994; Short, Cornelius, and Goldstone 1989; Short, Monheit, and Beauregard 1989).

Income plays an important role in influencing who has insurance in the United States. Despite Medicaid, 11.2 million, or 31.6 percent of the poor, had no health insurance in 1997 (Bennefield 1997). Hispanics suffer disproportionately (40.8%) from lack of insurance, both intermittently, during a given year and for an entire year. During 1997, poor African Americans (27.4%) and non-Hispanic whites (29.7%) experienced the lowest uninsured rates among the poor (Bennefield 1997).

Employment continues to be the highest predictor for having insurance in the United States (Fronstin 1997). Copeland's (1998) analysis of individuals' health insurance coverage from October 1994 to September 1995 found that approximately 77.6 percent of the nonelderly sample had health insurance. Of those with health insurance, 81 percent received coverage from employment-based sources. In 1997, among the general population of 15- to 64-year-old workers (full- and part-time), 53.0 percent of the workforce had employment-based insurance. However, poor workers were less likely to be insured than nonworkers. According to the Current Population Survey for 1997, about one-half of poor full-time workers were uninsured (49.2%). Among people without health insurance who worked in 1997, minority populations—especially Hispanics—were disproportionately represented. Among Hispanics who worked full time in 1997, 38.3 percent had no health insurance compared to African Americans and whites (22.1% and 15.8%, respectively). Almost half of all part-time workers of Hispanic origin had no health insurance (45.6%) compared to 33.7 percent of African Americans and 24.7 percent of whites (Bennefield 1998). In addition, Hispanics account for a disproportionate percentage of the recent growth in the uninsured population (Chapter 2; Berk, Albers, and Schur 1996; Short, Cornelius, and Goldstone 1989).

Increases Continue in Numbers of Uninsured

Several factors may contribute to this continued increase in the number of uninsured individuals and may also contribute to the impact of the lack of health insurance on access to health and medical care. Welfare reform has redefined the pool of the poor who are eligible for health insurance. Among those most affected by this redefinition, based on state prerogatives, are "qualified aliens," including refugees, asylees, people paroled in the United States for a period of one year, people who have had their deportation withheld, and people who have been given conditional entry. These groups of immigrants may no longer be eligible for specified federal public benefits. In addition, undocumented (illegal) aliens, family unity immigrants, temporary agricultural workers, asylum applicants, and people residing under "color of law" will no longer be eligible for federal public benefits as defined by PL 401C. Nor will they receive any state or local public benefits unless or until states enact laws to affirm their eligibility. The law further provides that only emergency medical treatment, short-term, non-cash, in-kind emergency disaster relief, or public health assistance in the form of immunization, testing, or treatment of communicable diseases, will be assured to both qualified and not qualified aliens (Hargraves 1996; National Conference of State Legislatures 1996; Quill et al. 1999).

The effect of welfare reform on American citizens has been to greatly alter their enrollment in traditional federal entitlement programs, such as Supplemental Securities Income (SSI) and Medicaid, by allowing greater state flexibility concerning who receives services and in what amounts. States have the latitude to determine potential limitations in the time of coverage for "temporary cash assistance" (TANF) programs. Welfare reform breaks the link between welfare (Aid to Families with Dependent Children [AFDC]) and Medicaid. The effect of this change in Medicaid eligibility and enrollment differs among the states, and its overall impact is yet to be determined.

The loss of jobs or fringe benefits, as the results of corporate downsizing, are also expected to affect the characteristics of and the number of uninsured people. The changing employment patterns of workers who are uninsured—from receiving fully paid health benefits to contributing more out-of-pocket costs for coverage—will result in fewer employees opting for full health care coverage. Other employment structural changes, indicated by the shift from manufacturing to services, increased part-time employment, behavioral preferences of the employed to prefer increased wages over benefits, and the decline in union membership, also explain why employed people remain uninsured (Monheit 1994).

Policies Attempt to Expand Access While Containing Costs

Recent public policy shifts have attempted to balance access to care with cost containment. While the goal of health insurance is to foster access to care, the goal of cost containment strategies is to limit health care costs. These strategies include diagnostic related groups (DRGs), certificate of need legislation, and most recently the introduction of managed care. Some planners have promoted managed care as a solution to the health care cost containment crisis. They believe that enrolling private and public insurance patients in managed care organizations (MCOs) will balance the commitment to providing access to the needy with controlling the costs of care.

However, there is some evidence that managed care unduly shifts the balance against providers' ability to care for the uninsured. Schlesinger, Dorwart, and Epstein (1996) note that managed care companies have been pressuring psychiatrists not to admit severely ill patients, the uninsured, or Medicaid recipients. In addition, psychiatrists have been pressured to limit the length of stay and the scope of treatment for these patients.

Increased strictures on primary health care and inpatient treatment have also accompanied the shift to MCOs. Meyer and Blumenthal (1996) report that the introduction of public managed care programs in the state of Tennessee (TennCare) has led to decreases in patient volume and revenue in academic medical centers, traditionally major health care providers for the uninsured. For example, Ross (1995) notes that the University of Southern California Medical Center in Los Angeles almost closed during the summer of 1995 because of a tightened managed care payment structure. Lipson and Naierman (1996) note that some MCOs, including hospitals, may not develop alternatives to traditional sources of primary care capacity quickly enough, leaving the Medicaid and uninsured populations without access to primary care. Thus, as a result of the growth of managed care as a cost-saving option, the uninsured population has even less access to health care. While the impact remains to be seen of continued reductions concerning the ability of academic medical centers and community health centers to provide the needed safety nets to the uninsured and poor, it is fair to expect that these same groups will be even more vulnerable in the future in light of socioeconomic trends and unprecedented levels of change in health care markets (Altman, Reinhardt, and Shields 1997). The "real" impact of welfare reform on the working poor provides little hope that minority populations will fare better within the health care marketplace.

Level of Uninsurance in Relation to Health Status

The lack of health insurance affects the health and well-being of Americans. Findings from The Commonwealth Fund Minority Health Survey (CMHS) suggest that health insurance plays an important role in the physical health and mental health of individual people of color (Chapters 2, 4, 6, 11), in individuals' level of satisfaction with the quality of their health care (Chapter 8), in the tendency for people to delay seeking needed health care (Chapter 6), in the ability to obtain appropriate preventive health services (Chapter 12), in the range of choices available to clients (Chapter 9), and in perceptions of discrimination (Chapter 10).

Short and Lair (1994) also found an inverse relationship between insurance status and perceived health. Individuals with private insurance reported themselves as the healthiest, followed by the uninsured, people who qualified for public insurance based on income, and finally, people who qualified for public insurance based on medical need. In addition, uninsured individuals who recently lost their private insurance or who live in working families are significantly healthier than the long-term, low-income, or nonworking uninsured. Holl et al. (1995) found that uninsured children lack usual sources of routine care, a usual source of sick care, and appropriate well-child care; they further note that uninsured children who have a chronic disease, such as asthma, face difficulties obtaining medical care and use substantially fewer outpatient and inpatient services.

Marquis and Long (1996) note that AFDC Medicaid beneficiaries use more outpatient and inpatient medical services than they would if they were uninsured. This does not mean that the uninsured are healthier. On the contrary, low-income working families without health insurance go without preventive care and tend to rely on emergency rooms; in one study four out of ten low-income adults experienced some time without insurance over a two-year period and were left with no choice but to forego needed care (Schoen and Puleo 1998). These findings imply that a lack of insurance can lead to delays in seeking care, poorer health, and more expensive health care because of the lack of continuity of care.

In sum, lack of insurance is a problem that cuts across vulnerable populations in society because having insurance is the portal of entry into the current system of health and medical services. The ongoing challenge to policymakers—to provide insurance for all—persists in the face of cost constraints that operate to reduce insurance coverage and health care access among the uninsured. In light of these findings, this chapter focuses on the impact of the lack of insurance on the access to care of the indigent. First, we determine who is disproportionately affected by a lack of insurance. Second, we examine the effects of lack of insurance on access. Third, we discuss policy implications for the delivery of health care to people who are uninsured. Data from the 1994 CMHS have been analyzed to address these issues.

METHODS OF ANALYSIS

This study focused on a subpopulation of 3,267 of the 3,789 adults between the ages of 18 and 64 in the CMHS.

Race and Ethnicity

Classification of survey respondents by ethnic/racial background was based on information reported for each respondent. We use the terms "Hispanics," "Latinos," and "Latino Americans" interchangeably to describe the experiences of those self-identified as Hispanics in the survey. We use the terms "African American" and "blacks" interchangeably to describe the experiences of those self-identified in the survey as non-Hispanic blacks or non-Hispanic African Americans.

Insurance

Survey respondents self-reported the insurance data presented here. Questions were asked to determine whether an individual was covered by health insurance on the interview date through work or union; through someone else's work or union; by health insurance purchased directly by the respondent or his/her family; or by some other group insurance, Medicare, or Medicaid. People under 65 years of age with Medicare insurance were excluded from this study. The category "private insurance only" represented respondents who had either health insurance through work or union, health insurance purchased directly by the respondent or his/her family, or some other group insurance, but who did not have Medicaid or some other public insurance. The category "any public insurance" represented those who had Medicaid on the date of the interview regardless of whether they also had some form of private insurance. The category "uninsured" represented the respondents who did not fall into any of the above insurance categories.

Tests of Significance

Tests of significance were conducted using SUDAAN (Shah et al. 1992) to determine the statistical significance of the findings. Two tests of statistical significance detected whether the data reported in these analyses were statistically significant. The first statistic used was the standard error of a percent. The second was a chi-square statistic, used in multiple logistic regression analyses, to determine if the odds ratio was significantly greater than one.

A major purpose of the 1994 CMHS was to allow the construction of population estimates based on sample data. Like all probability samples, there is a margin of error between the response given by a sampled respondent and what the actual response to a question would be if a census were taken. The "standard error" represents the difference between the reported results and what the results would have been if a census of the total population had been taken. Percentages displayed in tables and figures with a relative standard error of more than 30 percent are indicated in the tables with a footnote. This reflects that the actual response by the population for a given question may be at least 30 percent higher or lower than what is listed in the table.

DESCRIPTIVE ANALYSIS

Several characteristics of the uninsured population were described in Chapter 6, Tables 6.1 and 6.2. In the CMHS, respondents' age, race or ethnicity, country of origin, education, income, census region, marital status, and employment status were correlated with insurance status. Hispanics were by far the most likely of all ethnic groups to be uninsured in 1994 (35.1%), while Anglo Americans were the least likely to be uninsured (15.3%, p < 0.001). Foreign-born individuals were also significantly more likely than U.S.-born citizens to be uninsured (35.3% vs. 18.5%, p < 0.001). Older (ages 62–64) and younger Americans fared worse than individuals between the ages of 25 and 61 on their chances of having health insurance (p < 0.001; data not shown).

Previous chapters validate that large variations in insurance were associated with income and education levels. As income and education levels increased, the percent of uninsured decreased. The range was 50.6 percent for the lowest education level to 15.5 percent for the highest education level (p < 0.001). Individuals living in the Western region of the United States were almost twice as likely as those living in the Midwest to be uninsured (25.7% vs. 13.0%, p < 0.01).

Probably as a result of the linkage between AFDC and Medicaid and expanded Medicaid eligibility for low-income pregnant women, females of reproductive age were more likely than males to have insurance; one-third of males between the ages of 18 and 24 (33.7%) were uninsured versus 25.5 percent of females (p < 0.05) (Table 7.1). The percentage uninsured narrowed for respondents ages 25 to 50 (21% of males vs. 18% of females). For older people, the gender gap reversed, especially for women 51 to 61 years of age, who were 2.6 times as likely as males to be uninsured (22.8% vs. 8.7%).

Employed individuals are more likely than people not in the workforce to have insurance (Table 7.1). The beneficial effect of employment can be seen among virtually all subgroups of the population (data not shown). An exception is that people between 62 and 64 years of age who are unemployed are more likely than the employed to have insurance (93.3% vs. 75.6%). This may reflect early retirement due to disability, with consequent eligibility for Medicaid.

Within ethnic groups, education, income, marital status, and place of residence were correlated with being uninsured (data not shown). However, within socioeconomic groups, there were even larger variations in the percent of uninsured by race or ethnicity. Although numbers were too small to generalize, Native American men and women appeared to be more likely to have insurance. For all categories, white respondents were the least likely group to be uninsured. For example, three out of five Hispanics with less than a high school education were uninsured, while only slightly over 25 percent (25.2%) of whites with less than a high school education were uninsured. Close to 70 percent of the Hispanics in the lowest-income group were uninsured (69.8%), com-

Table 7.1   Percentage Distribution of Insurance Status by Gender, Ages 18–64

	Male		Female	
	Insured	Uninsured	Insured	Uninsured
Age	a		b	
18–24	60.3	33.7	74.5	25.5
25–50	70.5	20.5	82.3	17.7
51–61	91.3	8.7	77.2	22.8
≥62	80.8	19.2	73.8	26.2
Race	a		c	
Non-Hispanic white	83.2	16.8	86.2	13.8
Non-Hispanic African American	71.2	28.8	69.8	30.2
Non-Hispanic Native American	66.6	33.4[d]	23.8	76.2[b]
Non-Hispanic Asian	—	—	—	—
Hispanic	67.9	32.1	61.9	38.1
Hispanic origin				
Mexican	63.3	36.7	52.1	47.9
Puerto Rican	65.4	34.6	71.6	28.4
Cuban	71.3	28.7	49.5	50.5
Other Hispanic	53.0	47.0	54.1	45.9
Country of origin	a		a	
Born in U.S.	81.3	18.7	81.7	18.3
Foreign born	65.0	35.0	64.6	35.4
Education	a		a	
Less than high school	63.9	36.1	61.4	38.6
High school graduate	78.3	21.7	80.0	20.0
Some college+	84.7	15.3	84.4	15.6
Income	a		a	
<$15,001	48.6	51.4	50.1	49.9
$15,001–$25,000	72.9	27.1	72.1	27.9
$25,001–$50,000	86.2	13.8	90.2	9.8
≥$50,001	93.7	6.3	95.3	4.7
Census region	a		a	
Northeast	81.8	18.2	85.9	14.1
Midwest	86.8	13.2	87.2	12.8
South	77.3	22.7	74.8	25.2
West	73.5	26.5	75.1	24.9
Marital status	a		a	
Single	69.0	31.0	72.2	27.8
Married	86.2	13.8	85.2	14.8
Geographic area				
Urban	79.9	30.1	78.7	21.3
Suburban	79.1	20.9	82.8	17.2
Rural	81.4	18.9	77.7	22.3

(continues)

Table 7.1   (*Continued*)

	Male		Female	
	Insured	Uninsured	Insured	Uninsured
Employment status			c	
Employed	80.2	19.8	81.6	18.4
Unemployed	73.3	26.7	74.4	25.6

Source: Data from The Commonwealth Fund Minority Health Survey, 1994.

Note: "Single" is single, divorced, widowed, or separated; "married" is married or living as a couple; "unemployed" is unemployed, homemaker, student, or retired; "employed" is self-employed, employed full-time, or employed part-time.

[a]$p < 0.001$.

[b]$p < 0.01$.

[c]$p < 0.05$.

[d]Standard error ≥ 30 percent.

pared with 46.2 percent of the Anglo Americans in the lowest-income group (p < 0.001). Slightly over 45 percent (45.4%) of Hispanics living in urban areas were uninsured, compared with 31.4 percent of the African Americans and 11.0 percent of the whites (p < 0.001). In fact, within most sociodemographic or socioeconomic subgroups, the percentage of uninsured was highest for Hispanics, followed by African Americans, and lowest for whites.

The high rate of uninsurance among Hispanics varied somewhat within Hispanic subgroups (Table 7.2). For example, there was some evidence that Puerto Ricans were more likely to be insured than other Hispanics, especially among the least educated, the foreign born, and the wealthier individuals. Even among the employed, Mexicans and other Hispanics were less likely (albeit not significantly) to have insurance than were Puerto Rican or Cuban employed persons.

Multivariate Analysis

It is well known that a lack of insurance impedes access to health care. This association was also documented in the CMHS (Chapter 6). However, the question remains whether sociodemographic factors, race or ethnicity, socioeconomic factors, or geography affect access to health care, given insurance status. That is, do these factors create additional

Table 7.2   Percentage Distribution of Insurance Status by Employment Status, Ages 18–64

	Employed		Not Employed	
	Insured	Uninsured	Insured	Uninsured
Age	[a]		[b]	
18–24	65.8	34.2	84.4	15.6
25–50	82.1	17.9	73.0	27.0
51–61	87.8	12.2	60.3	39.7
≥62	75.6	24.4	93.3	6.7
Race	[a]		[a]	
Non-Hispanic white	85.1	14.9	82.0	18.0[c]
Non-Hispanic African American	72.7	27.3	55.8	44.2[c]
Non-Hispanic Native American	75.8	24.2	73.9	26.1
Non-Hispanic Asian	41.7	58.3[c]	45.4	54.6[c]
Hispanic	65.2	34.8	62.5	37.5
Hispanic origin				
Mexican	61.2	38.8	40.2	59.8
Puerto Rican	66.4	33.6	81.1	18.9
Cuban	65.7	32.5	28.6	71.4
Other Hispanic	54.6	45.4	47.8	52.2
Country of origin	[b]		[a]	
U.S. born	82.1	17.9	77.7	22.3
Foreign born	67.8	32.2	53.7	46.3
Education	[a]		[b]	
Less than high school	63.8	36.2	59.1	40.9
High school graduate	80.0	20.0	74.3	25.7
Some college +	85.5	15.0	81.1	18.9
Income	[a]		[a]	
<$15,001	50.3	49.7	45.3	54.7
$15,001–$25,000	72.1	27.9	74.4	25.6
$25,001–$50,000	88.8	11.2	84.1	15.9
≥$50,001	95.8	4.2	85.3	14.7
Census region	[a]		[b]	
Northeast	83.0	17.0	88.3	11.7
Midwest	88.5	11.5	76.8	23.2
South	77.5	22.5	66.7	33.3
West	75.2	24.8	69.0	31.0
Marital status	[a]		[a]	
Single	71.7	28.3	63.0	37.0
Married	86.7	13.3	80.0	20.0
Geographic area				
Urban	81.3	18.7	67.3	32.7
Suburban	81.1	18.9	79.5	20.5
Rural	80.3	19.7	75.4	24.6

(continues)

Table 7.2   *(Continued)*

	Employed		Not Employed	
	Insured	Uninsured	Insured	Uninsured
Gender				
Male	80.1	19.8	73.3	26.7
Female	81.6	18.4	74.4	25.6

Source: Data from The Commonwealth Fund Minority Health Survey, 1994.

Note: "Single" is single, divorced, widowed, or separated; "married" is married or living as a couple; "unemployed" is unemployed, homemaker, student, or retired; "employed" is self-employed, employed full-time, or employed part-time.

[a]$p < 0.001$.

[b]$p < 0.01$.

[c]Standard error ≥ 30 percent.

access barriers for the uninsured? Also, do these factors affect health care access among the insured? To answer these questions, two regression models—one for the uninsured and one for the insured—include demographic factors, race and ethnicity, socioeconomic factors, and geographic factors to examine the likelihood of seeing a physician. We conducted these analyses by stages to examine the relative contribution of different types of factors (such as geographic factors) on access to care. The chi-square statistics at the bottom of Table 7.3 are very helpful for examining the effect of each of these sets of factors on the relative odds of seeing a physician.

For the uninsured, while demographic, socioeconomic, and geographic factors add to the model, race, ethnicity, and citizenship do not contribute to the model (Table 7.3) (chi-square = 1.43, p = .7038). Some factors were consistent across all the steps of the analysis, while other factors only played a role in one of the analysis stages (Table 7.3). Youngest age (18–24), higher education level, and being unemployed were consistently correlated with the use of medical care for the uninsured. Also, among the uninsured, females were consistently more than twice as likely as males to see a physician in 1994.

Uninsured adults between the ages of 25 and 50 were more likely than others to see a physician only in the first two stages of the model (demographic factors and race and ethnicity). Income was not consistently correlated with the chances of seeing a physician (Table 7.3). Al-

Table 7.3   Predictors of a Physician Visit for Uninsured Persons (adjusted odds ratios)

	Race and Ethnicity			
	Demographic (Model 1)	Citizenship (Model 2)	Socioeconomic (Model 3)	Geographic (Model 4)
Demographic factors				
Age				
18-24	13.72[a]	14.66[a]	11.25[b]	10.19[b]
25-50	2.08[c]	2.08[c]	1.49	1.63
Gender				
Female	2.49[b]	2.38[b]	2.38[b]	2.31[b]
Marital status				
Single	1.43	1.42	1.32	1.34
Race				
Non-Hispanic African American		1.26	1.13	1.08
Hispanic		1.41	1.47	1.56
Country of origin				
Foreign born		0.65	0.51	0.63
Socioeconomic factors				
Education				
Less than high school			0.47	0.50
High school graduate			0.47[c]	0.50[c]
Income				
<$15,001			1.63	1.17
$15,001-$25,000			2.74[c]	2.03
$25,001-$50,000			1.38	1.42
Employment status				
Unemployed			3.78[c]	4.59[c]
Geographic factors				
Census region				
Northeast				0.55
Midwest				2.92
South				1.16
Geographic area				
Urban				1.03
Rural				0.69
Chi-square added	35.39	1.43	14.13	11.56
Degrees of freedom added	4	3	6	5
N	438	438	438	438
p value	.0000	.7038	.0281	.0412

Source: Data from The Commonwealth Fund Minority Health Survey, 1994.

Note: Referent categories are: ages $\geq$51, male, married, white, U.S. born, some college, income >$50,000, employed, West, and suburban. Chi-square in steps 2–4 of the model represent the effect of adding the variables from that step of the model to the variables from the previous step.

[a]$p < 0.001$.

[b]$p < 0.01$.

[c]$p < 0.05$.

though income was significant in predicting the probability of seeing a physician for the uninsured in stage three of the model, it was not significant when one also examined geographic factors. This may mean that income, in this situation, may be a proxy for geographic factors such as living in the Midwest.

We structured the models for the likelihood of the insured seeing a physician (data not shown) in the same fashion as those for the uninsured. What is different is that all of the sets of factors (demographic, geographic, etc.) are predictive of the probability of the insured seeing a physician. Gender, race and ethnicity, citizenship status, education, and income were consistently correlated with the use of medical care for the insured. Insured high school graduates were only three-fourths as likely as college-educated respondents to have seen a physician in 1994. The insured who earned less than $25,000 were only one-half as likely as those with incomes greater than $50,000 to have seen a physician in 1994. Insured females were almost three times as likely as insured males to have seen a physician. Insured Hispanic and insured foreign-born respondents were one-half as likely as whites and as U.S.-born individuals to have seen a physician.

Marital status was not consistently correlated with the chances of seeing a physician in 1994. In the second stage of the model (the inclusion of race or ethnicity and citizenship factors), insured single adults were less likely than married adults to see a physician in 1994. However, this was no longer the case in the other steps of the model. Geography was associated with access for the insured. People living in the South were less likely than people living in the West to see a physician. Also, people in rural and urban areas were more likely than suburbanites to see a health care provider.

CONCLUSIONS AND POLICY IMPLICATIONS

Solutions to the health insurance dilemma clearly come with contradictions. Because of sheer numbers, most uninsured people are white, employed, middle-to-upper-income Americans. This means that policies that focus on the numerical majority of the uninsured would help mainstream Americans more than Americans in minority populations.

However, higher proportions of the poor, unemployed, foreign-born, single, divorced, widowed, and separated individuals are uninsured. Thus, these disadvantaged populations would be helped more by initiatives targeted to a subpopulation of the uninsured (such as the uninsured poor). It is important to note, however, that there are distinctions by gender, employment status, and race and ethnicity that can result in variations among those who would be affected by interventions. For example, Latino Americans were more likely than others to be uninsured. In addition, this study discovered that country of origin and region of residence have some bearing on the chances of having insurance. These may be proxies for cultural barriers and regulatory barriers to obtaining needed health insurance, respectively. As a result, researchers and policymakers must account for these subtleties in addressing the needs of the uninsured.

Within the survey population of the uninsured, we found that a variety of factors contributed to the individual's decision to seek medical care or to go without it. Race and ethnicity and education played a role in the decision of uninsured men and uninsured, unemployed men to seek medical care. Income only played a role in the decision of the employed uninsured to seek or avoid medical care. Geography also played a role—for both employed and unemployed—in the decision to see a physician.

Regardless of whether the individual has insurance, far more women than men access health care. Although this is not a new finding, the consistency of results across health insurance statuses suggests that women's greater use of health care is more related to gender than to increased access to health insurance. In fact, in the CMHS, women were not more likely to have health insurance, despite their greater access to Medicaid. This increased access was no doubt offset for unmarried women by a decreased access to health insurance through a spouse's employment. For both the insured and the uninsured, higher education and income were positively correlated with seeing a physician in 1994.

These data highlight how a lack of insurance continues to pose problems for the needy. However, having insurance does not guarantee equal access, as indicated by socioeconomic and geographic differences among the insured in seeing a physician.

New Policies Must Target Disadvantaged Groups

The issue of being uninsured is critical because of its relationship to health and well-being. The fact that the uninsured are more likely than others to delay seeking medical care is very important because it creates a risk that indigent people, especially women and children, will not receive the health care they need. In the long run, this situation could lead to less-efficient and less-effective health care.

Certain populations may continue to be left out of the policy discussions for America unless we develop new policies to address their needs. Poverty and employment are intimately related to the problems of the uninsured and its consequences. Being poor creates a risk for uninsurance because of gaps in policies by income. With the elimination of AFDC and the move toward time limits for welfare assistance, it is likely that an even greater portion of the poor will become uninsured in the future. In a similar vein, the lack of coverage within the employment sector continues to pose problems for vulnerable workers. Further changes in the scope of fringe benefits for employees may force some people to choose between health insurance and take-home pay.

Our currently weakening "safety net" also has further implications for the uninsured. While national policy has shifted the responsibility for the care of the vulnerable to states and local communities, little evidence suggests that states have positioned themselves to respond to the contradictory challenges of welfare reform legislation, managed care, and public health.

To sort through the maze of contradictions related to the laws, practices, and responsibilities of health care "as a public good," we will require both new and renewed energy in deciding how we define the problematic situation posed by lack of insurance for a variety of subgroups within the U.S. population. Further, how institutions within the public arena (such as hospitals and public health professionals) design and provide prevention and intervention programs that improve the health status of vulnerable groups will depend on their abilities to handle the demands from purchasers of care and consumers alike.

Our continued use of the rational, instrumental approach to the complex problem of uninsurance without consideration of the contextual fabric that influences these groups and individuals will likely fail to meet their needs. Policymaking, research, and health care access must become a partnership in inquiry at both the macro (community), and micro (individual) levels. The normative processes that govern the lives, norms, and environments of those who work and live in America without health insurance must be discovered and used in the policy design process aimed at a remedy. In this way, we can ensure a more balanced approach to equity in the provision and distribution of health and medical care to all.

Acknowledgments

The author would like to thank Lee Cornelius for his advice and assistance with data analysis, John M. Cooks for gathering the important documentation needed for this work, and The Commonwealth Fund for its support in this analytic effort.

References

Aday, L. A., Anderson, R. M. 1981. Equity of access to medical care: a conceptual and empirical overview. *Medical Care* 19(Suppl. 12):4–27.

Altman, S., Reinhardt, U., and Shields, A. 1997. *The Future U.S. Health Care System: Who Will Care for the Poor and Uninsured?* Chicago, Ill.: Health Administration Press.

Bennefield, Robert L. 1995, 1996, 1997, 1998. Health Insurance Coverage: 1994, 1995, 1996, 1997. *Current Population Reports,* Census Bureau.

Berk, M. L., Albers, L. A., and Schur, C. L. 1996. The growth in the U.S. uninsured population: trends in Hispanic subgroups, 1977 to 1992. *American Journal of Public Health* 86(4):572–576.

Copeland, C. 1998. Characteristics of the nonelderly with selected sources of health insurance and lengths of uninsured spells. *Issue Brief, Employee Benefit Research Institute* 198(June):1–26.

Fronstin, P. 1997. Sources of health insurance and characteristics of the uninsured: analysis of the March 1997 Current Population Survey. *Issue Brief, Employee Benefit Research Institute* 192(Dec.):36–54.

Hargraves, M. 1996. Immigrants needing health care in Texas. *Texas Medicine* 96(10):64–77.

Holl, J. L., Szilagyi, P. G., Rodewald, L. E., Byrd, R. S., and Weitzman, M. L. 1995. Profile of uninsured children in the United States. *Archives of Pediatrics and Adolescent Medicine* 149(4):398–406.

Lipson, D. J., and Naierman, N. 1996. Effects of health system changes on safety-net providers. *Health Affairs* 15(2):33–48.

Marquis, M. S., and Long, S. H. 1996. Reconsidering the effect of Medicaid on health care services use. *Health Services Research* 30(6):791–808.

Meyer, G. S., and Blumenthal, D. 1996. TennCare and academic medical centers: the lessons from Tennessee. *Journal of the American Medical Association* 276(9):672–676.

Monheit, A. C. 1994. Underinsured Americans: a review. *Annual Review of Public Health* 15:461–485.

National Conference of State Legislatures. 1997. Medical assistance and health benefits under welfare reform. *Immigrant Policy Project Issue Brief.* Washington, D.C., pp. 1–7.

Quill, B. E., Aday, L. A., Hacker, C. S., and Reagon, J. 1999. Policy incongruence and public health professionals' dissonance: the case of immigrant and welfare policy. *Journal of Immigrant Health* 1:9–18.

Ross, J. 1995. A dangerous domino? *Hospitals and Health Networks* 69(17): 34–36, 38.

Schlesinger, M., Dorwart, R. A., and Epstein, S. S. 1996. Managed care constraints on psychiatrists' hospital practices: bargaining power and professional autonomy. *American Journal of Psychiatry* 153(2):256–260.

Schoen, C., and Puleo, E. 1998. Low-income working families at risk: uninsured and underserved. *Journal of Urban Health: Bulletin of the New York Academy of Medicine* 75:30–49.

Seccombe, K., Clarke, L. L., and Coward, R. T. 1994. Discrepancies in employer-sponsored health insurance among Hispanics, blacks, and whites: the effects of sociodemographic and employment factors. *Inquiry* 31(2):221–229.

Shah, B. V., Barnwell, B. G., Hunt, P. N., and LaVange., L. M. 1992. *SUDAAN Users Manual: Professional Software for Survey Data Analysis for Multistage Designs*. Research Triangle Park, N.C.: Research Triangle Institute.

Short, P. F., Cornelius, L. J., and Goldstone, D. E. 1990. Health insurance of minorities in the United States. *Health Care For the Poor and Underserved* 1:9–24.

Short, P. F., and Lair, T. J. 1994. Health insurance and health status: implications for financing health care reform. *Inquiry* 31(4):425–437.

Short, P., Monheit, A., and Beauregard, K. 1989. *A Profile for Uninsured Americans*. Rockville, Md.: U.S. Department of Health and Human Services, Agency for Health Care Policy and Research.

Starr, P. 1982. *Social Transformation of American Medicine*. New York: Basic Books.

8

Satisfaction with Care in Minority Populations

Lisa E. Harris, M.D.
Simon Mungai, M.A.
William M. Tierney, M.D.

THE VALUE OF MEASURING PATIENT SATISFACTION

Patients' experiences with the health care system relate to both the processes and outcomes of the care provided (Carmel 1985; Harris et al. 1995; Kane, Maciejewski, and Finch 1997; Linn, Linn, and Stein 1982; Thomas and Penchansky 1984; Wartman 1983; Wilson and McNamara 1982). To achieve quality in health care from the patient's perspective, the patient's needs and expectations must be met, with success measured not only in improved health status but also in increased patient satisfaction with care.

Patient satisfaction surveys have proliferated over the past two decades, targeting a variety of patient samples. However, socioeconomically disadvantaged and minority patients have generally been underrepresented in these efforts, at least in part because of perceived difficulties encountered in achieving desirable response rates (Acuff, Martin, and Andrulis 1994; Cleary et al. 1991; Walker and Restuccia 1984). But, when surveyed and compared with the majority population, these patients have reported higher rates of problems with care (Cleary et al. 1991). Further, it is precisely these disadvantaged patients, many with chronic diseases and related poor health status, for whom attempts to improve health care quality by inviting the patient's perspective might achieve the greatest results.

The Commonwealth Fund Minority Health Survey (CMHS) was the first comprehensive, nationally representative survey to focus specifically on minority populations concerning a wide range of issues related to health and health care. We analyzed items from the CMHS relating to patient experiences and satisfaction with care to help answer the following questions:

1. How does satisfaction with health care in minorities compare with satisfaction in Caucasians?
2. If minorities report less satisfaction with care, is this dissatisfaction related to minority status or socioeconomic status?
3. What can we learn from examining correlates of satisfaction that might help us improve patients' satisfaction with care?

METHODS OF ANALYSIS

The CMHS included one item that asked respondents to rate their overall satisfaction with the quality of their health care services on a four-point scale ranging from very satisfied to very dissatisfied. We used this item as our overall measure of satisfaction with services, reverse-coding the item so that the highest value (4) represented those most satisfied. In addition, for patients reporting having a regular doctor, the survey included three items related to overall satisfaction with their doctor: health care provided by their doctor overall, general satisfaction with their doctor, and the likelihood of recommending their doctor to a friend.

For our analysis, we created a single scale representing overall satisfaction with the doctor by first reverse-coding the three items so that a high value indicated a positive response. The scale was then created by computing the simple algebraic sum of the three item response values. Finally, we transformed the scale score to a 1 to 100 scale by subtracting the lowest possible score from the actual raw score, then dividing the difference by the possible raw score range, and finally multiplying the results by 100. The final score represents the percentage of the total possible score achieved (Ware et al. 1993).

To determine whether there is a difference in reported satisfaction between the racial groups, we performed our analysis of variance separately for "satisfaction with doctor" and "satisfaction with services." Then, to identify correlates of satisfaction, we constructed multiple linear regression models for each of these dimensions of satisfaction. Here we used as dependent variables our scale score for overall satisfaction with doctor (ranging from 1 to 100) and our single-item measure of overall satisfaction with services (ranging from 1 to 4). Independent variables were items from the CMHS chosen a priori for their face validity as potential correlates of satisfaction with doctor and satisfaction with services. We grouped candidate variables (see Table 8.1) into three categories describing characteristics of patients, of the office or health care delivery system, and of doctors.

The multiple linear regression models were constructed using SUDAAN statistical software designed for analyses of complex sample surveys (Shah, Barnwell, and Bieler 1996). For each model, we began by entering into the model those variables related to patients, followed by the set of variables related to the office/delivery system, and finally, the variables related to doctors.

RESULTS OF ANALYSIS

Satisfaction Varies between Racial Groups

The final respondent sample included 3,795 adults 18 years of age and older, representing an overall response rate of 60 percent. Of these, 1,114 were Caucasian, 1,048 African American, 1,001 Hispanic, and 632 Asian. (Asians, however, are not included in these particular analyses. Important differences in sampling for this group preclude meaningful comparisons with the remaining racial groups; see Technical Appendix.) Based on previous research, we constructed a list of forty-eight variables that might be associated with either satisfaction with doctor, satisfaction with services, or with both. We considered thirty-three variables for both models, four additional variables for only the doctor satisfaction model, and ten additional variables for the services satisfaction model. We further categorized these candidate variables as patient-related ($N = 19$, including race/ethnicity), personal barriers to health care ($N = 6$), office/system-related ($N = 4$), office/system barriers ($N = 6$), reported doctor's practice behavior ($N = 9$), and doctor's characteristics ($N = 4$) (Table 8.1).

For Caucasian, African American, and Hispanic respondents, the mean age was 43.4 ± 15.9 years; 49 percent were women; 21 percent had a household income of less than \$15,000; 46 percent reported that the last educational level achieved was less than or equal to high school graduation; and 73 percent reported having a regular doctor. We examined differences among race/ethnicity groups for each of the remaining 47 candidate variables (data not shown). Significant differences ($p < 0.05$ or smaller) emerged among the race/ethnicity groups for thirty-two of the forty-seven variables. The only patient-related variables

Table 8.1   Bivariate Comparisons between Independent Variables and Doctor/Service
Satisfaction Scales

Variable	Satisfaction Scale	
	Doctor (N = 2,367) (%)	Service (N = 3.163) (mean)
Patient related		
Race		a
African American	81.20	3.42
Hispanic	80.07	3.33
Caucasian	82.37	3.55
Age		b
<65 years	79.61	3.36
≥65 years	80.53	3.68
Gender		
Male	79.81	3.39
Female	79.70	3.41
Income categories		a
$7,500–$15,000	80.45	3.32
$15,001–$35,000	79.26	3.37
≥$35,001	79.80	3.46
Education categories		
Less than high school	79.56	3.40
High school or more	80.10	3.40
Self-reported health status	c	b
Excellent/good	80.37	3.44
Fair/poor	77.21	3.24
Self-reported mental health scale (0–100)(correlation coefficient)	−0.16	−0.23
Type of health insurance		a
No insurance	77.74	2.99
Public (Medicaid/other public insurance or Medicare)	77.63	3.35
Private (any private insurance, Medicare plus private, Medicaid plus private)	80.11	3.47
Membership in HMO	b	
Yes	77.61	3.44
No	91.12	3.47
Satisfied with health plan or insurance	b	b
Very / somewhat satisfied	80.99	3.55
Somewhat / very dissatisfied	73.67	2.90
Source of care when sick		b
ER	77.53	3.14
Other	79.89	2.90
Choice in site of care	b	b
A great deal / some	81.67	3.50
Very little / no choice	71.34	2.99

(*continues*)

Table 8.1 (*Continued*)

	Satisfaction Scale	
Variable	Doctor (N = 2,367) (%)	Service (N = 3.163) (mean)
Choose regular doctor	b	b
Yes	81.23	3.55
No	68.11	3.26
Times visited a doctor or medical facility in last 12 months	b	b
None	75.25	3.22
At least once	80.19	3.43
Trust doctor to help you	b	b
Very much / somewhat	80.51	3.44
Not very much / not at all	65.40	2.86
Follows doctor's advice	b	b
All the time / most of the time	80.97	3.45
Sometimes / rarely / never	69.66	3.04
Did not get needed care	b	b
Yes	70.21	2.85
No	80.77	3.47
Postponed seeking care	b	b
Yes	75.40	3.13
No	81.45	3.51
Used alternative medicine	c	b
Yes	78.57	3.31
No	80.76	3.47
Barriers		
Language differences	b	b
Major/minor problem	73.50	3.18
No problem at all	81.05	3.45
Being nervous or afraid	b	b
Major/minor problem	76.60	3.27
No problem at all	80.80	3.44
Transportation	b	b
Major/minor problem	75.80	3.14
No problem at all	80.52	3.46
Having to pay too much	b	b
Major/minor problem	77.51	3.21
No problem at all	82.25	3.62
Racial discrimination	b	b
Strongly/somewhat affected	72.53	3.14
Not at all affected	81.01	3.45
Better care if different race	b	b
Yes	71.50	3.04
No	80.70	3.44

(*continues*)

Table 8.1 (*Continued*)

	Satisfaction Scale	
Variable	Doctor (N = 2,367) (%)	Service (N = 3.163) (mean)
Office / delivery system related		
Number of different doctors seen	a	
1	76.43	3.22
≥2	80.42	3.45
Felt welcomed by doctor/staff	b	b
Very/somewhat welcome	80.20	3.43
Not welcome at all	45.04	2.16
Felt uncomfortable or treated badly while receiving health care	b	b
Yes	64.95	2.74
No	80.71	3.46
Had been refused care		b
Yes	73.40	2.83
No	79.88	3.41
Barriers		
Cannot get appointment	b	b
Major/minor problem	73.75	3.14
No problem at all	82.42	3.53
Wait time	b	b
Major/minor problem	75.28	3.20
No problem at all	83.64	3.60
Paperwork	b	b
Major/minor problem	77.15	3.23
No problem at all	80.82	3.49
Helpfulness of office staff	b	b
Very/somewhat satisfied	80.81	3.46
Somewhat /very dissatisfied	59.63	2.55
Convenience of office	b	b
Very/somewhat satisfied	80.70	3.47
Somewhat /very dissatisfied	65.14	2.71
Sensitivity about cost	b	b
Very/somewhat satisfied	81.99	3.54
Somewhat /very dissatisfied	67.05	2.79
Doctor related		
Doctor's sex	a	
Male	79.51	3.52
Female	81.53	3.53
Doctor's race	c	c
Asian	74.93	3.37
African American	83.71	3.62

(*continues*)

Table 8.1 (*Continued*)

Variable	Satisfaction Scale	
	Doctor (N = 2,367) (%)	Service (N = 3.163) (mean)
Hispanic	82.10	3.54
White	80.21	3.56
Received preventive care	b	b
Yes	81.48	3.48
No	80.24	3.43
Received second medical opinion		
Yes	79.90	3.44
No	80.24	3.43
Doctor advice on smoking/alcohol/drugs	c	c
Yes	81.01	3.45
No	78.90	3.38
Lifestyle counseling	b	b
Yes	82.39	3.48
No	75.11	3.30
Time spent with doctor	b	b
≤15 minutes	73.37	3.24
≥16 minutes	83.71	3.51
Barrier		
Access to specialty care	b	b
Major/minor problem	72.57	3.06
No problem at all	82.68	3.56
Skill of medical staff	b	b
Very/somewhat satisfied	80.85	3.46
Somewhat /very dissatisfied	48.61	2.34
Doctor		
Treating patient with dignity and respect	b	
Excellent/good	81.61	
Fair/poor	38.81	
Communication	b	
Excellent/good	82.51	
Fair/poor	43.83	
Listening	b	
Excellent/good	83.39	
Fair/poor	44.93	
Accessibility either by phone or in person	b	
Excellent /good	84.36	
Fair/poor	54.78	

Source: Data from The Commonwealth Fund Minority Health Survey, 1994.

[a] $p < 0.05$.

[b] $p < 0.001$.

[c] $p < 0.01$.

found not to be significantly different were gender, membership in an HMO, satisfaction with health plan or insurance, trusting doctor to help, not getting care when needed, postponing seeking care, and using alternative medicine. Three of the four office/system-related variables did not differ significantly by race/ethnicity; the one that did was whether the respondent had been refused care. Conversely, five of the six office/system-related barriers were significantly different by race/ethnicity; the only one not significantly different was the practice's sensitivity about cost. Doctor's gender did not differ significantly by respondent's race/ethnicity, but doctor's race/ethnicity did. Other, non-significant doctor-related variables were doctor's advice on smoking/alcohol/drugs and lifestyle counseling (see Chapter 12) and communication with the patient. All other doctor-related variables differed significantly by race/ethnicity of the respondents.

These racial/ethnic differences in factors potentially associated with patient satisfaction are somewhat mirrored in the satisfaction scales themselves. Analysis of variance demonstrated that there was a trend toward decreased overall satisfaction with doctors for Hispanics (mean scale score 80 $\pm$ 19.8) compared to African Americans (81.2 $\pm$ 18.79) and Caucasians (82.4 $\pm$ 18.9) (data not shown). However, the difference did not reach statistical significance ($p = 0.06$), and the effect size was minimal—.12—measured as the difference in overall satisfaction with services between each racial group and Caucasians, divided by the standard deviation of satisfaction for Caucasians (Cohen 1998). There was, however, a significant difference between racial groups in reported overall satisfaction with services. Satisfaction was the lowest for Hispanics (mean item score 3.3 $\pm$ 0.8), highest for Caucasians (3.6 $\pm$ 0.7), and intermediate for African Americans (3.4 $\pm$ 0.7, $p < 0.05$). The effect size for this difference was .32, representing a small-to-moderate effect (Cohen 1998).

Satisfaction with the Doctor and with Services Not Related to Demographics

We developed multiple linear regression models for satisfaction with doctor and with services (Tables 8.2 and 8.3). For each model, we present only those candidate variables demonstrating an independent association with satisfaction with doctor or with services. The models describing satisfaction with doctor (Table. 8.2) show that neither age, race, nor income was independently associated was satisfaction with doctor.

Table 8.2   Multiple Linear Regression Models for Satisfaction with Doctor (beta(SE))

Independent Variable	Model Including Patient Variables	Model Including Patient and Office/System Variables	Model Including Patient, Office/System, and Doctor Variables
Patient related			
Trust doctor	13.11 (5.39)[a]	8.14 (4.11)[a]	
Chose regular doctor	10.03 (2.71)[b]	8.82 (2.08)[b]	3.77 (1.65)[a]
Insurance (public vs. private)	7.10 (2.05)[b]	6.81 (2.21)[b]	
Self-reported mental health	−0.14 (0.04)[b]	−0.13 (0.03)[b]	−0.07 (0.02)[b]
Did not get needed care		−4.94 (2.21)[a]	
Postponed seeking care	−3.68 (1.38)[a]		
Choice in site of care	6.36 (2.18)[b]	4.23 (2.12)[a]	
Barrier			
Waiting time			−1.77 (0.87)[a]
Unable to get appointment		−2.92 (1.41)[a]	
Racial discrimination		−11.70 (2.84)[b]	
Felt welcomed by doctor/staff		21.65 (5.57)[b]	9.74 (4.91)[a]
Doctor related			
Regular doctor African American vs. Caucasian			3.40 (1.25)[a]
Treating patient with dignity/respect			9.69 (3.58)[a]
Communication			11.77 (2.74)[b]
Listening			21.00 (2.64)[b]
Accessibility			13.14 (2.64)[b]
Lifestyle counseling			3.37 (0.93)[b]
Time spent with doctor (>15 vs. ≤15 minutes)			4.50 (0.94)[b]
Skill of medical staff			12.51 (4.33)[b]
Multiple R^2	0.17	0.20	0.55

Source: Data from The Commonwealth Fund Minority Health Survey, 1994.
[a] $p < 0.05$.
[b] $p < 0.001$.

While patients with public insurance (Medicaid/other public insurance or Medicare) reported higher levels of satisfaction with the doctor compared to patients with private insurance, this variable lost its significance when we added independent variables related to the doctor. A respondent's having chosen his or her regular doctor was the only patient-related variable associated with increased satisfaction in the final model, describing satisfaction with the doctor and including variables related to the patient, the office/delivery system, and the doctor.

Table 8.3   Multiple Linear Regression Models for Satisfaction with Services (beta(SE))

Independent Variable	Model Including Patient Variables	Model Including Patient and Office/System Variables	Model Including Patient, Office/System, and Doctor Variables
Patient related			
Language differences	−0.09 (0.05)[a]		
Chose regular doctor	0.16 (0.07)[a]	0.16 (0.08)[a]	
Satisfied with plan	0.40 (0.07)[b]	0.25 (0.08)[b]	0.24 (0.08)[b]
Membership in HMO	−0.08 (0.03)[a]		
Mental health	−0.00 (0.00)[a]		
Did not get needed care	−0.28 (0.09)[b]	−0.21 (0.09)[a]	−0.22 (0.10)[a]
Paying too much	−0.11 (0.03)[b]		
Choice in site of care	0.34 (0.06)[b]	0.32 (0.06)[b]	0.29 (0.06)[b]
Office/delivery system related			
Waiting time		−0.10 (0.04)[a]	−0.10 (0.02)[a]
Helpful office staff		0.31 (0.11)[a]	0.22 (0.11)[a]
Office hours/location			0.16 (0.07)[a]
Office sensitive about cost of care		0.31 (0.07)[b]	0.29 (0.08)[b]
Doctor related			
Received preventive care			0.13 (0.04)[b]
Time spent with doctor (>15 vs. ≤15 minutes)			0.12 (0.04)[b]
Skill of medical staff			0.52 (0.18)[b]
Multiple R^2	0.27	0.31	0.34

Source: Data from The Commonwealth Fund Minority Health Survey, 1994.
[a] $p < 0.05$.
[b] $p < 0.001$.

Decreased overall satisfaction with doctor was also related to the belief that waiting time is a barrier to receiving care and to the feeling that they were not welcomed by the doctor and staff. The remainder of the variables independently associated with satisfaction with doctor were all doctor-related. These included the doctor's treating the patient with dignity and respect, communicating information regarding medical problems and medications effectively, listening to the patient's concerns and taking them seriously, and being accessible either by telephone or in person. Other variables were also independently associated with increased satisfaction in the final model describing satisfaction with doctor: the amount of time spent with the doctor (more than 15 minutes compared with 15 minutes or less), receiving lifestyle counseling (regarding weight management, healthy eating, or exercise), having a regular doctor who is African American, and being satisfied with the skill of the medical staff.

Models constructed for satisfaction with services (Table 8.3) show again that neither age, race, gender, nor income was independently associated with overall satisfaction with services. The only patient-related variables independently associated with satisfaction with services in the final model were increased satisfaction with the health plan or insurance and the choice in site of care (both of which were associated with increased satisfaction) and not getting needed care (which was associated with decreased satisfaction). Of the variables related to the office/delivery system, the reporting of waiting time as a barrier to receiving care was associated in the final model with decreased overall satisfaction with services, while several other variables were independently associated with increased overall satisfaction with services: increased happiness with the helpfulness of the office staff, with the convenience of the office hours/location, with the office's sensitivity regarding the cost of care, and with the skill of the medical staff. Additional predictors of satisfaction with services were a respondent's having received preventive care and reporting more time spent with the doctor (more than 15 minutes compared to 15 minutes or less).

To summarize, in the final models incorporating variables related to patients, the office and delivery system, and doctors, items that predicted increased satisfaction both with the doctor and with services were time spent with the doctor and reported satisfaction with the skill of the medical staff. Reported increased waiting time was associated with decreased satisfaction with both doctor and services. In addition, variables related to health maintenance (receiving preventive care and lifestyle counseling) were included in the final models representing satisfaction with services, and satisfaction with doctor, respectively. However, race, age, gender, and income had no independent association with overall satisfaction with either the doctor or with the services rendered, once intervening variables were included in the model.

POLICY IMPLICATIONS

This national survey, the first of its kind conducted specifically in minority populations, suggests that minority patients are less satisfied when compared to Caucasians, but the differences are minimal. In analyses that control for patients' experiences with the health care system, neither race nor measures of socioeconomic status (income, education, insurance status, cost or transportation barriers to health care) are independently associated with overall satisfaction with the doctor or with services. Rather, our results suggest that the prevailing concerns, regardless of race/ethnicity or SES, relate more to issues of health care access (being able to get needed care, choice in site of care, waiting times) and delivery (being able to choose one's doctor, time spent with the doctor, and satisfaction with the skill of the medical staff).

In addition, survey respondents valued a medical team's efforts at health promotion. Reports of having received preventive care emerged as an independent predictor of satisfaction with services, and having received lifestyle counseling as a predictor of satisfaction with the doctor. The remaining items associated with satisfaction with services were related primarily to the office/delivery system (satisfaction with the helpfulness of the staff, the convenience of hours and location, and sensitivity regarding the cost of care). Remaining items associated with satisfaction with the doctor were related largely to interpersonal skills (making patients feel welcomed, treating patients with dignity and respect, communicating and listening effectively, and being accessible).

Racial/Ethnic Differences

Although race did not demonstrate an independent relationship with satisfaction in the multivariable models, the modest differences in reported satisfaction with doctor and with services that we detected between racial/ethnic groups might be explained, in part, by important differences in the health care experiences of these patient groups. For example, African American and Hispanic respondents were more likely than Caucasians to report wait time as a barrier to receiving care and less likely to report having a choice in their doctor or site of care. Both minority groups also reported less time spent with the doctor compared to Caucasians, and Hispanics were less likely to report having received preventive care and less likely to rate their physicians' listening skills highly. In addition, although perceived racial discrimination emerged as an independent predictor of satisfaction with doctor when variables related to the patient and office/delivery system were included in the model, this variable lost its significance when variables related to the interpersonal skills of the physician as well as time spent with the physician were added to the model. It is reasonable to postulate that perceived racial discrimination can be overcome when the physician—through accessibility, effective communication, and adequate time spent with the patient—helps the patient feel valued as an individual.

We were further intrigued by our finding that having an African American doctor demonstrated an independent association with satisfaction with doctor. One plausible explanation is that African American physicians are more sensitive and attentive to the needs of minority patients and express this through increased accessibility, greater effort toward communication, and more time spent with patients. Indeed, bivariate comparisons that we performed as secondary analyses for patients having an African American physician versus those not having an African American physician demonstrated that patients in the former group (85% of whom were African Americans) were more likely to report having received preventive care, substance abuse and lifestyle counseling, and having spent more time with the doctor.

In addition, realizing that African American patients reported having African American physicians significantly more often than did the other racial/ethnic groups (20% for African Americans vs. < 2% for Hispanics and Caucasians), we thought that the variable describing race of the doctor might be masking the effect of race or perceived racial discrimination on satisfaction with care in the final model. Thus, we modeled satisfaction with the doctor (including independent variables related to the patient, the office/delivery system, and the doctor) excluding the variable describing race of the physician, and found that African American race achieved borderline significance (beta (SE) = -1.77 (0.97), $p = 0.07$), while racial discrimination retained its significance in the final model (beta (SE) = -4.49 (2.16), $p = 0.03$).

Effects on Mental Health and Effects of Other Aspects of Delivery

Finally, the observed negative correlation between self-reported mental health and reported satisfaction with the doctor deserves comment, especially when self-reported overall health status has generally demonstrated a positive relationship with satisfaction with care (Cleary and McNeil 1988). Although further studies are warranted to more fully explore this relationship, one possible explanation is that physicians spend more time with patients expressing symptoms of depression or anxiety.

This analysis of patients' reports of care, although limited by the cross-sectional nature of the data and the attendant inability to assign cause and effect relationships, does suggest that patient satisfaction might be favorably influenced by malleable attributes of health care organization and delivery. However, if prevailing trends under managed care persist (such as toward decreased choice of provider, limited access, and decreased time per patient visit), the most important patients' needs and expectations revealed by the survey (choice in doctor and site of care, appointment lengths of more than 15 minutes, and time devoted to preventive care and lifestyle counseling) may prove more difficult to satisfy. Managed care may be critical in reducing inappropriate health care utilization (and related costs) for wealthier patients with relatively unimpeded access to care, but the result could be devastating for poorer patients *already* experiencing barriers. Indeed, a number of national surveys have already pointed to the relative dissatisfaction with health care access reported by patients enrolled in managed care organizations as opposed to fee-for-service systems (Brown et al. 1993; Davis et al. 1995; Donelan et al. 1996; Mark and Mueller 1996; Nelson et al. 1996). They also point specifically to the higher number of reported problems in accessing care reported by sicker, older, and poorer Medicare beneficiaries (Nelson et al. 1996).

In addition to these effects of managed care, potential cutbacks in Medicaid and other public health programs threaten to bring about further declines in health care access and impose greater limits on choice of provider and site. These situations have the potential for poorer outcomes of care (Linn, Linn, and Stein 1982; Thomas and Penchansky 1984). Already vulnerable patients need increased appointment availability, rather than additional limitations, as well as opportunities to seek out providers with whom they feel comfortable. In addition, patients for whom communication with their provider might be difficult (because of language or cultural differences) need longer, not shorter, appointment times. Also, patients whose conditions of employment limit their access to "regular" office hours would likely benefit from increased access through evening and weekend hours.

The serious issues raised by this analysis highlight the importance of efforts such as this national survey to make known the needs of minority patients who, already vulnerable, risk becoming even more so unless their needs are first identified and then specifically addressed. Their needs, as indicated by this survey, include more rather than less flexibility in obtaining the medical services that will improve their health outcomes.

References

Acuff, K. L., Martin, V., and Andrulis, D. P. 1994. *Focus on the Patient: Public Hospitals and Patient-Centered Care.* Washington, D.C.: The National Public Health and Hospital Institute.

Brown, R. S., Clement, D. G., Hill, J. W., Retchin, S. M., and Bergeron, J. W. 1993. Do health maintenance organizations work for Medicare? *Health Care Financing Review* 15(2):7–23.

Carmel, S. 1985. Satisfaction with hospitalization: a comparative analysis of three types of services. *Social Science and Medicine* 21:1243–1249.

Cleary, P. D., Edgman-Levitan, S., Roberts, M., Moloney, T. W., McMullen, W., Walker, J. D., and Delbanco, T. L. 1991. Patients evaluate their hospital care: a national survey. *Health Affairs* 10:254–267.

Cleary, P. D., and McNeil, B. J. 1988. Patient satisfaction as an indicator of quality care. *Inquiry* 25(1):25–36.

Cohen, J. 1998. *Statistical power analysis for the behavioral sciences.* Hillsdale, N.J.: Lawrence Erlbaum.

Davis, K., Collins, S., Schoen, C., and Morris, C. 1995. Choice matters: enrollees' views of their health plans. *Health Affairs* 14:99–112.

Delbanco, T. L. 1991. Patients evaluate their hospital care: a national survey. *Health Affairs* 10:254–267.

Donelan, K., Blendon, R. J., Benson, J., Leitman, R., and Taylor, H. 1996. All payer, single payer, managed care, no payer: patients' perspectives in three nations. *Health Affairs* 15:257–265.

Harris, L. E., Luft, F. C., Rudy, D. W., and Tierney, W. M. 1995. Correlates of health care satisfaction in inner-city patients with hypertension and chronic renal insufficiency. *Social Science and Medicine* 41:1639–1645.

Kane, R. L., Maciejewski, M., and Finch, M. 1997. The relationship of patient satisfaction with care and clinical outcomes. *Medical Care* 35:714–730.

Linn, M. W., Linn, B. S., and Stein, S. R. 1982. Satisfaction with ambulatory care and compliance in older patients. *Medical Care* 20:606–614.

Mark, T., and Mueller, C. 1996. Access to care in HMOs and traditional insurance plans. *Health Affairs* 15:81–87.

Nelson, L., Gold, M., Brosn, R., Ciemnecki, A. B., Aizer, A., CyBulski, K. A. November 7, 1996. Access to care in Medicare managed care: results for a 1996 survey of enrollees and disenrollees. Report submitted by Mathematica Policy Research, Inc., to the Physician Payment Review Commission, Washington D.C.

Shah, B. V., Barnwell, B. G., and Bieler, G. S. 1996. *SUDAAN User's Manual.* Research Triangle Park, N.C.: Research Triangle Institute.

Thomas, J. W., and Penchansky, R. 1984. Relating satisfaction with access to utilization of services. *Medical Care* 22:553–668.

Walker, A. H., and Restuccia, J. D. 1984. Obtaining information on patient satisfaction with hospital care: mail vs. telephone. *Health Services Research* 19:291–306.

Ware, J. E., Snow, K. K., Kosinski, M., and Gandek, B. 1993. SF-36 Health Survey Manual and Interpretation Guide. The Health Institute, New England Medical Center. Boston, Mass.: Nimrod Press.

Wartman, S. A. 1983. Patient understanding and satisfaction as predictors of compliance. *Medical Care* 9:886–891.

Wilson, P., and McNamara, J. R. 1982. How perceptions of a simulated physician-patient interaction influence satisfaction and intended compliance. *Social Science and Medicine* 16:1699–1705.

9

Limited Choices for Medical Care among Minority Populations

Llewellyn J. Cornelius, Ph.D.

America's recent flirtation with health care reform centered around the notion of fostering consumer choice in provider selection (Enthoven 1978a, 1978b, 1980; Enthoven and Kronick 1989a, 1989b; Moffit 1994; Plaut and Arons 1994). The consumer choice model assumes that the current approach of provider selection is inefficient and denies health coverage to those who need it most (Enthoven and Kronick 1989a, 1989b). The consumer choice model of health care reform would give consumers more power in deciding what providers are best suited to address their health problems by increasing the number of providers a consumer could go to for health care. It is believed that by providing consumers with a greater range of choices, they would be more likely to select the best provider for their needs, within their fiscal constraints. Advocates of the consumer choice approach believe that fostering consumer choice could lead to improvements in the quality of care, increases in coverage for the underserved, and lower costs because of provider competition.

An earlier formulation of the consumer choice model was a publicly financed and administered model that emphasized the use of vouchers to enable people with private or public coverage to shop for their provider of choice. This plan relied on a uniform set of health benefits for enrollees. It also required that providers and insurers would care for enrolled patients regardless of their age, job status, or prior medical condition (Enthoven 1978a, 1978b, 1980; Winsten 1981). The most recent iteration of this plan was a model, publicly and privately financed and administered, that targeted the uninsured, the underinsured, people with limited health coverage, and those currently insured through the workplace (Enthoven and Kronick 1989a, 1989b).

The consumer choice approach had many critics. Some believed that consumer-oriented market reform would not work because it would lead providers and insurers to encourage consumers to underutilize medical care to save costs. This in turn would lead to a reduction in the quality of care. It was also believed that such a reform would organize providers and insurers, but not consumers, leaving them with fewer choices instead of more. Critics also suggested that consumer choice health care reform would require extensive governmental regulation, and this could reduce innovation and competition among providers (Hellinger 1982; Lynk 1982; Rushefsky 1981). The consumer option also might lead to higher copayment requirements and narrower coverage limits for enrollees (Lynk 1982).

Advocates for consumer choice stress the inability of the current system to care for disadvantaged groups, despite ongoing health policy interventions. Examples of these gaps in caring for the disadvantaged include: fewer physicians practicing in rural or urban areas (Friedman, McTernan, and Leiken 1985; Kindig et al. 1987; Knaap and Blohowiak 1989); fewer physicians accepting Medicaid patients (Perloff, Kletke, and Fossett 1995); a growth in the uninsured (see Chapter 6; Short, Cornelius, and Goldstone 1990); and the persistence in the percentage of Americans who are underinsured (Enthoven and Kronick 1989a, 1989b).

These gaps in services leave minority populations with fewer choices than others for obtaining needed medical care. Today, African and Latino Americans are more likely than other population groups to be uninsured, more likely to lack a usual source of care, and less likely to have a regular doctor at their usual source of care (Chapter 6; Cornelius, Beauregard, and Cohen 1991; Kasper and Barrish 1982). In addition, African and Latino Americans have been disproportionately dependent on hospital outpatient clinics and emergency rooms for their care (Cornelius, Beauregard, and Cohen 1991; Kasper and Barrish 1982).

Regular users of hospital outpatient departments and emergency rooms have lower continuity of care than regular users of physicians' offices (Fleming and Andersen 1986). They often have to wait longer to be seen than patients in physicians' offices, and they may see a different provider each time they visit. People with low continuity of health care are more likely than those with high continuity of care to require unnecessary laboratory tests, to have previous medical work duplicated, to use more ambulatory and inpatient medical care, to be less satisfied with the care they receive, and to report higher expenditures for their care (Becker, Dracchman, and Kirscht 1973; Breslau and Haug 1976; Cornelius 1997; Hochheiser, Woodward, and Charney 1971; Hurley, Freund, and Taylor 1989; Fletcher et al. 1983; Starfield et al. 1976; Weissman et al. 1991).

These studies suggest that consumer choice is an important issue because of its influence on access to the health care delivery system. The studies also suggest that the lack of choice in seeking medical coverage may be a significant problem for African and Latino Americans because of their greater dependency for their medical care on hospital emergency rooms or hospital outpatient departments. In addition, these studies suggest that a lack of choice in obtaining medical coverage may be related to negative health outcomes that stem from low continuity of care.

The purpose of this study is threefold: first, to examine which subpopulations of Americans are more likely to have limited choices for seeking medical care; second, to examine whether their chances of having limited choices for seeking health care vary by insurance, income or other factors; and third, to determine the extent to which having fewer choices is related to delays in seeing a provider for needed medical care or the dissatisfaction with the quality of health care received. Data from The Commonwealth Fund Minority Health Survey (CMHS), 1994, will be used to address these issues.

METHODS OF ANALYSIS

The terms "Hispanics," "Latinos," and "Latino Americans" are used interchangeably in this chapter to describe the experiences of respondents who identified themselves as Hispanics in the survey. The terms "African American" and "blacks" are used interchangeably to describe the experiences of those who identified themselves in the survey as non-Hispanic blacks or non-Hispanic African Americans.

Insurance

Insurance status as presented here relies on self-reported data from the survey respondents. Questions were asked to determine whether, on the interview date, a person was covered by health insurance through work or union; through someone else's work or union; through direct purchase by the respondent or the respondent's family; or through some other type of group insurance, or Medicare, or Medicaid. The category "private insurance only" represents respondents who had health insurance either through work or union, health insurance purchased directly by the respondent or a family member, or some other group insurance, but did not have Medicare, Medicaid, or some other public insurance. The category "any public insurance" represents people who had either Medicaid or Medicare on the date of the interview, regardless of whether they also had some form of private insurance. The category "uninsured" represents those who did not fall into any of the above insurance categories.

Usual Source of Care

Respondents were asked to indicate the location where they usually go when they are sick or need health care. The choices provided were: doctor's office, health maintenance organization (HMO) or physician group practice, hospital emergency room, hospital outpatient department, community health center, public clinic, military hospital, or other. For this analysis, the categories community health center, public clinic, and military hospital were combined with the "other" category. Respondents who indicated an HMO as their usual source of care did so independently of whether they were insured by an HMO.

Discrimination Levels

Questions regarding any discrimination experienced by the respondent rely on self-reports of mistreatment or discrimination. The variable "any discrimination" represents people who reported having health care experiences in the previous twelve months during which they were mistreated. It also includes respondents who felt they would have received better care had they belonged to a different race or ethnic group, or respondents who felt they were treated badly because of race/ethnicity, sex, age, health or disability, income level, or any other reason.

Other Measures

The variable "limited choices" will be used as a proxy for the concept of "consumer choice." People who reported having no choice, very little choice, or some choice about where they went for medical care are considered to suffer from a deficit of consumer choice. Persons who reported unlimited choice would be presumed to experience medical care in the same or similar ways as if the consumer choice model were in effect. Included in the group with no limited choices were people who responded that they were not sure whether they had limited choices (2.5%). The variable "satisfied with the quality of health care" represents respondents who reported being somewhat or very satisfied with the quality of health care services received. The variable "satisfied with the convenience of services" represents people who reported being somewhat or very satisfied with the convenience of their doctor's office or location.

Tests of Significance

We conducted tests of significance using SUDAAN (Shah et al. 1992) to determine the statistical significance of our findings. Two tests of statistical significance were used to detect whether the data reported in these analyses were statistically significant. The first statistic used was the standard error of a percent. A major purpose of the CMHS was to allow the construction of population estimates based on sample data. Like all probability samples, there is in this survey a margin of error between the response given by a sampled respondent and what the actual response to a question would be if a census were taken. The standard error represents the difference between the reported results and what the results would have been if a census of the total population were taken. Percentages displayed in tables and figures with a relative standard error of more than 30 percent are noted. This indicates that the actual response by the population for a given question may be at least 30 percent higher or lower than that listed in the table.

The second statistic used to perform tests of statistical significance in this study is the Student T test. The Student T test was used to determine the statistical significance of two percents or means being compared in the analysis and to test the significance of the coefficients reported in the regression analyses. Unless otherwise noted, we discuss only statistically significant differences ($p < 0.05$) in the text.

RESULTS OF ANALYSIS

Disparities in Choice

We found that approximately two out of every five (41.9%) working-age adults surveyed have some limitations in where they go for their medical care. African American and Latinos are more likely than whites (52.5%,

57.4%, and 38.4%, respectively) to be limited in where they can go for their medical care (p < 0.001). Respondents who are regular users of hospital outpatient departments (58.6%) or emergency rooms (61.5%) are more likely than respondents who regularly use a physician's office to have limited choices in where they can go for care (p < 0.001). People who are uninsured (61.6%) and those with incomes lower than $25,000 (> 50%) are more likely than people with insurance or those with incomes higher than $25,000 to be limited in where they can go for care (p < 0.001). Finally, people who perceive that they are discriminated against, who are more likely to delay seeking medical care when needed, and who are less likely to be satisfied with the quality of their health care or the convenience of the care are more likely to have limited choices (64.0%, 54.1%, and 78.3% respectively, p < 0.001).

The disparities in the percentage of people who have limited choices for medical care by income, insurance, and the usual source of care appear even larger when one examines ethnic and racial differences within these categories (Table 9.1). More than three-quarters of the uninsured African Americans and Latinos have limited choices concerning where they can go for medical care, compared with 57.6 percent of uninsured whites (p < 0.01). Slightly over half of the African Americans and Latinos with public insurance have limited choices for their health care needs, compared with 31.4 percent of whites with public insurance (p < .001). More than 70 percent (71.9%) of the Latinos who earn less than $25,000 have limited choices for seeking out medical care, compared with 47.8 percent of whites in the same income group (p < 0.05). Eight out of every ten Latinos (79.2%) who are regular users of hospital emergency rooms report having limited choices for seeking medical care, compared with 63 percent of African Americans and whites (p = 0.06).

Reasons for Limited Choices

A lack of insurance coverage is the most notable reason given by the survey respondents for having limited choices of where they can go for medical care (p < 0.001). Close to 20 percent (19.6%) indicate that they have a limited number of options available for seeking medical care because of insurance. Another 7.3 percent cite another financial issue as the reason why they have limited options available. Less than 7 percent report that they have limited options available for seeking medical care either because of the lack of availability of doctors (6.6%), transportation problems (2.9%), language problems (0.2%), or some other reason.

Table 9.1 Percentage Distribution of Choice in Seeking Medical Care, by Respondents' Race/Ethnicity and Insurance, and Usual Source of Care

	Unlimited Choice	Limited Choice
Private insurance only		
Latinos	52.0	48.0
Whites	62.4	37.6
African Americans	57.9	42.1
Any public insurance		
Latinos	47.7	52.3
Whites	68.6	31.4
African Americans	49.1	50.9
Uninsured		
Latinos	23.5	76.5
Whites	42.4	57.6
African Americans	23.0	77.0
Doctor's office		
Latinos	53.8	46.2
Whites	66.8	33.2
African Americans	53.5	46.5
Hospital OPD		
Latinos	29.6	70.4
Whites	39.0	61.0
African Americans	49.7	50.3
Hospital ER		
Latinos	20.8	79.2
Whites	37.8	62.2
African Americans	36.7	63.3
Income <$25,000		
Latinos	28.1	71.9
Whites	52.2	47.8
African Americans	41.1	58.9
Income ≥$25,001		
Latinos	54.5	45.5
Whites	67.3	32.7
African Americans	55.1	44.9

Source: Data from The Commonwealth Fund Minority Health Survey, 1994.

Latinos are more likely than whites to cite insurance as the reason why they have limited options for seeking medical care (28.2% vs. 17.9%, $p < 0.001$) (Table 9.2). There are also modest differences between whites, African Americans, and Latino Americans concerning other reasons reported for having limited choices, but these differences are not statistically significant.

Table 9.2   Reasons That Respondents Have Limited Health Care Choices, by Race/Ethnicity

	Financial (%)	Insurance (%)	Few Doctors (%)
Latinos	11.5	28.2	8.2
Whites	5.8	17.9	6.6
African Americans	10.8	24.0	6.0

Source: Data from The Commonwealth Fund Minority Health Survey, 1994.

MULTIVARIATE FINDINGS

Reasons for Delaying Medical Care

Our analysis investigated the probability of a person's delaying medical care in two logistic regression models, by whether the individual has some limitations in choice of medical care provider (Table 9.3). Race/ethnicity, income, perceived health, perceptions of discrimination, age, region of residence, and the physician's reputation were correlated with the decision to delay seeking medical care for people with unlimited choices for seeking medical care. In addition, race/ethnicity, insurance, educational level, income, the usual source of care, and perceptions of discrimination were correlated with the decision to delay seeking medical care for people with limited choices.

African Americans with choices were less likely than other ethnic groups to delay seeking medical care (log odds = 0.81, $p < 0.05$). People in fair or poor health who have choices were more likely than those in good or excellent health to delay seeking medical care (log odds = 1.68, $p < 0.01$). By contrast, older Americans with choices, and people living in the Midwest who have unlimited choices, were less likely than others to delay seeking medical care ($p < 0.05$). Finally, people with choices, who choose their regular doctor because of the doctor's reputation were less likely than others to delay seeking medical care (log odds = 0.62, $p < 0.05$).

Like African Americans with choices, African Americans with limited choices were less likely than other ethnic groups to delay seeking medical care (log odds = 0.59, $p < 0.01$). In addition, people who have limited choices who feel discriminated against were more likely than others to delay seeking medical care (log odds = 2.68, $p < 0.001$). Poor and uninsured people with limited choices were more likely than middle- and

Table 9.3　Predictors of Delaying Medical Care for Respondents with and without Limited Choices (adjusted odds ratios)

	Unlimited Choice of Care	Limited Choice of Care
Race/ethnicity[a]		
African Americans	0.81[b]	0.58[c]
Latino Americans	0.56	0.70
Insurance[a]		
Any public insurance	0.72	0.86
Uninsured	1.78	1.33[d]
Income[a]		
<$15,000	1.43	2.52[b]
$15,000–$25,000	1.74[b]	1.90
$25,001–$50,000	1.53	1.30
Employment status[a]		
Part-time worker	0.87	0.94
Not in labor force	1.38	0.85
Unemployed	0.78	0.88
Education level[a]		
Less than high school	0.92	0.56[c]
High school graduate	0.68	0.36[c]
Usual source of care[a]		
Doctor's office	1.35	0.92
HMO or group practice	0.75	0.23[b]
Hospital OPD	0.65	0.64
Hospital ER	1.77	1.07
Fair/poor perceived health[a]	1.68[c]	2.41
Any discrimination[a]	2.29[d]	2.68[d]
Gender—female[a]	1.35	1.34
Age[a]		
18–24	0.83	1.10
25–50	1.14	1.60
≥65	0.28[d]	0.46
Region[a]		
Northeast	0.85	0.82
Midwest	0.63[b]	1.07
South	0.82	0.92
Residence[a]		
Urban	0.86	0.72
Rural	0.87	0.81
Reasons for choosing regular doctor[e]		
Advertisements	0.63	0.89
Ease in getting appointments	1.16	1.17
Convenient location	1.12	0.74

(continues)

Table 9.3 (*Continued*)

	Unlimited Choice of Care	Limited Choice of Care
Medical credentials	0.84	0.69
Doctor recommended	1.24	1.10
Family recommended	0.84	0.81
Hospital affiliation	1.28	1.23
On approved list	0.78	0.65
ER referral	1.08	1.20
Doctor's race	0.96	1.58
Doctor's gender	1.17	0.54
Good reputation	0.62[b]	1.13
Doctor speaks language	0.89	1.06
Chi-square	208.89[d]	250.81[d]
N	1776	1381
Degrees of freedom	39	39

Source: Data from The Commonwealth Fund Minority Health Survey, 1994.

[a]Referent categories: whites, private insurance, income $>$\$50,001, employed full-time, college-educated, other sources of care, good/excellent health, no reported discrimination, males, ages 51–64, Western, suburban residents. Each column represents a separate multiple logistic model; within each model, odds ratios are adjusted for all independent variables.

[b]$p < 0.05$.

[c]$p < 0.01$.

[d]$p < 0.001$.

[e]Referent categories: statement listed was not a reason they selected their regular doctor.

upper-income Americans, or those with insurance, to delay seeking medical care when needed ($p < 0.05$). By contrast, respondents with less formal education and users of HMOs with limited choices were less likely than others to delay seeking medical care ($p < 0.05$).

Satisfaction with Quality and Convenience

We also investigated the probability of survey respondents being satisfied with quality of health care in two logistic regression models for those with and without limited choices in where they can go for medical care (Table 9.4). Among those with unlimited choices, we found that younger age, having a high school education, living in the South, and having no perceptions of discrimination were correlated with satisfaction with the quality of health care. However, controlling for these factors, race/ethnicity was not correlated. Among those with limited choices, satisfaction was correlated with perceived good health, no perception of discrimination, being female, and having a provider in a convenient location. Regardless of the amount of choice people had in where they went for care, people who perceive themselves as victims of discrimination were less likely than others to be satisfied with the quality of care (log odds = 0.15 and 0.25, p < 0.01).

A second indicator of the satisfaction with health care is satisfaction with the convenience of care (data not shown). Among those respondents who had choices, we found that race/ethnicity, the usual source of care, age, region of residence, location of provider, the use of advertisements, doctor's reputation, doctor's gender, recommendations from family members, and not having perceptions of discrimination were correlated with satisfaction with the convenience of care. African Americans with limited choices were more likely than other ethnic groups to be satisfied with the convenience of services (log odds = 2.01, p < 0.05). On the other hand, African Americans with choices were less likely than other ethnic groups to be satisfied with the convenience of services (log odds = 0.63, p < 0.05).

Although the issue of choice does not affect those people who choose their regular doctor based on advertisements or reputation, people who make their selection of a regular doctor based on these criteria were more likely than others to be satisfied with the convenience of care (log odds = 16.92, 9.36, 4.96, and 1.94, respectively, p < 0.05). Young adults and people living in the South who have choices were more likely than others to be satisfied with the convenience of care (p < .05). Finally, people with choices who choose their regular doctor because the provider practices in a convenient location, or because their family recommended that provider, were more likely than others to be satisfied with the convenience of care (p < 0.05).

CONCLUSIONS AND POLICY IMPLICATIONS

Two out of every five adults interviewed in the CMHS report having some limitation in choice of where they can go for medical care. African and Latino Americans are more likely than others to have limited choices, and they are also more likely to indicate that a lack of insurance is the reason why they have limited choices. Respondents with limited choices are disproportionately represented among those who delay seeking health care, who are not satisfied with the quality of health care, and who are not satisfied with the convenience of their care. The proportion

Table 9.4   Predictors of Respondent's Satisfaction with the Quality of Health Care, for Those with or without Limited Choices (adjusted odds ratios)

	Unlimited Choice	Limited Choice
Race/ethnicity[a]		
African Americans	0.54	1.52
Latino Americans	0.47	1.11
Insurance[a]		
Any public insurance	1.07	1.70
Uninsured	0.46	0.74
Income[a]		
<$15,000	0.74	0.52
$15,000–$25,000	0.98	0.58
$25,001–$50,000	2.58	0.98
Employment status[a]		
Part-time worker	0.83	0.81
Not in labor force	0.79	1.29
Unemployed	0.78	0.66
Education level[a]		
< High school	1.91	1.40
High school graduate	3.02[b]	1.40
Usual source of care[a]		
Doctor's office	0.25	1.11
HMO or group practice	4.01	1.29
Hospital OPD	1.77	2.21
Hospital ER	1.29	1.02
Fair/poor perceived health[a]	0.70	0.43[c]
Any discrimination[a]	0.15[e]	0.25[c]
Gender–female[a]	1.53	1.74[d]
Age[a]		
18 24	5.07[e]	1.20
25–50	1.64	0.82
≥65	0.88	0.48
Region[a]		
Northeast	1.84	1.13
Midwest	1.29	1.58
South	3.26[c]	1.96
Residence[a]		
Urban	0.97	0.96
Rural	0.50	0.64
Reasons for choosing regular doctor[c]		
Advertisements	1.12	0.99
Ease in getting appointments	1.41	0.90
Convenient location	1.25	2.14[a]
Medical credentials	2.71	1.12

(*continues*)

Table 9.4 (*Continued*)

	Unlimited Choice	Limited Choice
Doctor recommended	0.96	0.63
Family recommended	0.98	1.33
Hospital affiliation	2.25	1.21
On approved list	2.93	0.94
ER referral	0.95	3.13
Doctor's race	0.76	0.42
Doctor's gender	1.82	1.33
Good reputation	2.45	1.40
Doctor speaks language	2.24	1.04
Chi-square	163.95[c]	251.42[c]
N	1776	1381
Degrees of freedom	39	39

Source: Data from The Commonwealth Fund Minority Health Survey, 1994.

[a]Referent categories: whites, private insurance, income >$50,001, employed full time, college educated, other sources of care, good/excellent health, no reported discrimination, males, ages 51–64, Western, suburban residents. Each column represents a separate multiple logistic model; within each model, odds ratios are adjusted for all independent variables.

[b]$p < 0.05$.

[c]Referent categories: statement listed was not a reason they selected their regular doctor.

[d]$p < 0.001$.

[e]$p < 0.01$.

of respondents who have limited choices for obtaining medical care is even larger for African or Latino Americans who are uninsured or who earn less than $25,000.

For African Americans and Latinos, the availability of a minimum safety net is critical. The commitment for providing uncompensated health care for the indigent varies by community (Baxter and Mechanic 1997). For example, the top 10 percent of hospitals in Detroit and New York account for less than 35 percent of the debt and charity care, while in Dallas, Houston, Los Angeles, and San Antonio the top 10 percent account for more than 65 percent of debt and charity care. The same 10 percent of hospitals accounted for less than 35 percent of the Medicaid payments in New York, Detroit, and San Diego, compared to more than 70 percent in Los Angeles and Dallas. Thus on some level, the ability to seek out medical care is influenced by the strength of the safety net.

In addition to showing that African and Latino Americans are more likely to have limited choices for seeking medical care, this study also concludes that discrimination, insurance, education, and the usual source of health care play a role in the decision to delay seeking medical care for those with limited options. Discrimination is also correlated with satisfaction with the quality of care and the convenience of care. It may be that provider discrimination in effect creates barriers to care for minorities by limiting where they can go for health care. In addition, factors related to why a person chooses his or her regular doctor is correlated with both delays in seeking medical care and with satisfaction with medical care. In short, limited choices are more correlated with negative health outcomes (delaying medical care or not being satisfied with the quality of care), and having more choices available is positively correlated with not delaying medical care and being satisfied with the quality of care. African and Latino Americans appear to fall among those individuals who are more at risk of adverse outcomes because they have limited health options.

This study reaffirms the finding that African and Latino Americans are at greater risk of poor health outcomes because of their lack of choice among health providers. Providing consumer choice was originally thought to help improve access to care for the disadvantaged. It was hoped that the passage of appropriate health legislation would ensure a system of health care that would guarantee all Americans some minimum level health coverage, with a choice of providers. Given that legislation for health care reform failed in Congress, coupled with an increasing emphasis on health care cost containment through managed care, which may serve to reduce choice even further, the situation may have deteriorated further since 1994 when this survey was conducted.

Providing More Choices to Consumers

There is still some hope for including consumer choice in health care policy. First, some aspects of the consumer choice plan survived. The Health Insurance Portability and Accountability Act of 1996 (PL 104-191) is an example of a law designed to improve consumer choice. This law allows people to: (a) change jobs and take their health insurance with them; (b) limit providers' use of pre-existing conditions to exclude people from health plans; and (c) provide incentives to small employers to create coalitions to negotiate with providers and health plans (U.S. Congress 1995, 1996b). This ensures that people who select their providers can maintain the continuity of care established by virtue of having health insurance.

Second, there has been a large growth in managed care organizations (MCOs). There are now more than 52 million Americans enrolled in some type of managed care entity (National Center for Health Statistics 1997). Employers and agencies who offer managed care plans are expected to provide the consumer with several choices of plans, as well as a choice of providers within a plan. They are also expected to sponsor annual open enrollment periods to encourage consumer choice among several health plans. It is hoped that the process of providing consumers with a choice of health plans will allow them a chance to examine the benefits of specific plans, the range of providers, limitations in coverage, and costs of coverage before they select a plan.

Providing choice among plans by itself, however, does not lead an individual to select the most optimal plan. In a recent Congressional hearing it was noted that some elderly Americans had up to thirty-seven different plans for supplemental medical coverage (Shearer 1990). A second study reported that elderly people from better socioeconomic backgrounds made better supplemental insurance purchase decisions than others (Rice, McCall, and Boismier 1991). This would suggest that, although having a variety of choices is important, access to complete information about those choices is also important.

In the end, it appears that two interventions would foster more consumer choice for minorities: (1) give the disadvantaged more choice in the type of provider and the settings for care; and (2) widely disseminate information about these options throughout the African and Latino American community.

Some health planners may see the recent promotion of Medicaid MCOs as an attempt to provide consumer choice for the poor. As of 1996, slightly over 13.3 million Medicaid patients were enrolled in an MCO (Long and Liska 1998). While the evaluation of these programs is at best anecdotal, some analysts claim that these options provide access to medical services (such as health education, preventive health services, and immunizations) that were formerly unavailable to the poor (who are disproportionately African and Latino American).

Using Culture-Specific Communication Approaches to Explain Choices

Providing easy-to-understand information about plans may also be seen as a gateway to consumer choice. However, a strong emphasis on cultural sensitivity, creativity, planning, and innovation in the development of information dissemination campaigns may increase the chance of successfully reaching out to African and Latino Americans. To succeed in this outreach effort, planners will need to think more creatively about how to inform specific communities about their choice of health plans. This may include examining how information is disseminated through the community and by whom. It may also include using audio, video, and written materials to describe the details of possible choices. Information disseminated to Latino and African Americans may need to incorporate underlying cultural traditions, values, and belief systems that are relevant to specific subgroups. Information targeted to Latinos will also require the translation of brochures and documents into Spanish (using "forward and backward translation" to ensure that cultural nuances are retained in the document translation process).

These two suggested strategies for improving the health of minority populations—providing more choices and educating people about those choices—are interdependent variables. Attempts to succeed in providing consumer choice among minority populations will require both—offering more care options and thinking more creatively about how to inform the community about the differences and similarities among these options in ways they will comprehend.

References

Baxter, R. J., and Mechanic, R. E. 1997. The status of local health care safety nets. *Health Affairs* 16(4):7–23.

Becker, M. H., Dracchman, R. H., and Kirscht, J. P. 1973. A field experiment to evaluate various outcomes of continuity of physician care. *American Journal of Public Health* 64:1062–1070.

Breslau, N., and Haug, M. R. 1976. Service delivery structure and continuity of care: a case study of pediatric practice in the process of re-organization. *Journal of Health and Social Behavior* 17:339–352.

Breslau, N., and Reeb, K. G. 1975. Continuity of care in a university based practice. *Journal of Medical Education* 50(10):965–969.

Cornelius, L. J. 1997. The degree of usual provider continuity for African and Latino Americans. *Journal of Health Care for the Poor and Underserved* 8(2):170–186.

Cornelius, L. J, Beauregard, K., and Cohen, J. 1991. *Usual Sources of Medical Care and Their Characteristics.* DHHS Pub. No. (PHS) 91-0042. Rockville, Md.: U.S. Department of Health and Human Services, Agency for Health Care Policy and Research.

Enthoven, A. C. 1978a. Consumer-choice health plan (first of two parts). Inflation and inequity in health care today: alternatives for cost control and an analysis of proposals for national health insurance. *New England Journal of Medicine* 298:650–658.

Enthoven, A. C. 1978b. Consumer-choice health plan (second of two parts). A national-health insurance proposal based on regulated competition in the private sector. *New England Journal of Medicine* 298:709–720.

Enthoven, A. C. 1980. Consumer-centered vs. job-centered health insurance. *Journal of Nursing Administration* 10:19–27.

Enthoven, A., and Kronick, R. 1989a. A consumer-choice health plan for the 1990s. Universal health insurance in a system designed to promote quality and economy (first of two parts). *New England Journal of Medicine* 320:29–37.

Enthoven, A., and Kronick, R. 1989b. A consumer-choice health plan for the 1990s. Universal health insurance in a system designed to promote quality and economy (second of two parts). *New England Journal of Medicine* 320:94–101.

Fleming, G. V., and Andersen, R. M. 1986. *The Municipal Health Services Program: Improving Access While Controlling Costs?* Chicago: Pluribus Press.

Fletcher, R. H., O'Malley, M. S., Earp, J. A., Littleton, T. A., Fletcher, S. W., Greganti, M. A., Davidson, R. A., and Taylor, J. 1983. Patients priorities for medical care. *Medical Care* 21(2):234–242.

Friedman, E., McTernan, E. J., and Leiken, A. 1985. A historiography of a model statewide allied health manpower supply/demand study. *Journal of Allied Health* 14:129–139.

Hellinger, F. J. 1982. Perspectives on Enthoven's consumer choice health plan. *Inquiry* 19:199–210.

Hochheiser, L. I., Woodward, K., and Charney, E. 1971. Effects of the neighborhood health center on the use of pediatric emergency departments in Rochester, New York. *New England Journal of Medicine* 285:148–152.

Hurley, R. E., Fruend, D. A., and Taylor, D. R. 1989. Emergency room use and primary care case management: evidence from four Medicaid demonstration programs. *American Journal of Public Health* 79:843–846.

Kasper, J. A., and Barrish, G. 1982. *Usual Sources of Medical Care and Their Characteristics.* DHHS Pub. No. (PHS) 82-3324. Rockville, Md.: U.S. Department of Health and Human Services, National Center for Health Services Research.

Kindig, D. A., Movassaghi, H., Dunham, N. C., Zwick, D. I., and Taylor, C. M. 1987. Trends in physician availability in 10 urban areas from 1963 to 1980. *Inquiry* 24:136–146.

Knaap, G. J., and Blohowiak, D. 1989. Intraurban physician location. New empirical evidence. *Medical Care* 27:1109–1116.

Long, P., and Liska, D. 1998. *State Facts: Health Needs and Medical Financing.* Washington, D.C.: Kaiser Commission on Medicaid and the Uninsured.

Lynk, W. J. 1982. Regulation and competition: an examination of "the consumer choice health plan." *Journal of Health Politics, Policy and Law* 6:625–636.

Moffit, R. E. 1994. Personal freedom and responsibility: the ethical foundations of a market-based health care reform. *Journal of Medicine and Philosophy* 19:471–481.

National Center for Health Statistics. 1996. *Health, United States, 1995.* Hyattsville, Md.: U.S. Department of Health and Human Services, Public Health Service.

Perloff, J. D., Kletke, P., and Fossett, J. W. 1995. Which physicians limit their Medicaid participation, and why. *Health Services Research* 30:7–26.

Plaut, T. F., and Arons, B. S. 1994. President Clinton's proposal for health care reform: key provisions and issues. *Hospital and Community Psychiatry* 45:871–876.

Rice, T., McCall, N., and Boismier, J. M. 1991. The effectiveness of consumer choice in the Medicare supplemental health insurance market. *Health Services Research* 26:223–246.

Rushefsky, M. E. 1981. A critique of market reform in health care: the "consumer-choice health plan." *Journal of Health Politics, Policy and Law* 5:720–741.

Shah, B. V., Barnwell, B. G., Hunt, P. N, and LaVange, L. M. 1992. *SUDAAN Users Manual: Professional Software for Survey Data Analysis for Multistage Designs.* Research Triangle Park, N.C.: Research Triangle Institute.

Shearer, G. 1990. Testimony before the Subcommittee on Health, Committee on Ways and Means. U.S. Congress. House. 101st Cong., 2nd sess., March 12.

Short, P. F., Cornelius, L. J., and Goldstone, D. E. 1990. Health insurance of minorities in the United States. *Journal of Health Care for the Poor and Underserved* 1:9–24.

Starfield, B., Simborg, D. W., Horn, S. D., and Yourtes, S. A. 1976. Continuity and coordination: their achievement and utility. *Medical Care* 14:625–636.

Starr, P. 1982. *The Social Transformation of American Medicine.* New York: Basic Books.

U.S. Congress. 1995. The Health Insurance Reform Act of 1995. *Congressional Record.* Washington, D.C.: U.S. Congress, S9906.

U.S. Congress. 1996a. The Health Insurance Reform Act of 1996. *Congressional Record.* Washington, D.C.: U.S. Congress, S3492–S3493, S3503–S3569.

U.S. Congress. 1996b. The Health Insurance Portability and Accountability Act of 1996. *Congressional Record.* Washington, D.C.: U.S. Congress, H2867–H2870, H2951–H2965, H3045–H3083, H3112–H3126, H3836–H3864, H9473–H9569.

Weissman, J. S., Stern, R., Fielding, S. L., and Epstein, A. M. 1991. Delayed access to health care: risk factors, reasons and consequences. *Annals of Internal Medicine* 114(4):325–331.

Winsten, J. A. 1981. Competition in health care: is "consumer choice" in the consumer's interest? *New England Journal of Medicine* 305:1280–1282.

10

Social Status and Perceived Discrimination

Who Experiences Discrimination in the Health Care System, How, and Why?

Thomas A. LaVeist, Ph.D.
Chamberlain Diala, Ph.D.
Nicole C. Jarrett, B.S.

The Commonwealth Minority Health Survey (CMHS) revealed racial and ethnic differences in the use of medical care services (see Chapters 2–5). Racial differences in utilization of medical care services persist (Blendon et al. 1989; Charatz-Litt 1992), despite the remarkable gains that have been made from the times when African Americans were denied admission to hospitals. Civil rights litigation did much to increase access to appropriate medical care by making it unlawful for health care facilities to deny access on the basis of race. However, although some studies show that Medicare and Medicaid in the 1970s had ostensibly eliminated racial differences in health care utilization (Aday and Eichhorn 1972; Aday, Fleming and Andersen 1984), there is compelling evidence to the contrary (Blendon et al. 1989; Davis and Roland 1983; Wolinsky et al. 1990).

Perhaps the most well-documented racial differences in medical care utilization are in coronary procedures. African American patients are less likely than white patients to undergo diagnostic, invasive, and therapeutic coronary procedures after a myocardial infarction. African American patients also undergo fewer cardiac catheterizations, angioplasties, coronary angiographies, and bypass graft surgeries (Carlisle et al. 1995; Giles et al. 1995; Peterson et al. 1994; Wenneker and Epstein 1989; Whittle et al. 1993). Observed racial differences in amputation, renal transplantation, surgical treatments for breast cancer, discretionary surgery, orchiectomies for prostate cancer, and many other major diagnostic and therapeutic procedures highlight the necessity to understand why unequal access to medical care services persists (Alexander and Sehgal 1998; Diehr et al. 1989; Ford and Cooper 1995; Gittelsohn et al. 1991; Guadagnoli et al. 1995; Satariano et al. 1992; Yergan et al. 1987).

Disparities in selected procedures and treatments do not occur only along racial lines. Less access to appropriate levels of medical care has also been observed for women and low-income patients (Alexander and Sehgal, 1998; Diehr et al. 1989; Harris, Andrews, and Elixhauser 1997; Miller et al. 1997).

Researchers who believe there *are* race differences in medical care utilization have paid little attention to the reasons these differences exist. Results in previous chapters suggest that more exposure to the health care system is related to having experienced discrimination in care (see Chapters 2 and 3). Once discriminated against, however, individuals may postpone or forgo needed care. The matter of the degree and variety of sources of discrimination experienced by patients has not been previously addressed in the scientific literature. Here we use data from the CMHS to address this issue. To understand such processes, we need to conclusively establish the meaning of race and the pathways through which race and other social status indicators affect the use of medical services (LaVeist 1994, 1996). Some have speculated that there may be factors within health care settings that lead individuals not to use services (Dutton 1978). The specific research questions to be addressed are to what extent patients feel they have experienced discrimination in their dealings with the health care system, and who is most likely to perceive discrimination?

METHODS OF ANALYSIS

Our analysis will examine the subsample of the CMHS consisting of African American, Hispanic, and white respondents ($N = 3,080$). Racial status and Hispanic heritage were obtained through respondent self-reporting. Respondents were first asked "Are you of Hispanic origin or descent?" A total of 1,001 (26.4%) respondents reported they were Hispanic. They were next asked to indicate a country of origin. Analyses to examine the specific Hispanic subgroups are not displayed in this chapter because, counter to our expectations, these analyses did not yield significant differences among the groups.

Respondents were then asked to indicate their racial status as either white, black, African American, Asian or Pacific Islander, Native American, or some other race. Some 1,695 respondents (44.7%) indicated they were white; 665 respondents (17.6%) reported they were black; and 383 respondents (10.1%) reported that they were African American. The black and African American groups were combined, yielding 1,048 (27.7%) respondents. Accordingly, African American, Hispanic, and white were not treated as mutually exclusive groups in this analysis. There were thirteen black Hispanics (2.9% of blacks) and 170 white Hispanics (5.7% of whites).

We conducted univariate, bivariate and multivariate analyses. The univariate analysis focused on the degree and magnitude of the perception of discrimination experienced by respondents. This analysis also examined the sources of discrimination. The bivariate analysis examined the racial and ethnic differences in perceived discrimination and the effects of other social status indicators on discrimination. The multivariate analysis used weighted logistic regression to determine if the relationships found in the bivariate analysis persisted once other factors were included in the analysis.

Dependent Variables

The dependent variable in the bivariate and multivariate analyses was "perceived discrimination" experienced within the health care system. Discrimination was measured by first asking "Thinking of your experiences with receiving health care in the past twelve months, have you felt uncomfortable or been treated badly, or not?" Of the 3,080 total number of respondents, 241 (7.8%) African American, Hispanic, and white respondents reported they had. These 241 respondents then answered a series of follow-up questions related to the various sources of discrimination they perceived. The follow-up questions were "Do you think you felt uncomfortable or were treated badly because of your (1) race or ethnicity, (2) sex, (3) age, (4) health or disability, or (5) income level?" Finally, each respondent was asked "Do you think there was ever a time when you would have gotten better medical care if you had belonged to a different race or ethnic group, or not?"

Social Status Variables

The independent variables referred to as social status variables correspond to the causes of discrimination inquired about in the dependent variables (i.e., race/ethnicity, sex, age, health/disability, and income level). Race and ethnicity were measured by a set of binary variables indicating African American, Hispanic, and white. Sex was specified by a binary variable indicating female. Age was specified as a set of binary variables representing ages: 18–30, 31–50, 51–65, and older than 65. In the multivariate analysis, "older than 65" was the referent in the analysis. Income was specified as a set of binary variables, as follows: less than $7,500; $7,501–$15,000; $15,001–$25,000; $25,001–$50,000; and greater than $50,000. The comparison category for the multivariate analysis was less than $7,500. In this analysis, health status is considered a social condition, which can lead to discrimination. We measured self-rated health status by a set of binary variables representing poor, fair, good, or excellent health. Poor health status was the category omitted for comparison in the multivariate analysis.

DISCRIMINATION AND THE HEALTH CARE SYSTEM

Summarizing the responses to questions relating to discrimination experienced within the health care system (Table 10.1), we see that for the total sample, as well as each racial/ethnic group, income discrimination was the most frequently cited cause of perceived discrimination. Just over 30 percent of all respondents who perceived discrimination felt it was due to their income level. In each case, fewer than 20 percent of re-

Table 10.1 Percentage of African Americans, Hispanics, Whites, and All Groups Perceiving Discrimination within the Health Care Setting

Variable	Total Sample (N = 5,292)	African Americans (N = 445)	Hispanics (N = 453)	Whites (N = 4,573)
Ever felt treated badly?[a]	7.7	9.1	11.1	7.4
Because of				
Race/ethnicity[b]	9.1	42.5	28.0	4.7
Sex[b]	11.3	17.5	8.0	10.9
Age[b]	14.5	12.5	18.0	13.9
Health/disability[b]	16.5	32.5	16.0	15.2
Income level[b]	30.5	50.0	42.0	28.9
Would receive better care if different race?[a]	7.6	22.6	15.1	5.6

Source: Data from The Commonwealth Fund Minority Health Survey, 1994.
[a]Percentages based on the total number of respondents within the race/ethnic group.
[b]Percentages based on the number of respondents reporting having experienced discrimination within a health care setting.

spondents within the total sample experienced the other causes of discrimination (race, age, and health/disability). In addition, only 7.6 percent of the respondents reported that they felt they would have received better medial care if they had belonged to a different race/ethnic group.

Observing the responses to these questions across race/ethnic groups, we find several interesting patterns. One-half of the African Americans who reported discrimination felt they had been discriminated against because of their income level. More than 40 percent felt they had been discriminated against owing to race, and nearly one third (32.5%) reported being discriminated against because of their health or disability status. Hispanic respondents also reported income and race discrimination as the two most common causes of discrimination. However, Hispanics were more likely to report age discrimination (18%) than either sex (8%) or health/disability discrimination (16%). These patterns contrast with those of white respondents, who also reported income discrimination most commonly but did not report race as a significant cause of discrimination.

With the exception of age discrimination, African American respondents were more likely than either Hispanic or white respondents to report each cause of discrimination. African Americans were 1.5 times as likely as Hispanics and 9 times as likely as whites to report race discrimination. They were also 2.2 times as likely as Hispanics and 1.6 times as likely as whites to report sex discrimination. African Americans reported health/disability discrimination at about double the frequency of Hispanics or whites, who reported roughly equal levels. African Americans were 1.2 times as likely as Hispanics and 1.7 times as likely as whites to report discrimination based on income.

African Americans who reported having been discriminated against in the health care system reported a mean of 2.0 causes of discrimination (Table 10.2). This is compared to 1.6 causes for Hispanics and 1.8 causes for whites. In fact, although no Hispanics and whites reported all five causes of discrimination, 1.8 percent of African Americans did. Also, although fewer than one-half of Hispanics and whites reported more than one cause of discrimination, 57.8 percent of African Americans reported multiple causes.

WHO IS DISCRIMINATED AGAINST?

This analysis examines predictors of perceived discrimination for the five causes of discrimination (race/ethnicity, sex, age, health/disability, and income). The results of bivariate logistic regression analysis, in which we

Table 10.2   Percentage Distribution of the Number of Sources of Perceived Discrimination among African American, Hispanic, and White Survey Respondents

Number of Sources of Discrimination	Total Sample (N = 5,292)	African Americans (N = 445)	Hispanics (N = 453)	Whites (N = 131)
1	58.7	42.2	51.3	61.7
2	23.2	26.0	24.7	23.4
3	14.3	24.5	20.6	11.8
4	3.4	5.5	3.3	3.2
5	0.3	1.8	0.0	0.0
Mean	1.6	2.0	1.8	1.6

Source: Data from The Commonwealth Fund Minority Health Survey, 1994.

regressed each cause of discrimination on the set of social status variables, show that African Americans were more likely to report perceived racial discrimination than non-African Americans (Table 10.3). Each entry represents a separate bivariate regression analysis. Because the variables were not entered simultaneously, this information should not be interpreted as a multiple logistic regression.

In this analysis, African Americans were more than four times as likely (odds ratio = 4.82) than non-African Americans to perceive that they would have received better care had they been of another race. And, with an odds ratio of 8.15, African Americans were far more likely to perceive racial discrimination. African American heritage also placed respondents at double the risk of discrimination based on health/disability. They were more than twice as likely as non-African Americans to have experienced discrimination based on income status (odds ratio = 2.14). Compared to older respondents, the youngest patients were at significantly increased risk of discrimination from their age (odds ratio = 3.15), race (odds ratio = 2.69), and sex (odds ratio = 3.13).

Hispanic respondents were also at greater risk of racial discrimination. They were more than twice as likely as non-Hispanics to report feeling they would have received better care if they belonged to another race (odds ratio = 2.28), and they were more than three time as likely to report being discriminated against because of race (odds ratio = 3.55). In addition, Hispanic respondents were almost twice as likely as non-Hispanics to perceive income discrimination (odds ratio = 1.93).

Table 10.3 Bivariate Odds Ratio for Each Source of Discrimination and Each Independent Variable

Variable	Age	Better Care If Different Race	Health/ Disability	Income	Race	Sex
Age						
18–30 years	3.15[a]	2.14[b]	ns	ns	2.69[a]	3.13[a]
31–50 years	ns	0.69[a]	ns	ns	0.41[b]	ns
51–65 years	ns	ns	ns	ns	ns	ns
≥65 years	ns	0.55[a]	ns	ns	0.18[a]	0.03[b]
African American	ns	4.82[b]	2.01[a]	2.14[b]	8.15[b]	ns
Hispanic	ns	2.28[b]	ns	1.93[a]	3.55[b]	ns
Income						
≤$7,500	ns	ns	ns	ns	6.10[b]	ns
$7,501–$15,000	ns	ns	ns	ns	ns	ns
$15,001–$25,000	ns	ns	ns	0.39[b]	ns	ns
$25,001–$50,000	ns	0.63[a]	ns	0.34[b]	ns	ns
≥$50,001	ns	ns	ns	0.01[b]	ns	ns
Female	ns	ns	2.32[a]	ns	ns	3.29[a]
Self-rated health status						
Poor	ns	2.52[b]	4.70[b]	6.49[b]	3.75[a]	ns
Fair	3.58[a]	2.05[b]	ns	ns	ns	ns
Good	ns	ns	ns	0.46[a]	ns	ns
Excellent	0.16[a]	0.46[b]	0.07[b]	ns	0.33[a]	ns

Source: Data from The Commonwealth Fund Minority Health Survey, 1994.

Note: The analysis presented should not be interpreted as a multiple logistic regression. Each entry in the table represents a separate logistic regression. The referent category for each analysis is all not in that category (e.g., for 18–30 years of age, referent is all older). ns = not significant.

[a]$p \leq 0.05$.
[b]$p < 0.01$.

Income was a potent predictor of discrimination. Lower-income respondents were 6.10 times as likely to report feeling they would have received better care if they had belonged to a different race; more affluent respondents reported less discrimination related to race, health, and income discrimination. Females were more than three times as likely to report sex discrimination (odds ratio = 3.29).

Subjective health status was also a consistent predictor of respondents' experiencing discrimination. For each cause of discrimination, except for income and sex, respondents who reported they were in "excellent" health were significantly less likely to have experienced discrimination in their interactions with the health care system. The relative risk for experiencing discrimination for respondents with excellent health ranged from 0.07 for discrimination based on health/disability to 0.46 for those who believed they would have received better care if they had been of a different race. Conversely, those in poorest health were significantly more likely to have experienced discrimination in their interactions with the health care system. They were 6.5 times as likely to perceive income discrimination, compared with healthier respondents; 4.7 times as likely to report health discrimination; and 3.8 times as likely to report racial discrimination.

These bivariate findings lead to two important questions. Does being in multiple risk categories lead to increasing risks? And do the findings in Table 10.3 persist once the social status variables are entered simultaneously in a multivariate model? Each of these questions will be addressed in turn.

Multiple Risk Models

To examine the issue of multiple risk, we computed a variable that counted the number of high-risk social status categories each respondent belonged to. This included (1) young age (18–30), (2) African American, (3) Hispanic, (4) low income (income less than $25,000), (5) female, and (6) poor self-rated health. Most (78.5%) reported at least one high-risk category. Although respondents could have up to six risk factors, the highest number of risk factors reported by any respondent was four (2.2%). The mean number of risk factors was 1.38. About one-third (34.8%) reported one risk category. Some 44 percent of respondents were in two or more risk categories, and 13.2 percent were in three or more.

We tested the bivariate effect of multiple risk status on discrimination by specifying a set of bivariate weighted logistic regression models by which each risk factor category is compared with all other risk factor groups (Table 10.4). A general pattern can be seen where belonging to multiple risks categories leads to more discrimination. This pattern shows up best in the model where the dependent variable is "receive better care if belong to a different race group." This model displays a dose-

Table 10.4   Bivariate Odds Ratio of Multiple Social Status Risk Factors on Discrimination

Number of Risks	Age	Better Care If Different Race	Health/ Disability	Income	Race	Sex
1	ns	0.48[a]	0.26[a]	ns	0.26[b]	ns
2	3.12[a]	1.53[a]	2.60[a]	ns	ns	4.42[b]
3	ns	2.63[b]	ns	2.42[b]	7.26[b]	ns
4	ns	3.18[b]	ns	ns	4.05[a]	ns

Source: Data from The Commonwealth Fund Minority Health Survey, 1994.

Note: The analysis presented in this table should not be interpreted as a multiple regression. Each entry represents a separate logistic regression model with each independent variable. Thus, for example, persons with one risk factor are compared with those with none or two or more risk factors. ns = not significant.

[a] $p \leq 0.05$.

[b] $p < 0.01$.

response effect where an increasing number of risk factors leads to a higher relative risk of experiencing discrimination. The models that specify race and income discrimination as the dependent variable deviate somewhat from this pattern among respondents in four risk categories. However, it is important to remember that only 2.2 percent of respondents reported belonging to four risk categories, so that analysis is based on a relatively small number of respondents.

Multivariate Models

To test the findings reported based on our bivariate logistic regression analysis, to see whether they would persist within multivariate analysis, the social status variables examined in bivariate analysis were examined in multivariate models (Table 10.5). These analyses are weighted, and we controlled for design effects. We present only statistically significant findings. The only predictor of age discrimination that is significant within a multivariate model is excellent health. Respondents who are in excellent health report significantly less age discrimination compared to other respondents.

African Americans and Hispanics are significantly more likely to report race discrimination than are non-African Americans and non-Hispanics. Overall, income status is not a potent predictor of discrimination, but there is a general pattern where respondents with higher incomes report less discrimination.

Table 10.5 Multivariate Logistic Regression Models of Each Source of Discrimination on Social Status Variables (adjusted odds ratios)

Variable	Age	Better Care If Different Race	Health/ Disability	Income	Race	Sex
Age						
18–30	ns	0.35[a]	9.30[b]	17.47[a]	ns	20.94[a]
31–50	ns	ns	ns	10.23[a]	ns	16.70[a]
51–65	ns	ns	ns	8.52[a]	ns	10.67[a]
African American	ns	4.79[a]	ns	1.73[b]	8.16[a]	ns
Hispanic	ns	2.47[a]	ns	ns	4.43[b]	ns
Income	ns	ns	ns	ns	ns	ns
$7,501– $15,000	ns	ns	ns	ns	0.16[b]	ns
$15,001– $25,000	ns	ns	ns	ns	ns	ns
$25,001– $50,000	ns	0.54[b]	ns	ns	0.12[a]	ns
≥$50,000	ns	ns	ns	0.01[a]	ns	ns
Female	ns	ns	2.26[b]	ns	ns	3.48[b]
Self-rated health status						
Fair	ns	ns	ns	ns	0.22[a]	ns
Good	ns	0.42[b]	ns	0.14[a]	ns	ns
Excellent	0.05[b]	0.25[a]	0.03[a]	0.24[c]	0.22[a]	ns
Chi-square for overall model	883.16[a]	983.93[a]	621.90[a]	848.34[a]	1,418.71[a]	978.68[a]

Source: Data from The Commonwealth Fund Minority Health Survey, 1994.

Note: Referent categories: age ≥65, income ≤$7,501, male, poor health. ns = not significant. Each column represents a separate multiple logistic model; within each model, odds ratios are adjusted for all independent variables.

[a]$p < 0.01$.
[b]$p \leq 0.05$.

There is a pattern, across the various causes of discrimination, where younger respondents report more discrimination. Specifically in the case of income and sex discrimination, there is a linear effect where older age is associated with less reporting of discrimination. Female respondents are more than twice as likely as males to report being discriminated against because of health/disability status, and are more than three times as likely to perceive having been discriminated against because of sex.

We summarize the results of analyses that test the effect of

(1) Medicare, (2) Medicaid, (3) race of physician the same as race of patient, and (4) sex of physician the same as sex of patient. The effect of each of these variables on each of the six types of experienced discrimination was tested after controlling for the six social groups at increased risk of experiencing discrimination—younger age, African American, Hispanic, lower income, female, and poorer subjective health. Here each table entry represents a separate multiple logistic regression model of one of the four variables and one of the six types of experienced discrimination, controlling for the six risk factors. Accordingly, the table should not be read as a simultaneous model. Only models with statistically significant results are presented.

Although Medicare recipients were at lower risk of experiencing age, health, and race discrimination, Medicaid recipients were at significantly increased risk of race discrimination (Table 10.6). When physicians and patients are of the same race, patients were significantly less likely to feel they would receive better care if they belonged to a different race. However, concordance between the race of the physician and patient did not significantly reduce the risk of experiencing racial discrimination. And, interestingly, if the physician and patient were of the same sex, this did not lead to a reduced risk of sex discrimination.

Table 10.6   Separate Logistic Regression Models, Each Controlling for Social Status Variables (adjusted odds ratios)

Variable	Age	Better Care If Different Race	Health/ Disability	Income	Race	Sex
Medicare	0.31^a	ns	0.27^b	ns	0.03^b	ns
Medicaid	ns	ns	ns	ns	3.47^a	ns
Race concordance	ns	0.64^a	0.35^a	ns	ns	ns
Sex concordance	ns	ns	ns	ns	ns	ns

Source: Data from The Commonwealth Fund Minority Health Survey, 1994.

Note: Each entry in this table represents an odds ratio from a separate logistic regression model controlling for the social status variables: Hispanic, African American, age, income, female, and subjective health status. This table should not be interpreted as a simultaneous multiple logistic regression model. ns = not significant.

[a] $p \leq 0.05$.

[b] $p < 0.01$.

SOCIAL STATUS AND HEALTH CARE DISCRIMINATION

This chapter examines the effect of social status on experiencing discrimination within the health care system. The primary social status groups of interest are race/ethnicity, age, income, sex, and health status. As one might imagine, each social status category places respondents at greater risk of experiencing discrimination that is based on the corresponding cause of discrimination. That is, younger respondents are more likely to experience age discrimination; African Americans and Hispanics are more likely to experience race discrimination; low-income individuals are more likely to experience class discrimination; females are more likely to experience sex discrimination; and individuals who report being in poor health are more likely to suffer discrimination based on health or disability status.

We also find, however, that various social status categories are predictors of causes of discrimination that are not as closely associated with the status category. African Americans were more likely to have perceived discriminatory treatment based on income than non-African Americans. Younger patients were substantially more likely to have perceived themselves to have been victimized by race and sex discrimination. Low-income respondents perceived experiencing discrimination based on race and disability status. Women were more likely than men to report health/disability discrimination. Individuals with poor health were at increased risk of being victimized by age, health/disability, race, and income discrimination. And, finally, respondents who report excellent health were substantially less likely to report discrimination based on four out of five causes of discrimination.

In the analysis that tests whether belonging to more than one of the social status categories places individuals at increased risk of experiencing discrimination, we find that being in multiple risk categories places individuals at increased jeopardy of experiencing discrimination. The general pattern of this analysis reveals that belonging to two or more risk categories leads to discrimination victimization within the health care system.

Controlling for all of the social status categories, we find that receipt of Medicare leads to a reduced risk of discrimination, whereas receipt of Medicaid leads to an increased risk of racial discrimination. This difference may be caused by differences in the sources of care used by Medicare and Medicaid patients. Many physicians refuse to see Medicaid patients in their private offices, preferring to treat them at clinics—and patients may perceive more discriminatory treatment in such health care settings. If the patient and physician are of the same race group, the amount of perceived discrimination seems to be somewhat reduced. However, a concordance between the sex of the patient and the sex of the physician does not have a similar effect.

IMPLICATIONS FOR FUTURE RESEARCH

This chapter has dealt with the perception of discrimination within health care settings. Surely, the perception of discrimination does not equal validation of discrimination in the health care system. It is certainly possible that the "true" level of discrimination is over- or underestimated by the misperceptions of respondents. However, as a first step in conducting research on the consequences of discrimination on health services utilization, it is important to examine perceptions, because perceptions influence behavior.

Workers in health care settings are not immune from the failings and frailties that afflict other humans. This includes prejudice and stereotyping based on superficial characteristics such as race, ethnicity, age, disability, social class, or sex. However, the consequences of these human failings are magnified in their importance because of the sensitive nature of the relationship between patients and health care providers. It is unlikely that strategies such as sensitivity or diversity training can do much to change the hearts and minds of individuals. But it is less important that hearts and minds be changed than it is that professional behavior be maintained—and that patients be made to feel they are receiving care in a nondiscriminatory setting.

Future research on discrimination within health care settings must be designed to probe thoroughly individual discrimination experiences to determine whether patterns exist that can lead to suggested changes in the organization and delivery of medical care or changes in health policy.

References

Aday, L., and Eichhorn R. 1972. *The Utilization of Health Services: Indices and Correlates*. DHEW (HSM) 73-3003. Rockville, Md.: National Center for Health Services Research and Development.

Aday, L., Fleming, G., and Andersen, R. 1984. *Access to Health Care in the U.S.: Who Has It, Who Doesn't*. Chicago: Pluribus Press.

Alexander, G. C., and Sehgal, A. R. 1998. Barriers to cadaveric renal transplantation among blacks, women, and the poor. *Journal of the American Medical Association* 280(13):1148–1152.

Blendon, R. J., Aiken, L., Freeman, H., and Corey, C. 1989. Access to medical care for black and white Americans: a matter of continuing concern. *Journal of the American Medical Association* 261(2): 278–281.

Carlisle, D. M., Leake, B. D., and Shapiro, M. F. 1995. Racial and ethnic differences in the use of invasive cardiac procedures among cardiac patients in Los Angeles County, 1986 through 1988. *American Journal of Public Health* 85:352–356.

Charatz-Litt, C. 1992. A chronicle of racism: the effects of the white medical community on black health. *Journal of the National Medical Association* 84:717–725.

Davis, K., and Rowland, D. 1983. Uninsured and underserved: inequities in health care in the United States. *Milbank Memorial Fund Quarterly* 61 (2):149–176.

Diehr, P., Yergan, J., Chu, J., Feigl, P., Glaefke, G., and Moe, R., et al. 1989. Treatment modality and quality differences for black and white breast-cancer patients treated in community hospitals. *Medical Care* 27:942–958.

Dutton, D. B. 1978. Explaining the low use of health services by the poor: costs, attitudes or delivery system? *American Sociological Review* 43(3):348–368.

Ford, E. S., and Cooper, R. S. 1995. Racial/ethnic differences in health care utilization of cardiovascular procedures: a review of the evidence. *Health Services Research* 30(1 Part 2):237–252.

Giles, W. H., Anda, R. F., Casper, M. L., Escobedo, L. G., and Taylor, H. A. 1995. Race and sex differences in rates of invasive cardiac procedures in US hospitals. Data from the National Hospital Discharge Survey. *Archives of Internal Medicine* 155:318–324.

Gittelsohn, A. M., Halpern, J., and Sanchez, R. L. 1991. Income, race, and surgery in Maryland. *American Journal of Public Health* 81:1435–1441.

Guadagnoli, E., Ayanian, J. Z., Gibbons, G., McNeil, B. J., and LoGerfo, F. W. 1995. The influence of race on the use of surgical procedures for treatment of peripheral vascular disease of the lower extremities. *Archives of Surgery* 130:381–386.

Harris, D. R., Andrews, R., and Elixhauser, A. 1997. Racial and gender differences in use of procedures for black and white hospitalized adults. *Ethnicity and Disease* 7(2):91–105.

LaVeist, T. 1994. Beyond dummy variables and sample selection: what health services researchers ought to know about race as a variable. *Health Services Research* 29(1):1–16.

LaVeist, T. 1996. Why we should continue to study race . . . but do a better job: an essay on race, racism and health. *Ethnicity and Disease* 6 (winter/spring):21-29.

Miller, B., Campbell, R. T., Furner, S., Kaufman, J. E., Li, M., Muramatsu, N., and Prohaska, T. 1997. Use of medical care by African American and white older persons: comparative analysis of three national data sets. *Journals of Gerontology. Series B, Psychological Sciences and Social Sciences* 52 (6):S325–S335.

Peterson, E. D., Wright, S. M., Daley, J., and Thibault, G. E. 1994. Racial variation in cardiac procedure use and survival following acute myocardial infarction in the Department of Veterans Affairs. *Journal of the American Medical Association* 271:1175–1180.

Satariano, E. R., Swanson, G. M., and Moll, P. P. 1992. Nonclinical factors associated with surgery received for treatment of early-stage breast cancer. *American Journal of Public Health* 82:195–198.

Wenneker, M. B., and Epstein, A. M. 1989. Racial inequalities in the use of procedures for patients with ischemic heart disease in Massachusetts. *Journal of the American Medical Association* 261:253–257.

Whittle, J., Conigliaro, J., Good, C. B., and Lofgren, R. P. 1993. Racial differences in the use of invasive cardiovascular procedures in the Department of Veterans Affairs medical system. *New England Journal of Medicine* 329:621–627.

Wolinsky, F., Aguirre, B., Fann, L-J., Keith, V., Arnold, C., Mederhauer, J., and Dietrich, K. 1990. Ethnic differences in the demand for physician and hospital utilization among older adults in major American cities: conspicuous evidence of considerable inequalities. *Milbank Memorial Fund Quarterly* 67(3–4):412–449.

Yergan, J., Flood, A. B., LoGerfo, J. P., and Diehr, P. 1987. Relationship between patient race and the intensity of hospital services. *Medical Care* 25(7): 592–603.

11

Race, Stress, and Mental Health

David R. Williams, Ph.D., M.P.H.

MINORITY STATUS AND MENTAL HEALTH

This chapter examines social conditions linked to the lives of minority group members and the larger social context within which mental health problems emerge. We will systematically examine the extent to which racial categorization and stratification predict variations in people's experiences of stress and mental health functioning.

One of the most critical issues in the study of the mental health of minority populations in the United States is to identify whether minority status predicts an increased risk for mental health problems (Vega and Rumbaut 1991). This research is contingent on an enhanced understanding of what race is, as well as the delineation of the specific factors linked to race that influence health status. Because the categories of race and ethnicity are not the cause of variations in health status, health researchers should avoid reifying these terms (Williams 1997). They are descriptive labels that reflect the variations in risk factors that could lead to ill health. Studies of minority health status should rest on a clear understanding of what racial and ethnic labels actually measure.

The Meaning of Race

Statistical Directive No. 15 of the Office of Management and Budget (OMB) requires federal agencies to report statistics for four racial groups (American Indian and Alaskan Native, Asian or Pacific Islander, African American, and white) and one ethnic category (Hispanic origin). In terms of biological characteristics and genetics, these categories are more alike than different. Irrespective of geographic origin or race, all human beings are identical in 75 percent of known genetic factors (Lewontin 1984). In addition, some 95 percent of human genetic variation exists within racial groups, with relatively small and isolated populations, such as Eskimos and Australian Aborigines, contributing most of the between-group variation (Lewontin 1972). Moreover, there are no specific scientific criteria that will unambiguously distinguish different racial groups. Rather, the officially recognized racial categories in the United States may capture ethnic differences between population groups. An *ethnic group* is a group within the larger society that can be identified on the basis of common geographic origins, family patterns, language, religion, values, traditions and symbols, literature, music, dietary preferences, and employment patterns.

The development of the concept of race predates modern scientific theories of genetics. Historically, race was used to classify human variation as well as to develop an apparently scientific rationale for the exploitation of groups that were regarded as inferior (Montagu 1965). Three of the five categories currently used in OMB Statistical Directive No. 15 were in the first census. As required by Article I of the U.S. Constitution, this census enumerated whites, black slaves (recorded as three-fifths of a person), and Indians who paid taxes (Anderson and Fienberg 1995). Thus, from the beginning, racial categories reflected a hierarchy of racial preference: whites at the top, blacks at the bottom, and other groups in the middle. Although the three-fifths rule was eventually abandoned by the Thirteenth Amendment, there has been a history of racial oppression in the United States. Current racial categories capture some of the inequalities that emerged as attitudes and beliefs about racial groups became policies and societal arrangements to limit the opportunities and life chances of stigmatized groups.

Historical events and political factors, such as the influx of immigrants, shaped the development of new racial categories (Anderson and Fienberg 1995). The 1870 Census added "Chinese" as a new racial group because of the Chinese immigrants who entered the United States in the mid-nineteenth century. However, immigration and naturalization laws barred Chinese immigrants from becoming U.S. citizens. Only white immigrants could be citizens, and in 1882, the Chinese Exclusion Act barred further immigration. The 1890 Census added "Japanese" as a new category to the race or color question. The 1920 Census added "Filipino," "Hindu," and "Korean." The 1930 Census added "Mexican" as a new racial category.

Current categories do not capture all of the presumed racial and ethnic variation in the United States. Rather, they identify only the *minority* racial and ethnic groups. Instead of indicating the numerical size of a population, the term *minority* reflects stratification and access to power and resources (Nelson and Tienda 1985). Minority status reflects the convergence of ethnic origin and socioeconomic disadvantage. A *minority group* is one whose members are subjected to unequal treatment through prejudice and discrimination by a dominant group. Historically, only a select few ethnic groups have become minority groups.

History suggests that current racial and ethnic categories will change, and there is no consensus, even within minority groups, on preferred labels or terminology. A national survey of 60,000 adults in 1995 confirmed this (Tucker et al. 1996). Some 58 percent of Hispanics indicated that "Hispanic" was the term they preferred; 12 percent preferred "Latino"; 20 percent preferred some other term; and 10 percent had no preference. Almost two-thirds of whites preferred "white," while 44 percent of African Americans preferred "black" and 28 percent preferred "African American." Given that the racial/ethnic terms used should be those broadly recognized by a wide variety of people and those that respect individual dignity, the terms *African American* or *black* and *Hispanic* or *Latino* can be used interchangeably.

Race and Stress

There is growing recognition that stress is not randomly distributed in society. Rather, the social conditions in which a group is embedded are important determinants of the level of exposure to stress (Pearlin 1989; Williams and House 1991). Minority racial and ethnic status thus become crude proxies for exposure to both higher levels of stress and fewer resources to cope with stress, when compared to the white population. Challenges resulting from the need to adapt to mainstream American culture, in addition to socioeconomic disadvantage, can lead minority group members to experience higher levels of those stressful experiences captured by standard stress scales.

Additionally, there is growing interest in the extent to which stressors unique to minority status might also adversely affect the mental health status of these groups. The most frequently nominated stressors of this kind (Williams 1996a; Williams et al. 1997) are experiences of racial discrimination and blocked opportunity. These high levels of stress could adversely affect mental health status, although only a few recent attempts in the literature systematically examine the variation in general measures of stress and race-related stressors across minority populations.

Stress is an important risk factor for mental health problems (Brown and Harris 1989; Elliot and Eisdorfer 1982), and there are important suggestions in the literature that discrimination might also adversely affect the mental health of minority group members. In the National Study of Black Americans, a global measure of racial discrimination was adversely related to physical and mental health status (Jackson et al. 1996; Williams and Chung, in press). Similarly, two studies of Hispanic women found reports of ethnic discrimination positively related to psychological distress (Amaro et al. 1987; Salgado de Snyder 1987). In a study of Puerto Ricans in New York, Rogler et al. (1994) found that people who scored high on a particular scale (one that captured the extent to which Puerto Ricans were treated unjustly because of discrimination against them) were more likely to be receiving mental health services than people who scored low on the scale. It has also recently been argued that racial discrimination is an important risk factor for the mental health of Asian Americans (Kuo 1995).

Race/Ethnicity and Mental Health

Mental health researchers have commonly used scales of psychological distress because they are easy to administer, do not consume much time, and provide a distribution of mental health status on a continuum (Vega and Rumbaut 1991). The scales consist of symptoms that are typically more prevalent at lower levels of socioeconomic status (SES) and relate to measures of stress and physical problems. These symptoms do not capture a clinical diagnosis; rather, they relate to demoralization.

Symptom checklist scales typically assess depressed mood, psychological distress, and a level of dysfunction (Link and Dohrenwend 1980; Vega and Rumbaut 1991). It is also important when analyzing mental health status to distinguish between somatic (and other symptoms of depression) and more cognitive and evaluative-oriented dimensions of mental health status, such as life satisfaction (Vega and Rumbaut 1991). Measures of subjective well-being attempt to capture an individual's overall perception of the quality of life (George 1992). Life satisfaction is the most frequently used measure in this regard, and it is closely related to other concepts that measure subjective well-being, such as morale and happiness. In addition, life satisfaction is a fairly stable indicator of an individual's long-term perception of the overall quality of his or her life.

The mental health literature indicates that racial/ethnic status might predict variations in mental health outcomes. Most of this research has focused on black-white differences in mental health. Early studies of treated populations tended to show that African Americans had more mental health problems than whites (Neighbors 1984; Williams and Fenton 1994). However, studies of more broad-based populations have been inconsistent. In an early review of eight community-based studies, Dohrenwend and Dohrenwend (1969) indicated that half showed higher rates of mental health problems for African Americans—and the other half showed higher rates for whites. Subsequent studies have frequently found higher rates of psychological distress for blacks than whites, with the racial difference reduced to non-significance when adjusted for SES (Neighbors 1984; Vega and Rumbaut 1991; Williams and Fenton 1994). However, the pattern is not uniform.

In a comprehensive review of the literature on minority mental health status, Vega and Rumbaut (1991) concluded that some recent studies find higher levels of distress for African Americans, while others find lower levels for African Americans compared to whites. These inconsistencies may be linked to regional variation or measurement error. Other studies have found no racial differences in psychological well-being. For example, in a large national study, race was found to be unrelated to self-esteem, and African American and white respondents did not report differences in experiencing an impending nervous breakdown (Veroff et al. 1981). Levels of psychological anxiety and physical health were also equivalent across race, and these researchers found no signs of demoralization in blacks' assessment of their lives. They concluded that African Americans probably handle stress in ways that do not translate into psychological problems.

Inconsistent Distribution of Mental Health Problems by Race/Ethnicity

Studies of psychiatric disorders suggest that African Americans are not disadvantaged compared to whites. The large Epidemiologic Catchment Area (ECA) study found few racial differences in psychiatric illness (Robins and Regier 1991). More recently, in the first national study of psychiatric disorders in the United States, Kessler et al. (1994) found that African Americans have lower rates of mental illness than whites in all major diagnostic categories.

The pattern of black-white differences in life satisfaction has also not been consistent. On the one hand, Bracy (1976) found that African

Americans consistently report lower levels of life satisfaction than whites, and this relationship persists even after adjustment for a broad range of SES and demographic characteristics. Clemente and Sauer (1976) report similar findings. Thomas and Hughes (1986), in an analysis of the relationship between race and life satisfaction in the General Social Survey between 1972 and 1985, found that African Americans consistently reported lower scores than whites, even after controlling for SES, age, and marital status. In contrast, Herzog et al. (1982) found that there were no racial differences in life satisfaction after adjustment for SES and demographic variables.

Research on the mental health of the Hispanic population to date does not provide a clear picture of the distribution of mental health problems for Hispanics when compared to the major racial groups or for subgroup variations within the Hispanic category (Vega and Rumbaut 1991; Rogler et al. 1989). For example, in the Hispanic Health and Nutrition Examination Survey (Hispanic HANES), Puerto Ricans had higher rates of depression than Cubans and Mexican Americans, as measured by the Center for Epidemiologic Studies Depression (CES-D) scale (Shrout et al. 1992). In some studies, Mexican Americans have higher symptoms than non-Hispanic whites or African Americans, but in the Hispanic HANES, Mexican Americans have low rates of depressive symptoms (Vega and Rumbaut 1991).

Our understanding of the distribution of psychological distress and psychiatric disorders in the Asian population is very limited (Sue et al. 1995; Vega and Rumbaut 1991). Sue et al. (1995) have argued that large-scale studies of Asian populations outside of the United States can provide useful information in the absence of good U.S. data. They reviewed studies conducted in Singapore, Taiwan, China, and Korea. Some of these studies found that the rates of psychiatric disorders are similar to those found for the U.S. population, while others found lower rates.

Early studies of U.S. treatment data report very low levels of mental health problems in the Asian population. However, several community-based studies have found high levels of psychological distress. Kuo (1984) conducted the first community study of the prevalence of CES-D-defined depression among Asians. Asians had a higher level of depression than non-Hispanic whites. There was significant variation among the Asian groups, with Koreans having the highest rates of depressive symptoms. Chinese and Japanese had the lowest rates, with Filipinos having rates in the middle. A study of Korean immigrants in Chicago found that this group had high scores on the CES-D depression scale (Hurh and Kim 1988). Using the same measure, Ying (1988) found high mean scores for Chinese Americans in San Francisco. The recently conducted Chinese American Psychiatric Epidemiologic Study is the most comprehensive study of the mental health of any Asian American group. Involving a probability sample of Chinese Americans in Los Angeles, this study found that the rates of mental disorders are low for this population, with anxiety rates especially low (Sue et al. 1995).

Migration and Mental Health

Minority populations are very diverse, as some of the findings indicate, and many researchers argue that greater attention should be paid to this heterogeneity (Vega and Rumbaut 1991; Williams et al. 1994; Zane et al. 1994). Social circumstances such as the timing of migration and processes of incorporation into the United States vary, and they may affect importantly both the distribution of risk factors and the vulnerability of minority populations to mental health problems. Prior research in the mental health field indicates that socially disadvantaged people are likely to experience higher levels of stress than more advantaged individuals, and they are also likely to be more adversely affected by stressors. Refugees, especially those from Southeast Asia, might be particularly vulnerable in this regard (Lum 1995). Several studies have found high rates of mental health problems among Southeast Asian refugees (Buchwald et al. 1993; Kinzie et al. 1990; Lum 1995).

The literature reflects a concern about the ways that migration to the United States and acculturation can affect mental health status. The migration experience can include loss of social relationships, difficulties in finding new social ties, and problems of acquiring a new language and adapting to a new culture. The need to find one's way in a new and unfamiliar economic system, with possible changes in social status, can be a special source of stress. Vega and Rumbaut (1991) also emphasize that immigration to the United States brings important transitions in role behaviors. Role conflicts in parenting and role inconsistencies in employment status (working at jobs with lower status than in one's home country) are very common.

The relation of immigrant status to the health of Hispanics is not clear, and the relationship appears to vary for specific Hispanic groups. In the Hispanic HANES, immigrants from Cuba and Mexico seemed to have lower levels of depressive symptoms than non-Hispanic whites.

On the other hand, the opposite pattern existed for immigrants from Puerto Rico to the mainland. Puerto Ricans studied in New York reported higher CES-D scores than other studies reveal for Puerto Ricans on the island (Vega and Rumbaut 1991). Recent research by Shrout et al. (1992) compared rates of psychiatric disorders for island Puerto Ricans with Mexican immigrants and native-born Mexican Americans in Los Angeles. These investigators found that immigrant Mexican Americans had the fewest mental health problems, native-born Mexican Americans had the most problems, and Puerto Rican respondents fell in between.

Research reviewed by Sue et al. (1995) indicate that Asian American students, regardless of acculturation level, have higher levels of psychological distress than whites. However, less-acculturated Asian American students have more psychological problems than their more-acculturated peers. Several other studies suggest that foreign-born Asians, even those who have resided in the United States for ten years or more, have higher levels of distress than their white peers (Sue et al. 1995). In contrast, research on Southeast Asian refugees reviewed by Vega and Rumbaut (1991) indicate that the first three years after immigration is the period of greatest psychological impact. This period is characterized by initial euphoria, then disenchantment (with high rates of psychological distress), and, finally, recovery by the end of three years. Vega and Rumbaut (1991) also indicate that similar patterns have been found for Cuban, Eastern European, Korean, and Chinese immigrants. Rogler et al. (1991) report that negative, positive, and curvilinear relationships have been found for the relationship between acculturation and mental health status for Hispanics.

METHODS OF ANALYSIS

The goals of this study, using data from the CMHS, are to (1) assess the extent to which race/ethnicity predicts variations in levels of stress; (2) examine the extent to which mental health problems are differentially distributed across racial/ethnic status; and (3) identify the nature of the association between generational status and mental health. One of the important strengths of this study is that it uses a set of common measures of both stress and mental health status across a broad range of minority populations. Studies of this kind are rare in research on minority mental health (Vega and Rumbaut 1991).

Measures of Mental Health Status and Stress

The same measures were used in both survey samples. All single items and indices are coded in the direction of the variable name so that a high score reflects a high value of that variable. Two measures of mental health status are considered in the analyses. Psychological distress was assessed by the five-item mental health subscale of the SF-36 (Ware et al. 1995). This scale (Cronbach's alpha = .76) sums the frequency with which the respondent felt (a) calm and peaceful, (b) downhearted and blue, (c) so down in the dumps that nothing could cheer him or her up; (d) had been a very nervous person in the previous 30 days, and (e) had been a happy person in the previous 30 days. These items are typical of the symptoms of depression and anxiety and are commonly used in health surveys to measure psychological distress. The second measure of mental health status is a global indicator of general well-being, with "life satisfaction" being a single-item rating of the respondent's satisfaction with life on a five-point scale, ranging from very satisfied to very dissatisfied.

The survey recorded five measures of stress. "Global stress" is a summary measure of the general undesirable life events that a respondent experienced during the previous year. The eleven items constituting the global stress scale are divided into four types of stress: relationship (illness or death of a close family member, problems with aging parents, problems with children, and problems with spouse or partner); occupational (hassles at work and trouble balancing work and family demands); financial (problems with money and loss of one's job or of spouse's job); racial bias (respondent or family treated badly because of race or cultural background), and violence (fear of crime or violence in one's community and knowing someone who was a victim of violence). For each of these items of stress, respondents indicated the extent to which they were affected by them. The coding scheme (for creating the index) gave a value of 2 for respondents who indicated that they were affected strongly, a value of 1 for those who indicated that they were affected somewhat, and a value of 0 for those who indicated that they were not affected at all.

For analyses that use the main sample, where the focus is on differences between blacks, whites, and Hispanics, the analytic categories, black and white, exclude persons of Hispanic origin. When we performed analyses for the Asian or black population, we included all respondents who self-identified with these categories, irrespective of their responses on the ethnicity question. Given a central interest in the heterogeneity of racial and ethnic minority populations, an attempt was made whenever possible to look at ethnic variation within each of the categories. Accordingly, in selected analyses, we further divided Hispanics into Mexican, Puerto Rican, and "other Latinos" (a residual category that consists of Cubans, Dominicans, Costa Ricans, and an "Other" category). Similarly, we divided blacks into those who indicated that they were of Caribbean heritage versus those who were not, and we divided the Asian category into Chinese, Vietnamese, and Korean.

Sociodemographic Control Variables

Age (in years), gender (1 = female, 0 = male), and marital status are sociodemographic control variables used in our analyses. Given that prior research indicates considerable variation in mental health status among unmarried groups (Williams, Takeuchi, and Adair 1992), we divided marital status into a set of four dummy variables: single, widowed, separated and divorced, and married (reference category).

Two measures of SES are used. Education, based on formal years of schooling, is divided into four categories that capture meaningful differences in educational credentials: less than high school completion, high school completion, some college, and college graduate (which is the reference category in the regression analyses). Income is our second measure of SES. It describes the total household income in the previous year. We divided income into four dummy variables: less than $7,500; $7,501–$25,000; $25,001–$50,000; and greater than $50,000 (the reference category in the regression analyses). Because the meaning of a given level of household income is related importantly to the number of people dependent on it, we control for household size whenever we use household income. Household size is a count of the number of people living in the household, ranging from 0 to 10 or more.

The issue of adaptation to American society is a significant factor when considering the health experience of minority populations that have a large number of immigrants. We employ a measure of generational status that combines length of stay in the United States with generation in the United States. This variable consists of four categories. Respondents who were not born in the United States (first-generation immigrants) were divided into recent immigrants (five years or less in the

United States) and long-term immigrants (six years or more in the United States). The third category, second-generation, consists of U.S.-born individuals with at least one parent born outside the United States. The third-generation category (reference category in the regression analyses) consists of the remaining respondents who were born in the United States—as were their parents.

Data Analysis

The data for both the main and Asian samples were weighted to take into account different probabilities of selection and to adjust the demographics of the sample to the Current Population Survey's latest parameters on the basis of gender, race, age, educational attainment, and health insurance status. Simple descriptive analyses present racial differences in the distribution of stress. We report an overall F-test for the mean differences between the categories, and Duncan's Multiple Range Test to determine the sample means that differ significantly from one another. However, we rely primarily on ordinary least-squares regression analyses to examine the relationship between race and mental health status and to assess the impact of stress on health. The regression models allow us to test for statistical significance and to control simultaneously for age, gender, SES, and household size. These statistical procedures assume simple random sampling and tend to underestimate variances and overestimate statistical significance when the sampling design is complex. Accordingly, for analyses with the main sample, we use the SUDAAN software (Shah et al. 1992) to make the appropriate adjustments to standard errors and p values.

We ran a set of hierarchical regression models in which the major classes of potential explanatory variables were entered in separate blocks. Model 1 in Tables 11.2 through 11.5 presents the association between race/ethnicity and health, controlled for age. Model 2 adds gender and marital status, while model 3 adds the two measures of socioeconomic status (income and education) and household size. Model 4 considers the additive contribution of stress to health status. A fifth model, consistently run, is not presented in these tables. This fifth model assessed the extent to which stress might have a more adverse impact on the mental health functioning of some racial/ethnic groups than others. Here we created interaction terms that capture the multiplicative relationship between stress and racial or ethnic status, and we added these to the previous model.

SUMMARY OF FINDINGS

Racial/Ethnic Differences in Stress

Mean scores on stress measures for whites, African Americans, and Latinos indicate that survey respondents from the two minority populations tend to have higher levels of stress than whites (Table 11.1). The scores for African Americans and Latinos on the summary measure of stress (global stress) are significantly higher than that of whites. African Americans have the highest overall score, with a recorded level of stress significantly higher than that of Latinos.

This pattern, indicating higher levels of stress for the two minority groups, is evident across all of the subtypes of stress. However, the overall F-test for differences is significant only for financial stress and racial bias. African Americans and Latinos have identical mean scores on financial stress, with their level of stress significantly higher than that of whites. Large differences are evident concerning racial bias. Compared to whites, scores on racial bias are seven times as high for African Americans and four times as high for Latinos. The differences between African Americans and Latinos are also statistically significant, while racial/ethnic differences in relationship and occupational stress are not statistically significant.

Because of the different sampling strategy for the Asian sample of survey respondents, we did not perform tests of significant differences

Table 11.1 Mean Levels of Stress for Racial Groups

Race/ Ethnicity	Global	Relationship	Occupational	Financial	Racial Bias	Violence
Whites (W)	4.45	1.74	0.97	0.94	0.04	0.75
Blacks (B)	5.81	1.90	1.02	1.26	0.30	1.33
Latinos (L)	5.28	1.78	1.01	1.26	0.17	1.07
F Ratio	31.95[a]	1.75	0.46	24.79[a]	138.91[a]	65.81
Duncan's Test	B&L>W			B&L>W	B&L>W	B&L>W
	B>L				B>L	B>L
Asians	5.10	1.80	0.89	1.03	0.41	0.97

Source: Data from The Commonwealth Fund Minority Health Survey, 1994.
[a]$p \leq 0.01$.

with the other racial/ethnic groups. Nonetheless, we can offer an overall descriptive profile of the distribution of specific types of stress for this group (see Table 11.1). Overall, Asian respondents report high levels of stress. In general, Asians reported higher levels of stress than do whites, and similar levels to Hispanics. Racial bias is a significant stressor for Asians. This is interesting because the mean level for Asians exceeds that of all other groups, including African Americans. This pattern is noteworthy because stereotypic images of Asians as the "model minority" could lead to the conclusion that Asian Americans do not experience racial discrimination. The sampling strategy used in this study for selecting Asians, however, based on readily identified Asian surnames, could have over-represented Asians who are at higher risk for experiencing discrimination.

There is heterogeneity in each of the minority populations (data not shown). For each group, the major subgroups of that population experience differences in levels of stress. For Hispanics, we record mean levels of stress for Mexicans, Puerto Ricans, and other Latinos. A consistent pattern appears for Hispanics across all of the types of stress. Puerto Ricans have the highest level of stress (5.99), and the category "other Latinos" tends to show higher levels of stress than Mexicans (for global stress, 5.43 vs. 5.02). The F-test is significantly different for the following stress indicators: global, relationship, occupational, and violence. Puerto Ricans have higher means than Mexicans on global and relationship stress and violence, while other Latinos have higher occupational stress scores than Mexicans.

Stress levels differ between the native-born black population and blacks of Caribbean ancestry (data not shown). Interestingly, the mean on the global stress measure for Caribbean blacks (6.66) is higher than that of American blacks (5.72). This pattern is consistent across all types of stress, but it is statistically significant only for financial stress (1.56 vs. 1.23); it is marginally significant for violence. The high level of financial stress for Caribbean blacks is surprising because recent research documents that Caribbean immigrants continue to have a higher socioeconomic status than other African Americans (Kalmijn 1996).

Among Chinese, Vietnamese, and Koreans, there is a pronounced pattern of significant differences in levels of stress (data not shown). Chinese have the highest levels of stress (6.50); Koreans, the lowest levels (3.37); and Vietnamese are in-between (5.46). Chinese have a higher score than Vietnamese and Koreans on global and occupational stress. The Chinese also surpass Koreans on relationship, financial, and violence stress. Stress levels for the Vietnamese exceed those of the Koreans for violence, as well as global, relationship, and financial stress.

Psychological Distress

Concerning psychological distress in the main sample, model 1 shows the association between race/ethnicity and psychological distress adjusted for age (Table 11.2). Age is inversely related to psychological dis-

Table 11.2   The Association to Psychological Distress of Race, Sociodemographic Factors, Socioeconomic Status, and Stress (unstandardized regression coefficients)

	Model 1	Model 2	Model 3	Model 4
Age				
45–64	−0.09	−0.01	−0.11	−0.07
≥65	−0.68[a]	−0.55	−0.66	−0.65
Race/ethnicity				
African Americans	−0.41	−0.41	−0.34	−0.09
Latinos	−0.64[b]	−0.64[b]	−0.31	−0.22
Gender–female		0.02	−0.07	−0.05
Marital status				
Single		0.26	0.24	0.32
Widowed		−0.16	−0.30	−0.19
Separated/divorced		−0.07	−0.13	0.09
Education				
<High school			0.61	0.35
High school			0.12	0.06
Some college			0.17	0.23
Income				
<$7,500			3.89[b]	2.93[b]
$7,501–$25,000			1.90[b]	1.45[b]
$25,001–$50,000			1.15[b]	0.88[b]
Household size			0.12	−0.16[a]
Global stress				0.66[b]
Intercept	12.14	12.04	10.21	8.04
R^2	0.00	0.00	0.04	0.22
N	3,080	3,080	3,080	3,080

Source: Data from The Commonwealth Fund Minority Health Survey, 1994.

Note: Referent categories: age 18–44, whites, married, college graduate, income >$50,000.

[a] $p \leq 0.10$.

[b] $p \leq 0.01$.

tress, with a marginally significant tendency for people over age 65 to have lower levels of distress than adults under age 45. For race/ethnicity, it is interesting that Latinos report significantly *lower* levels of distress than whites. Also, although not statistically significant, the direction of the association is for African Americans to have lower levels of psychological distress than whites.

Model 2 considers the contribution of gender and marital status. Surprisingly, both of these variables are unrelated to psychological distress. Model 3, presenting the contribution of education, income, and household size, shows a strong graded inverse relationship between income and psychological distress, with each higher income category having lower levels of distress than the preceding category. Although people who did not complete high school tend to have higher levels of distress than college graduates, this pattern is not statistically significant. Interestingly, consideration of the SES variables and household size reduces the relationship between race and distress; the coefficient for Latinos is reduced by more than 50 percent, to non-significance.

Model 4, which adds the global measure of stress, indicates a strong positive relationship between stress and psychological distress. The addition of stress produces a dramatic increase in the R^2 of the overall model (from 4% to 22%) and also affects some of the other variables. First, the consideration of stress weakens the relationship between SES and psychological distress. The coefficients for income diminish somewhat, but they remain significant when stress is added to the model. Second, the association for household size becomes marginally significant and reverses direction after adjustment for stress. In contrast to a non-significant positive association between household size and distress noted in model 3, model 4 shows a weak inverse relationship between household size and distress. This suggests that, in the face of stress, people residing in larger households may be able to mobilize enough social support to reduce the negative effects of stress on their mental health status.

In additional analyses (not shown), we assessed the relationship of each of the subtypes of stress to psychological distress in a model that adjusted for age, race/ethnicity, gender, marital status, SES, and household size. Considered singly, all of the stress measures are positively related to psychological distress. However, when all of the subtypes of stress are entered simultaneously into the regression model, the association of racial bias and violence with distress becomes non-significant. Williams et al. (1995) have noted that a single-item measure of racial discrimination can overlap with other measures of stress on a standard life events inventory, and that adjusting racial bias for other stress reduces its association with mental health status.

Hispanics. Similar model analyses, conducted for the Hispanic population only, focus on the heterogeneity of this population. These analyses contrast Puerto Ricans and other Latinos with Mexican Americans. Model 1 shows that both Puerto Ricans and other Latinos tend to have higher levels of distress than Mexican Americans, but this pattern is significant for Puerto Ricans only (Table 11.3). For Hispanics, age is unrelated to psychological distress, and gender and marital status are also unrelated to distress. Model 3 reveals a strong inverse relationship between income and psychological distress for Latinos, with household size and education also related to distress. Hispanic survey respondents who have not completed high school, as well as those with some college education, have higher levels of distress than college graduates. There is also a strong positive relationship between household size and psychological distress, with respondents in larger households reporting higher levels of distress. Unlike the pattern for psychological stress in the main sample (Table 11.2), where consideration of SES reduces the association between race and distress, the significant coefficient for Puerto Ricans increases slightly when SES is taken into account (Table 11.3).

Model 4 reveals that global stress for Hispanics is strongly related to psychological distress. The addition of this stress variable reduces dramatically, but does not completely eliminate, the higher levels of distress for Puerto Ricans when compared to Mexicans. This suggests that the higher levels of stress for Puerto Ricans, compared to Mexican Americans, play a major role in accounting for the elevated levels of psychological symptoms among Puerto Ricans. The consideration of stress reduces the association between household size and distress to nonsignificance, and this also mediates the association between income and psychological distress. The pattern reported for the subtypes of stress in the main sample is identical, in additional analyses, to that observed for Latinos. All of the stress measures are individually related to distress, but the associations with discrimination and violence do not remain significant when all of the stress measures are considered simultaneously.

African Americans. We present the association between ethnicity, stress, and psychological distress for U.S. respondents of African descent by contrasting respondents of Caribbean ancestry with other African Americans (Table 11.4). Model 1 shows that Caribbean blacks have significantly higher levels of psychological distress than other blacks. How-

Table 11.3   The Association to Psychological Distress of Ethnicity, Sociodemographic Factors, Socioeconomic Status, and Stress, for Hispanics Only (unstandardized regression coefficients)

	Model 1	Model 2	Model 3	Model 4
Age				
45-64	−0.42	−0.47	−0.49	−0.35
≥65	−0.35	−0.08	−0.35	−0.06
Ethnicity				
Puerto Ricans	1.34[a]	1.35[a]	1.38[a]	0.78[b]
Other Latinos	0.30	0.33	0.47	0.11
Gender—female		0.46	0.53	0.48
Marital status				
Single		0.30	0.31	0.24
Widowed		1.07	0.87	0.15
Separated/divorced		0.90	0.75	0.47
Education				
<High school			1.31[c]	0.66
High school			0.53	0.72[b]
Some college			1.03[c]	1.18[a]
Income				
<$7,500			3.23[c]	2.30[a]
$7,501-$25,000			1.60[a]	0.78[b]
$25,001-$50,000			0.81	0.11
Household size			0.24[c]	0.13
Global stress				0.62[a]
Intercept	12.28	11.84	9.06	7.12
R^2	0.01	0.02	0.06	0.24
N	1,001	1,001	1,001	1,001

Source: Data from The Commonwealth Fund Minority Health Survey, 1994.

Note: Referent categories: age 18–44, Mexicans, married, college graduate, income >$50,000.

[a] $p \leq 0.01$.

[b] $p \leq 0.10$.

[c] $p \leq 0.05$.

ever, similar to the pattern observed for Latinos, age is unrelated to distress. Model 2 shows the incremental contribution of gender and marital status. The association between Caribbean ancestry and distress is unchanged by adjustments for these demographic variables. However, here we note for the first time that there is a significant association between gender and psychological distress: black women report higher levels of distress than black men.

Table 11.4 The Association to Psychological Distress of Ethnicity, Sociodemographic Factors, Socioeconomic Status, and Stress, African Americans Only (unstandardized regression coefficients)

	Model 1	Model 2	Model 3	Model 4
Age				
45–64	0.69	0.55	0.20	0.05
≥65	−0.62	−0.77	−0.97	−1.00[a]
Ethnicity				
Caribbean ancestry	1.56[b]	1.60[b]	1.44[b]	1.06[c]
Gender–female		0.94[c]	0.74	0.76[a]
Marital status				
Single		−0.46	−0.65	−0.67
Widowed		0.15	0.53	0.41
Separated/divorced		1.28	1.22	1.03
Education				
<High school			0.28	0.35
High school			−0.35	−0.33
Some college			0.25	0.46
Income				
<$7,500			3.82[b]	3.20[b]
$7,501–$25,000			2.35[b]	1.47[b]
$25,001–$50,000			0.12	−0.17
Household size			0.21[c]	0.11
Global stress				0.52[b]
Intercept	12.27	11.82	9.96	7.76
R^2	0.01	0.02	0.08	0.21
N	1,048	1,048	1,048	1,048

Source: Data from The Commonwealth Fund Minority Health Survey, 1994.

Note: Referent categories: age 18–44, American blacks, married, college graduate, income >$50,000.

[a]$p \leq 0.10$.

[b]$p \leq 0.01$.

[c]$p \leq 0.05$.

Model 3 adds the SES variables and household size. Of the two SES indicators, only income is associated with distress. The two lowest income categories have higher levels of distress than the highest income category. There is also a positive association between household size and psychological distress. Adjustment for SES and household size reduces the association of both ethnicity and gender to psychological distress, with gender no longer being significant.

As we have seen in our earlier analyses, model 4 shows a strong positive relationship between the global stress measure and psychological distress. The significant association between household size and distress shown in model 3 is now reduced by almost one-half and is no longer significant. In contrast, the coefficients for ethnicity and income in model 3 are reduced but remain significant in model 4. Thus, similar to the pattern among Hispanics, differential exposure to stress accounts for a substantial part of subgroup variations in distress. In additional analyses (not shown here), we entered all of the subtypes of the global stress variable into a regression model that contained all of the model 3 variables. We found that relationship, occupational, and financial stress are all significantly related to high levels of distress. When all of the subtypes of stress are simultaneously considered, racial discrimination and fear of violence are unrelated to distress for African Americans.

Asians. For the Asian sample, the focus is on ethnic variations between Vietnamese, Koreans, and Chinese concerning the relationship between stress and psychological distress. Consistent with the literature, which documents important variations in mental health status for ethnic groups within the Asian population, we find that levels of psychological distress vary for these three Asian groups. Compared to the Chinese, Vietnamese report lower levels of distress, and Koreans report higher levels (data not shown).

This pattern of the distribution of mental health problems is not parallel to the earlier observed distribution of stress, which showed that Chinese had the highest level of stress, Koreans the lowest, with Vietnamese in between. In model 2, gender and marital status are unrelated to psychological distress, while in model 3, income is significantly associated with psychological distress. Here Asians at the two lowest levels of income report greater distress than those at the highest level. Education is also related to mental health status, but the pattern is somewhat surprising. Asians with some college, when compared to Asian college graduates, have elevated levels of psychological distress. The other educational categories do not differ from college graduates in terms of psychological distress.

Model 4 for the Asian subgroups reveals a strong positive relationship between global stress and psychological distress. Asians with higher levels of stress are more likely to have mental health problems. Adjustment for global stress reduces the coefficient for Vietnamese to non-significance. Although Koreans have the lowest levels of stress, they have the highest levels of mental health problems. Moreover, adjustment for stress produces a classic suppression effect, with the coefficient for Koreans becoming larger than in the previous model. When adjusted for global stress, the association between income and distress is reduced, especially for the second-lowest income group. Analyses (not shown) of subtypes of stress reveal the now familiar pattern of each kind of stress being positively related to distress: relationship, occupational, and financial stress are significant when we consider all simultaneously.

Differential Vulnerability. We find consistently that stress is strongly related to psychological distress for all of the racial/ethnic groups studied. Based on prior theory and research, we were interested in whether the relationship between stress and psychological distress varies for either the major racial/ethnic minority populations considered or for the subgroups within each of the populations. We systematically evaluated this hypothesis of differential vulnerability. In analyses not shown, we created multiplicative interaction terms between global stress and the relevant racial or ethnic status category. We added these interaction terms to a new model that included age, race or ethnicity, gender, marital status, education, income, household size, and global stress. We found none of the interactions between global stress and race or ethnicity to be significant.

In addition, in similar analyses we explored interactions between each of the subtypes of stress (relationship, occupational, financial, racial discrimination, and fear of violence) and race and ethnic status. We found few significant associations. In the main sample, there was a marginally significant tendency for relationship stress and occupational stress to be more strongly related to psychological distress for African Americans than for whites, and a significant pattern for violence to have a weaker association with distress for African Americans than for whites. There were no significant interactions between the subtypes of stress and ethnicity for African Americans or Asians. For Hispanics, there was one significant association: financial stress was less strongly related to distress for Puerto Ricans than for Mexican Americans.

Our findings suggest that stress has uniform adverse effects on the mental health status of the major racial/ethnic groups surveyed. However, there is no overwhelming support for a clear and consistent pattern of differential vulnerability.

Race, Stress, and Life Satisfaction

We systematically evaluated the relationship between race, sociodemographic factors, SES, and stress to life satisfaction. Here we used regression models very similar to those just described for psychological distress to demonstrate the relationship between race/ethnicity, stress, and life satisfaction for African Americans, whites, and Latinos (Table 11.5). Model 1 shows that age is unrelated to life satisfaction. There is a marginally significant relationship between race/ethnicity and our indicator of psychological well-being: African Americans have higher levels of life satisfaction than whites, but Latinos have lower levels. The addition of gender and marital status in model 2 makes little incremental contribution to explained variance, and this addition does not reduce the relationship between race and life satisfaction.

Table 11.5   The Association to Life Satisfaction of Race, Sociodemographic Factors, Socioeconomic Status, and Stress (unstandardized regression coefficients)

	Model 1	Model 2	Model 3	Model 4
Age				
45–64	−0.00	−0.03	−0.02	−0.03
≥65	−0.02	−0.10[a]	−0.09	−0.09
Race/ethnicity				
African Americans	0.09[a]	0.10[a]	0.10[a]	0.04
Latinos	−0.09[a]	−0.09[a]	−0.05	−0.04
Gender–female		−0.06[a]	−0.05	−0.05
Marital status				
Single		−0.06	−0.06	−0.07
Widowed		0.19[a]	0.21[b]	0.19[a]
Separated/divorced		−0.06	−0.05	−0.08[a]
Education				
<High school			−0.05	−0.02
High school			−0.05	−0.04
Some college			0.01	0.01
Income				
<$7,500			−0.60[c]	−0.48[c]
$7,501–$25,000			−0.34[c]	−0.28[c]
$25,001–$50,000			−0.16[c]	−0.13[c]
Household size			0.00	0.04[b]
Global stress				−0.08[c]
Intercept	4.31	4.37	4.60	4.87
R^2	0.00	0.01	0.04	0.13
N	3,080	3,080	3,080	3,080

Source: Data from The Commonwealth Fund Minority Health Survey, 1994.
Note: Referent categories: age 18–44, whites, married, college graduate, income >$50,000.
[a]$p \leq 0.10$.
[b]$p \leq 0.05$.
[c]$p \leq 0.01$.

There is a marginally significant tendency for women to report lower levels of life satisfaction than men. In addition, marital status is weakly related to well-being. Widowed individuals report only marginally significant higher levels of life satisfaction than the married. Of the two SES variables considered in model 3, only income is related to life satisfaction. Money may not buy happiness, but there is a strong positive relationship between income and life satisfaction. People at each higher level of income report more life satisfaction than those in the income category beneath them. It is also worth noting that adjustment for SES reduces the marginally significant coefficient for Latinos to non-significance, but it leaves the coefficient for African Americans unchanged.

Model 4 considers the contribution of stress to life satisfaction. There is a significant inverse relationship between global stress and life satisfaction. Consistent with the pattern observed for psychological distress, global stress is also associated with reduced levels of psychological well-being. The addition of global stress in model 4 also changes some of the relationships observed in model 3. The marginally significant coefficient for race (black) is reduced by more than one-half to non-significance, and new patterns emerge in the relationship between marital status and life satisfaction. The earlier observed pattern (marginally significant) of widowed individuals having higher levels of life satisfaction than the married is unchanged. But, in addition, there is a marginally significant tendency for the separated/divorced to report lower levels of life satisfaction than the married. The association between income and distress is now reduced, but it remains significant when adjusted for stress. Similar to the pattern observed for psychological distress, the association between household size and life satisfaction becomes positive when adjusted for global stress. Instructively, the variables considered here explain less of the variance in life satisfaction (13%) than the variance observed earlier for psychological distress (22%).

Hispanics. Concerning the relationship between ethnic variation, stress, and life satisfaction for Hispanics, when adjusted for the demographic variables, Puerto Ricans and other Latinos tend to have lower levels of life satisfaction than Mexican Americans—but this relationship is only marginally significant for other Latinos (data not shown). Women also report lower levels of life satisfaction than males, but marital status is unrelated to life satisfaction. The association of gender and ethnicity to life satisfaction remains significant when adjusted for SES. Of the two SES variables considered, only income is significantly related to life satisfaction for Hispanics. As noted previously (Table 11.5), there is a strong positive relationship between income and life satisfaction. And similar to the analyses conducted for the main sample, we see a strong inverse relationship between global stress and life satisfaction. The addition of global stress makes an important contribution to explained variance, increasing the R^2 from 5 percent in model 3 to 20 percent in model 4. Household size becomes marginally significant in model 4. That is, there is a tendency for larger households to report lower levels of life satisfaction. When adjusted for stress, the association of life satisfaction with both ethnicity and marital status are reduced to non-significance. Global stress also mediates a substantial part of the association between income and psychological well-being.

African Americans. Concerning the relationships between stress and life satisfaction for African Americans, the association is similar to the one observed for psychological distress. Model 1 indicates that blacks of Caribbean ancestry report lower levels of life satisfaction than other African Americans (data not shown). This relationship is unchanged when adjusted for gender and marital status. Gender and marital status are unrelated to levels of life satisfaction. Model 3 shows that the consideration of SES and household size has minimal impact on the significant relationship of ethnicity to life satisfaction observed in model 2. Also, there is a strong inverse relationship between household size and life satisfaction. Respondents who reside in larger households report lower levels of life satisfaction. As expected, model 4 reveals a significant inverse relationship between global stress and life satisfaction.

Asians. Concerning the relationships among ethnicity, sociodemographic factors, SES, stress, and life satisfaction for Asians only, significant variation with life satisfaction emerges (data not shown). This variation for the Asian subgroups is similar to the pattern observed for psychological distress. Compared to the Chinese, Vietnamese have higher levels of life satisfaction and Koreans have lower levels. This pattern remains unchanged when adjusted for the sociodemographic variables and SES. When controlled for global stress, the coefficient for Vietnamese is reduced to non-significance but the coefficient for Koreans becomes larger. In addition, only the SES variables and global stress are significantly related to life satisfaction. There is the expected positive relationship between income and life satisfaction, with people in the two lowest-income categories tending to report lower levels of life satisfaction than those in the highest category. This relationship is reduced and remains marginally significant only for the lowest-income group when adjusted for global stress. Similar to the Asian pattern for psychological distress, Asians with some college education have lower levels of life satisfaction. Global stress is also significantly related to life satisfaction: reports of higher levels of stress among Asian Americans are predictive of lower levels of life satisfaction.

In other analyses (not shown), we disaggregated the subtypes of global stress and examined their relationships with life satisfaction singly and in combination. Considered individually, all of the measures of stress were inversely related to life satisfaction in the main sample and in the subgroups (African Americans, Hispanics, and Asians), with one exception. That is, violence was unrelated to life satisfaction for African Americans. When considered simultaneously, relationship stress, occupational stress, and financial stress are associated with lower levels of life satisfaction in the main sample as well as for African Americans, Latinos, and Asians. In addition, for African Americans and Asians, violence becomes positively related to life satisfaction when controlled for the other measures of stress.

Differential Vulnerability. Similar to the analyses reported earlier for psychological distress, we performed a series of analyses to evaluate systematically the extent to which stress might have a differential impact on life satisfaction for the racial and ethnic groups in the survey. We found only one significant association. The coefficient representing the interaction of global stress and Vietnamese ethnicity was positively related to life satisfaction. That is, global stress has a smaller negative impact on life satisfaction levels of Vietnamese Americans than on other racial/ethnic groups. In additional analyses (not shown) where the global stress measure was disaggregated, this pattern was evident for racial bias as well as relationship, occupational, and financial stress.

Analyses for the association between generational status and psychological stress for the main survey sample, as well as for each of the major minority groups (Table 11.6), show that generational status does not predict variations in psychological distress. In the main sample and for the African American and Asian samples, recent immigrants (five years or less in the United States) tend to have higher levels of psychological distress than third-generation residents, but these differences are not statistically significant.

Summarizing a similar set of analyses for the life satisfaction variable, we found that generational status is unrelated to life satisfaction in the main sample, but there are important subgroup differences (Table 11.6). For Hispanics, recent immigrants report higher levels of psychological well-being than their third-generation counterparts. An opposite pattern is evident for Asians, with all recent and longer-term immigrants

Table 11.6   The Association between Generational Status and Psychological Distress[a] and between Generational Status and Life Satisfaction[a] (unstandardized regression coefficients)

	Main Sample	Hispanics	African Americans	Asians
Psychological distress				
First generation				
≤5 years	1.83	−0.32	1.65	1.40
≥6 years	0.53	0.05	0.88	1.06
Second generation	−0.39	0.07	−1.41	0.54
Constant	8.08	7.08	7.85	7.46
R^2	0.22	0.24	0.21	0.27
Life satisfaction				
First generation				
≤5 years	0.01	0.32[b]	−0.59	−0.62[c]
≥6 years	−0.00	0.04	0.01	−0.50[b]
Second generation	0.04	0.02	0.15	−0.50[d]
Constant	4.86	4.96	4.77	5.11
R^2	0.13	0.20	0.12	0.16

Source: Data from The Commonwealth Fund Minority Health Survey, 1994.

Note: Referent category: third generation. Each column represents two separate regression models—one each for psychological distress and for life satisfaction.

[a]Adjusted for age, gender, marital status, race or ethnicity, SES, household size, and global stress.

[b]$p \leq 0.05$.

[c]$p \leq 0.01$.

[d]$p \leq 0.10$.

having lower levels of well-being than third-generation Asian Americans. Among African Americans, recent immigrants tend to have lower levels of life satisfaction than their third-generation peers, but this difference is not significant. Consistent with the literature, then, we find some evidence of poorer mental health status for recent immigrants, but this pattern varies depending on the minority group and the health status indicator.

Limitations of the Study

The CMHS provides a unique opportunity to consider risk factors for mental health status and for overall levels of mental health status for whites and a broad range of minority populations in the United States.

Many of our results are consistent with prior research, but others are not. We must consider carefully the extent to which potential sample limitations might shed light on some of the observed discrepancies between our findings and other research. This issue is particularly relevant because the CMHS is a probability-based sample of households with telephones in the United States.

It has been known for some time that telephone coverage is not uniform in terms of region and SES. Households in the South and low SES households, more generally, have lower levels of telephone coverage. Because at least some minority populations are over-represented in Southern states, and because most minority populations contain a disproportionate number of lower SES persons, this issue becomes especially relevant in minority health research.

Over the last few years, the telephone has become a major alternative to face-to-face interviews. For the most part, primarily because of cost considerations, survey researchers have adopted the telephone as a research instrument (Groves and Kahn 1979). Much of the preliminary evidence comparing the relative efficacy of telephone versus face-to-face interviews suggests that there may be little or no major differences (Groves and Kahn 1979). Early studies of this kind either focused on predominantly white populations or did not assess racial differences. Some recent evidence indicates that African Americans and Hispanics (unlike whites) substantially under-report the frequency of alcohol problems in telephone interviews, when compared to personal interviews (Aquilino 1994). We do not know to what extent this phenomenon may generalize to other sensitive health topics, conditions, and experiences. At the same time, experience with multiple waves of data collection over a twelve-year period in the National Study of Black Americans (with wave 1 being a personal interview and all other waves being telephone interviews) suggests that under-reporting is unlikely to be a major problem in studies of stress and mental health for African Americans.

For African Americans, Asians, and Hispanics, the CMHS differs in important ways from the 1990–1994 Current Population Survey (see Technical Appendix) population characteristics. Most relevant for our findings is the tendency for most of these populations in the CMHS sample to be higher in SES than the populations from which they were drawn. Given a very strong relationship between SES and health, and the interaction of SES with minority health status (Williams 1996b; Williams and Collins 1995), caution should be used when generalizing these findings to the larger minority populations in the United States. At the same time, the fact that we can document important racial/ethnic differences in stress and health, even with a relatively advantaged sample of minority group members, emphasizes the power of racial/ethnic status as a critically important determinant of life chances and well-being.

DISCUSSION AND RESEARCH IMPLICATIONS

Minority Groups Handle Stress Differently

The analyses reported here offer additional evidence that racial/ethnic status is a crude proxy for uncovering differences in living and working conditions for major subgroups in the U.S. population. We have found that the major minority groups, compared to whites, report higher levels of a broad range of stressors. Our measurement of stress attempts to capture stress related to minority status itself. As expected, we find that the gap between whites and minority group members on racial bias is larger than that of any other type of stress. Traditional inventories used to elicit stress in the population do not include measures of racial discrimination. This finding highlights the importance of this source of stress, and it suggests that researchers must give more systematic attention to the conceptualization and measurement of race-related stressors (Williams 1996a; Williams et al. 1997).

Our analyses show that levels of health status vary by racial/ethnic group, but the pattern is complex. Compared to whites, African Americans do not differ on psychological distress, and they tend to have higher levels of life satisfaction. In contrast, Hispanics report poorer health status than whites on both mental health measures. It is possible that these data understate mental health problems for both African Americans and Latinos. First, as noted earlier, given the higher SES profile of the sample in the CMHS, compared to the overall U.S. African American and Hispanic population, the CMHS could under-represent disadvantaged segments of the African American and Latino population—those groups known to have higher levels of health problems. Moreover, it is well documented that the U.S. Census is less successful in counting minority populations than the white population, and that individuals omitted from the census are more likely to be of low SES (Notes and Comments 1994; Williams 1996b).

Second, the measure of psychological distress used in this study could also understate mental health problems. The symptoms of depression and anxiety assessed in the psychological distress scale used in this study are similar to those commonly used in surveys like the Center for Epidemiologic Studies Depression (CES-D) scale to assess psychological distress. However, a comparison of the scale in the CMHS with the CES-D reveals that the CMHS scale lacks items that capture hopelessness, self-concept, and somatic symptoms such as problems with sleeping, eating, or crying. Given that other research indicates that minority patients tend to somatize their symptoms of psychological distress (Buchwald et al. 1993; Kinzie et al. 1990; Rogler et al. 1989), the under-representation of somatic symptoms in this scale may underestimate the degree of psychological distress in minority populations.

At the same time, the patterns of findings reported here are consistent with other research that finds few racial differences in psychological distress (Vega and Rumbaut 1991; Williams et al. 1997) and no racial difference in or better mental health status when psychiatric disorders are considered (Kessler et al. 1994; Robins and Regier 1991). At any rate, these particular findings emphasize the need to pay greater attention to those health-enhancing cultural resources that minority group members have and that may shield them from some of the adverse consequences of stress (Mirowsky and Ross 1980; Rogler et al. 1989; Williams and Fenton 1994). It has been suggested that a broad range of cultural resources, including family support and religious involvement, may play an important role in buffering minority populations from the negative effects of stress.

Our analyses also provide compelling evidence that all of the major minority populations are characterized by considerable heterogeneity. We documented these variations not only for the Hispanic and Asian populations but also for the African American population. In particular, we found a consistent and surprising pattern, with people of Caribbean ancestry scoring worse on psychological distress and life satisfaction than other African Americans. This is an intriguing and unexpected pattern, and it should receive attention in future research. In addition, length of stay in the United States appears to be a useful indicator of variations in health status. Future research on the relationship between acculturation and mental health status should also give greater attention to the use of bicultural strategies (participating in *both* the culture of origin *and* that of the new society). Several studies reviewed by Vega and Rumbaut (1991) suggest that immigrants who use bicultural strategies seem to do better in terms of mental health status than those who exclusively remain tied to their culture of origin or become Americanized.

Policy Implications

The literature on the use of mental health services in the United States indicates that sociodemographic characteristics predict demand (Crow et al. 1994). Generally, whites use mental health services at a higher level than non-whites, women are more likely to use mental health services than men, SES is positively related to health services utilization, people older than 40 use fewer mental health services than younger adults, and the use of services varies by region.

Although our findings provide an important snapshot of the mental health status of racial and ethnic minority populations in the United States, the data do not provide a firm basis for identifying the need for mental health services, developing cost-effective care, or reducing uncertainty in determining the appropriate levels of use for various demographic subgroups.

In an attempt to contain spiraling health care costs, a number of managed care strategies have been implemented to reduce unnecessary medical care utilization while assuring the provision of needed adequate medical and mental health services (Mechanic et al. 1995). Some of these managed care plans are concerned about the implications of sociodemographic variations for managed care. However, neither the findings of this study nor the larger literature provides enough information to use demographic data to calibrate precisely the actual need or demand for a specific population.

Estimates based on patterns of use do not capture the level of need that exists within a population. In the National Comorbidity Survey, only 40 percent of the people who had a psychiatric illness had ever received treatment, while almost half of all people in treatment did not meet the criteria for psychiatric illness (Kessler et al. 1994). Accordingly, there is a critical need for broad-based population data that can better identify the characteristics of people with serious mental health problems, whether or not they are in treatment. The available data from large studies like the Epidemiologic Catchment Area Study and the National Comorbidity Survey provide some representation of the African American population, but they offer limited coverage of Hispanics and virtually no coverage of Asian Americans.

Stress and Socioeconomic Status: Predictors of Poorer Health

Our analyses also indicate that the social context is not benign; it can have a broad range of pathogenic consequences. For both of the mental health outcomes considered (psychological distress and life satisfaction) for all of the subgroups included, two classes of variables consistently predict poorer health status: stress and SES. Both of these constructs capture important aspects of the social environment and highlight the role that the social context can play in enhancing or impairing health status.

Our findings here are consistent with the larger body of literature that finds stress to be an important determinant of adverse changes in physical and mental health status. Similarly, one of the strongest known predictors of physical health is socioeconomic position. Interestingly, we consistently find that income is a stronger predictor of stress than education. This finding is particularly significant in view of a growing body of evidence that indicates widening income inequality in the United States and other western countries, plus the worsening of the health status of both poorer populations and at least some minority groups (Williams and Collins 1995). Note, however, that income is one aspect of SES that is readily amenable to intervention through policy. Thus, there is an urgent need for more efforts at a societal level to reduce income inequalities and thereby improve the overall health status of populations.

Efforts to understand the distribution of mental health problems within the population must give more attention to the measurement of the construct. First, researchers should not take constructs developed and normed on one population and apply them indiscriminately to other populations. Second, efforts to understand the distribution of psychopathology must give careful attention to measuring the appropriate dimension of mental health status. Evidence to date indicates that scales of psychological distress capture qualitatively different phenomena than measures of psychiatric disorder. Therefore, these measures cannot be substituted for each other (Downey and Coyne 1991).

These data also suggest that there may be considerable unmet need for mental health services within the U.S. population. Economic status affects mental as well as physical health. Consistent with other research, we found that economic status is one of the strongest predictors of variations in mental health. Importantly, we uncovered economic status variations in mental health for each of the minority populations considered. Thus, there may be considerable need for outreach and targeted recruitment efforts to ensure that these groups have appropriate access to mental health services. This is critically important, especially given that many members of minority populations are unlikely to have health care insurance. Moreover, many of them receive primary medical care in hospital emergency rooms and other non-optimal organized care settings. The receipt of this type of care is often associated with a loss of dignity, the absence of continuity, and a lack of incentives to seek preventive and primary care in a timely manner.

The vast majority of American adults enter the health care system at least once each year (see Chapter 1). Our findings and other data suggest that there may be a serious need to instigate appropriate screening for mental health services at whatever points that people enter the health care system. Screening procedures should then be coordinated to the delivery of a comprehensive set of services, including mental health services, to address the needs of minorities. Any program of comprehensive health care must include the unmet mental health needs of minority populations. The delivery of care must also be sensitive and culturally appropriate.

Acknowledgments

The author wishes to thank Michelle Harris-Reid, Mercedes Rubio, and especially Colwick Wilson for assistance with data analysis and Car Nosel for preparing the manuscript.

References

Amaro, H., Russo, N. F., and Johnson, J. 1987. Family and work predictors of psychological well-being among Hispanic women professionals. *Psychology of Women Quarterly* 11:505–521.

Anderson, M., and Fienberg, S. E. 1995. Black, white and shades of gray (and brown and yellow). *Chance* 8:15–18.

Aquilino, W. S. 1994. Interview mode effects in surveys of drug and alcohol use: a field experiment. *Public Opinion Quarterly* 58:210–240.

Bracy, J. H. 1976. The quality of life experience of black people. In A. Campbell, P. E. Converse, and W. L. Rodgers, eds., *The Quality of American Life: Perceptions, Evaluations, and Satisfactions.* New York: Russell Sage Foundation.

Brown, G. W., and Harris, T. O. 1989. *Life Events and Illness.* New York: Guilford Press.

Buchwald, D., Manson, S. M., Dinges, N. G., Keane, E. M., and Kinzie, J. D. 1993. Prevalence of depressive symptoms among established Vietnamese refugees in the United States: detection in a primary care setting. *Journal of General Internal Medicine* 8:76–81.

Clemente, F., and Sauer, W. J. 1976. Life satisfaction in the United States. *Social Forces* 54:621–631.

Crow, M. R., Smith, H. L., McNamee, A. H., and Piland, N. F. 1994. Considerations in predicting mental health care use: implications for managed care plans. *Journal of Mental Health Administration* 21:5–23.

Dohrenwend, B. P., and Dohrenwend, B. S. 1969. *Social Status and Psychological Disorder: A Casual Inquire.* New York: John Wiley.

Downey, C., and Coyne, J. 1991. Social factors and psychopathology: stress, social support and coping processes. *Annual Review of Psychology* 42: 401–425.

Elliott, G., and Eisdorfer, C. 1982. *Stress and Human Health.* New York: Springer.

George, L. K. 1992. Economic status and subjective well-being: a review of the literature and an agenda for future research. In N. E. Cutler, D. W. Gregg, and M. P. Lawton, eds., *Aging, Money and Life Satisfaction.* New York: Springer.

Groves, R. M., and Kahn, R. L. 1979. *Surveys by Telephone: A National Comparison with Personal Interviews.* New York: Academic Press.

Herzog, A. R., Rodgers, W. L., and Woodworth, J. 1982. *Subjective Well-Being among Different Age Groups.* Ann Arbor, Mich.: Institute for Social Research, University of Michigan.

Hurh, W. M., and Kim, K. C. 1988. *Uprooting and Adjustment: A Sociological Study of Korean Immigrants' Mental Health.* (Final report to the National Institute of Mental Health.) Macomb, Ill.: Department of Sociology and Anthropology, Western Illinois University.

Jackson, J. S., Brown, T. N., Williams, D. R., Torres, M., Sellers, S. L., and Brown, K. 1996. Racism and the physical and mental health status of African Americans: a thirteen year national panel study. *Ethnicity and Disease* 6:132–147.

Kalmijn, M. 1996. The socioeconomic assimilation of Caribbean American blacks. *Social Forces* 74:911–930.

Kessler, R. C., McGonagle, K. A., Zhao, S., Nelson, C. B., Hughes, M., Eshleman, S., Wittchen, H. U., and Kendler, K. S. 1994. Lifetime and 12-month prevalence of DSM-III-R psychiatric disorders in the United States. *Archives of General Psychiatry* 51:8–19.

Kinzie, J. D., Boehnlein, J. K., Leung, P. K., Moore, L. J., Riley, C., and Smith, D. 1990. The prevalence of posttraumatic stress disorder and its clinical significance among Southeast Asian refugees. *American Journal of Psychiatry* 147:913–917.

Kuo, W. H. 1984. Prevalence of depression among Asian-Americans. *Journal of Nervous Mental Disorders* 172:449–457.

Kuo, W. H. 1995. Coping with racial discrimination: the case of Asian Americans. *Ethnic and Racial Studies* 18(1):109–127.

Lewontin, R. C. 1972. The apportionment of human diversity. *Evolutionary Biology* 6:381–398.

Lewontin, R. C. 1984. *Not in Our Genes: Biology, Ideology and Human Nature.* New York: Pantheon.

Link, B., and Dohrenwend, B. P. 1980. Formulation of hypotheses about the true prevalence of demoralization. In B. P. Dohrenwend, ed., *Mental Illness in the United States: Epidemiological Estimates.* New York: Praeger.

Lum, O. M. 1995. Health status of Asians and Pacific Islanders. *Ethnogeriatrics* 11:53–67.

Mechanic, D., Schlesinger, M., and McAlpine, D. D. 1995. Management of mental health and substance abuse services: state of the art and early results. *Milbank Quarterly* 73:19–55.

Mirowsky, J., and Ross, C. 1980. Minority status, ethnic culture, and distress: a comparison of blacks, whites, Mexicans and Mexican-Americans. *American Journal of Sociology* 86:479–495.

Montagu, A. 1965. *The Idea of Race.* Lincoln: University of Nebraska Press.

Neighbors, H. W. 1984. The distribution of psychiatric morbidity in black Americans. *Community Mental Health Journal* 20:169–181.

Nelson, C., and Tienda, M. 1985. The structuring of Hispanic ethnicity: historical and contemporary perspectives. In R. D. Alba, ed., *Ethnicity and Race in the USA.* New York: Routledge.

Notes and Comments. 1994. Census undercount and the quality of health data for racial and ethnic populations. *Ethnicity and Disease* 4(1):98–100.

Pearlin, L. I. 1989. The sociological study of stress. *Journal of Health and Social Behavior* 30:241–256.

Robins, L. N., and Regier, D. A. 1991. *Psychiatric Disorders in America: The Epidemiologic Catchment Area Study.* New York: Free Press.

Rogler, L. H., Cortes, D. E., and Malgady, R. G. 1991. Acculturation and mental health status among Hispanics. *American Psychologist* 46:585–597.

Rogler, L. H., Cortes, D. E., and Malgady, R. G. 1994. The mental health relevance of idioms of distress. *Journal of Nervous and Mental Disease* 182:327–330.

Rogler, L. H., Malgady, R. G., and Rodriguez, O. 1989. *Hispanics and Mental Health: A Framework for Research.* Malabar, Fla.: Robert E. Krieger Publishing.

Salgado de Snyder, V. N. 1987. Factors associated with acculturative stress and depressive symptomatology among married Mexican immigrant women. *Psychology of Women Quarterly* 11: 475–488.

Shah, B. V., Barnwell, B. G., Hunt, P. N., and LaVange, L. M. 1992. *SUDAAN Users Manual: Professional Software for Survey Data Analysis for Multistage Designs.* Research Triangle Park, N.C.: Research Triangle Institute.

Shrout, P. E., Canino, G. J., Bird, H. R., Bravo, M., Rubio-Stipec, M., and Burnam, M. A. 1992. Mental health status among Puerto Ricans, Mexican Americans, and non-Hispanic whites. *American Journal of Community Psychology* 20:729–754.

Sue, S., Sue, D. W., Sue, L., and Takeuchi, D. T. 1995. Psychopathology among Asian Americans: a model minority? *Cultural Diversity and Mental Health* 1:39–51.

Thomas, M. E., and Hughes, M. 1986. The continuing significance of race: a study of race, class, and quality of life in America, 1972–1985. *American Sociological Review* 51:830–841.

Tucker, C., McKay, R., Kojetin, B., Harrison, R., de la Puente, M., Stinson, L., and Robison, E. 1996. Testing methods of collecting racial and ethnic information: results of the Current Population Survey Supplement on Race and Ethnicity. *Bureau of Labor Statistical Notes* 40:1–149.

U.S. Office of Management and Budget. 1978. *Directive No. 15: Race and Ethnic Standards for Federal Statistics and Administrative Reporting.* Washington, D.C.: Office of Federal Statistical Policy and Standards, U.S. Department of Commerce.

Vega, W. A., and Rumbaut, R. G. 1991. Ethnic minorities and mental health. *Annual Review of Sociology* 17:351–383.

Veroff, J., Douvan, E., and Kulka, R. A. 1981. *The Inner American: A Self-Portrait from 1957 to 1976.* New York: Basic Books.

Ware, J. E., Kosinski, M., Bayliss, M. S., and McHorney, C. A. 1995. Comparison of methods for the scoring and statistical analysis of SF-36 health profile and summary measures: summary of results from the medical outcomes study. *Medical Care* 33(Suppl. 4):264–279.

Williams, D. R. 1996a. Racism and health: a research agenda. *Ethnicity and Disease* 6(1,2):1–6.

Williams, D. R. 1996b. Race/ethnicity and socioeconomic status: measurement and methodological issues. *International Journal of Health Services* 26(3):583–605.

Williams, D. R. 1997. Race and health: basic questions, emerging directions. *Annals of Epidemiology* 7(5):322–333.

Williams, D. R., Brown, T. N., Sellers, S. L., Forman, T. A., and Jackson, J. S. 1995. Racism and the health status of African Americans: resources and risk factors. Presented at the August 1995 annual meeting of the American Sociological Association, Washington, D.C.

Williams, D. R., and Chung, A. M. In press. Racism and health. In R. Gibson and J. S. Jackson, eds., *Health in Black America.* Thousand Oaks, Calif.: Sage Publications.

Williams, D. R., and Collins, C. 1995. Socioeconomic and racial differences in health. *Annual Review of Sociology* 21:349–386.

Williams, D. R., and Fenton, B. 1994. The mental health of African Americans: findings, questions, and directions. In I. L. Livingston, ed., *Handbook of Black American Health: The Mosaic of Conditions, Issues, Policies, and Prospects.* Westport, Conn.: Greenwood.

Williams, D. R., and House, J. S. 1991. Stress, social support, control and coping: a social epidemiologic view. In B. Badura and I. Kickbusch, eds., *Health Promotion Research: Towards a New Social Epidemiology.* Copenhagen: World Health Organization.

Williams, D. R., Lavizzo-Mourey, R., and Warren, R. C. 1994. The concept of race and health status in America. *Public Health Reports* 109(1):26–41.

Williams, D. R., Takeuchi, D., and Adair, R. 1992. Socioeconomic status and psychiatric disorder among blacks and whites. *Social Forces* 71:1791–1794.

Williams, D. R., Yu, Y., Jackson, J. S., and Anderson, N. B. 1997. Racial differences in physical and mental health: socioeconomic status, stress, and discrimination. *Journal of Health Psychology* 2:335–351.

Ying, Y. W. 1988. Depressive symptomatology among Chinese-Americans as measured by the CES-D. *Journal of Clinical Psychology* 44:739–746.

Zane, N. W. S., Takeuchi, D. T., and Young, K. N. S. 1994. *Confronting Critical Health Issues of Asian and Pacific Islander Americans.* Thousand Oaks, Calif.: Sage Publications.

12

Eating Well, Exercising, and Avoiding Smoking

Health Promotion among Men and Women in Minority Populations

Carol J. R. Hogue, Ph.D., M.P.H.

People can do much to maintain their own health status through avoiding smoking and other addictive behaviors, eating a healthy diet, and getting enough exercise to prevent obesity and assure cardiovascular fitness. The harmful effects of smoking are well documented and widely understood. The benefits of an active lifestyle are also well established and broadly understood. The role of specific foods in disease prevention is somewhat more controversial. However, it is generally agreed that at least one-third of all cancer deaths are related to diet, and as many as 60 percent of cancers in women are related, at least in part, to dietary factors (Cotunga et al. 1992).

STUDIES ON MINORITY HEALTH BEHAVIORS

Prevalence of Smoking

Especially for African Americans and Hispanics, much has been written about the prevalence of smoking—but analyses are often simplistic and do not address the question of the interaction of race and ethnicity with socioeconomic status (SES). Further, much that is written assumes that the racial/ethnic gap in health is related to excess smoking among minorities, despite evidence to the contrary. Historically, surveys in this country have found that African American men smoked more than white men, but this difference disappeared or was reversed when SES was held constant (Escobedo et al. 1991; Feigelman and Gorman 1989). Trends in smoking prevalence from the mid-1970s suggested that even crude black-white differences among men would disappear; younger African American men were not beginning to smoke as much as compared to younger white men, and African American women continued to smoke less than white women (Bachman et al. 1991; Fiore et al. 1989; Feigelman and Lee 1995; Flint and Novotny 1998). This convergence became apparent by 1990 (Anonymous 1992c).

The prevalence of smoking among Hispanics falls between that for African Americans and whites (Gritz et al. 1998). Past studies of racial and ethnic differences in smoking prevalence have found that Hispanic women smoke less than white women, after adjustment for SES (Perez-Stable, Marin, and Marin 1994; Winkleby et al. 1995), and also smoke less than African American women of similar social status (Sanders-Phillips 1994). However, Hispanic women who do smoke may be less likely to receive counseling from their health care provider (Winkleby et al. 1995). Findings are mixed regarding whether Hispanic men smoke more or less than white men of comparable SES (Perez-Stable, Marin, and Marin 1994; Winkleby et al. 1995), but there is little disagreement that Hispanic men smoke more than Hispanic women.

Less is known about the smoking habits of Asian Americans. Among adolescents in Worcester, Massachusetts, and adults in Seattle / King County, older Vietnamese men smoked more than older white men, and Vietnamese boys smoked as heavily as did white boys, but Vietnamese women and girls rarely smoked (Anonymous 1992d; Wiecha 1996). Vietnamese American and Chinese American men in California reported higher smoking prevalence (35% and 28%, respectively) than white men in California (Anonymous 1992a, 1992b).

Prevalence of Eating Well and Exercising

Diets that are high in calories and sodium but low in potassium and calcium are thought to contribute to the higher prevalence and severity of hypertension among African Americans as compared with whites (Adrogue and Wesson 1996). It has also been hypothesized that the excess risk of cancer among African Americans is related to racial and ethnic differences in diets. However, there is limited evidence that African Americans consume foods that increase cancer risk (Swanson et al. 1993). Some representative samples of adults indicate few differences between African Americans and whites in frequencies of fruit, vegetable, and fat consumption, although differences in the way that food is prepared might affect cancer risk (Swanson et al. 1993). Other studies suggest that African Americans consume more fat, especially by eating more fried food (Patterson et al. 1995).

Hispanics may eat less fat and consume fewer calories, but their diets may also be deficient in essential micronutrients such as vitamin A, phosphorous, calcium, niacin, and vitamin C (Lopez et al. 1995; Patterson et al 1995). Among Hispanics, older Puerto Rican and Cuban Americans report healthier diets than younger Hispanics and Mexican Americans (Loria et al. 1995). It is not clear how much these differences reflect levels of acculturation or SES and educational differences. Better-educated people, regardless of race or ethnicity, tend to eat healthier diets (Shimakawa et al. 1994; Swanson et al. 1993).

More women than men report healthy eating habits, including a more diverse diet, with more fruits and vegetables (Patterson et al. 1995). However, racial and ethnic differences have been observed among women. Despite similarities in reported diets, more African American than white women have a high body mass index (Burke et al. 1992; Boardley et al. 1995; Shimakawa et al. 1994). This may be related to higher energy intake, differences in food preparation techniques, and lower levels of energy consumption—differences that remain after adjustment for educational attainment and income.

Evidence of Leisure-time Physical Activity

Leisure-time physical activity declines with increasing age and with decreasing education (Anderssen et al. 1996; Crespo et al. 1996). In a national survey, African American and Hispanic women—but not men—reported lower levels of energy consumption than were reported by whites (Crespo et al. 1996); this negative association was found for women in regional studies, even after adjustment for socioeconomic and other variables (Bild et al. 1993; Perez-Stable, Marin, and Marin 1994; Washburn et al. 1992). However, in one study of older Americans, differences in educational attainment explained differences in physical activity between African Americans and whites (Clark 1995). Reasons for racial and ethnic differences in leisure-time activity prove to be complex and poorly understood. Factors found to be associated with increased physical activity include a sense of personal control, regular participation in organizations and groups, interpersonal support (Felton and Parsons 1994), and belief in the efficacy of preventive health behavior (Broman 1995).

Evidence That Health Care Advice Makes a Difference

Randomized trials of provider advice indicate that people change their behaviors when they receive targeted and well-planned messages from their health care providers. For example, 14.2 percent of smokers who were enrolled in a cessation program incorporating the National Cancer Institute physician intervention program and follow-up counseling by a study nurse remained abstinent one year after the intervention. When this intervention was supplemented with nicotine patch therapy for a random sample of patients, 27.5 percent of smokers were abstinent one year later (Hurt et al. 1994). Advice on improving dietary habits also helps. Compared with men diagnosed with hypertension who received only blood pressure monitoring, men diagnosed with hypertension who were randomly assigned to receive dietary advice from a clinical nutritionist lowered their blood pressure measures and increased weight loss by one year after the intervention (Beckman et al. 1995).

Health promotion counseling has been demonstrated to help members of minority populations living under high-stress conditions to reduce smoking and obesity and to increase leisure-time activity. In a primary care clinic in Harlem, New York, physicians were trained in the National Cancer Institute physician intervention program. African American adults who received advice from those physicians were significantly more likely to report having cut down on the amount they smoked seven months after having received the advice (Royce et al. 1995). Among poor African American and white women in Virginia, those receiving cancer-prevention lessons and dietary counseling reported significantly greater reductions in fat consumption and increases in vitamin E intake than those in a control group who received money-management lessons (Cox et al. 1995). In a longitudinal study of African American and white South Carolinians who reported being physically inactive in 1987, significantly more reported having increased their activity level four years later if they had received advice on physical activity from their physician (Macera et al. 1995).

Despite the evidence and the considerable pressure from professional groups to include health promotion messages in routine care, many providers do not. Among adults in Missouri with at least one modifiable risk factor (smoker, obese, inactive), fewer than one-half reported hearing health promotion advice from their physicians (Friedman et al. 1994). In Pennsylvania, separate surveys of physicians and residents revealed that, although providers report that they advise virtually all their smoking patients to stop smoking and that they provide some action (such as setting a quit date or prescribing nicotine gum), one-third of the smokers who reported having seen a physician in the previous year did not remember that they were asked if they smoked, and less than one-half received specific advice or counseling about stopping (Brink et al. 1994). Even in hospitals with no-smoking policies, hospitalized smokers may receive no counseling on how to stop or how to remain abstinent after their release from the hospital (Neighbor, Stoop, and Ellsworth 1994).

Few physicians counsel their patients regarding exercise. For example, in a random sample of Massachusetts primary care internists, only one-third reported that they counseled at least 75 percent of their patients (Sherman and Hershman 1993). Provider characteristics, such as older age, perceived importance of exercising, and expected level of success with patient advice, as well as their own fitness level, were positively associated with giving fitness advice to their patients.

METHODS OF ANALYSIS

The Commonwealth Fund Minority Health Survey (CMHS) provides an opportunity to examine what people say about behaviors that affect their health and what health promotion messages they remember hearing from their health care provider. A strength of this study is that it uses one set of health promotion measures for large samples of men and women across a broad range of race/ethnicity groups. This approach permits a national estimate, with across-group comparisons while adjusting for contextual variables. With this study, it is possible to explore the relationship between race/ethnicity and SES as we explain differences in health promotion behaviors.

The purposes of these analyses are (1) to determine whether race/ethnicity and gender are associated with avoiding smoking, eating well, and exercising sufficiently, and, if so, whether such associations are independent of socioeconomic factors and health care structural variables; and (2) for similar factors, to determine whether race/ethnicity or gender is associated with health care providers' advice on addictive behaviors and on fitness.

Measures of Health Promotion Behaviors

Respondents in the CMHS were asked "Do you smoke cigarettes now, or not?" Those responding "yes" were classified as self-reported smokers, and others were classified as nonsmokers. Because smoking status was not validated through a biochemical marker, this study does not have the precision of clinic-based studies that incorporate biochemical markers. Misclassification would be in the direction of smokers being misclassified as nonsmokers; minority and less-educated smokers may be more under-reported than majority and better-educated smokers (Wagenknecht et al. 1992). Thus, misclassification bias would tend to create underestimates of differences between the groups being studied. Any observed differences are likely to be real and may be greater than actually observed.

The survey included the following question on diet: "How often do you maintain a healthy diet, that is, a diet that is low in fat and high in fruits and vegetables?" The National Academy of Sciences first published dietary guidelines supporting the consumption of a diet that is low in fat and high in fruits and vegetables in 1982. Most adults know these guidelines and believe that diet and disease are related (Cotunga et al. 1992).

Respondents were also asked "How often do you exercise hard—that is, so you breathe heavily and your heart and pulse rate are increased for a period lasting at least 20 minutes?" Responses for both questions were categorized into frequencies of never, less than 1 day a month, 1–3 days a month, 1 day a week, 2 days a week, 3 days a week, 4–5 days a week, 6–7 days a week, and not sure ($< 2\%$ of responses). We classified respondents reporting that they eat a healthy diet "4 or more days a week" as eating well. Likewise, we classified those responding that they exercise hard "4 or more days a week" as routinely and vigorously exercising. Other studies have used less stringent cut-off points for these behaviors, but we chose a more stringent criterion. Our purpose was to counteract as much as possible the effects of a potential "response bias" toward answering the question in the desirable way.

Measures of Provider Advice

Respondents were asked "During your care in the past year, did the doctor (health professional) talk to you about: (i) smoking, or the use of alcohol or other drugs; (ii) being the right weight, healthy eating or exercise; (iii) birth control or the use of condoms?" For each of these three groupings of advice, respondents could answer "yes," "no," "not applicable," or "not sure." We limited our analysis to respondents who indicated that they had accessed health care within the twelve months prior to their interview, and compared respondents with a "yes" response to the others.

Statistical Methods

Cross-tabulated variables were tested by chi-square for differences by race/ethnicity and by gender. Odds ratios and confidence intervals for multiple logistic regression models were estimated with SUDAAN.

Independent Variables

Race/ethnicity were self-reported and, for this analysis, were categorized as African American, Hispanic, Asian, and white. We examined gender, age (in three categories: 18–39, 40–64, and ≥ 65 years), and marital status. In the multivariate analyses, these variables were entered as a set of sociodemographic variables.

Socioeconomic variables were entered second in the hierarchical, multivariate models. These included employment status (employed, unemployed, and not in the labor force), income (in six levels), home ownership, and education (in three levels). Individuals not in the workforce included homemakers, retired people, and disabled people. Number in the household was included to adjust the income variable.

Healthy behaviors may be related to an awareness of the importance to one's health of regular access to preventive and curative health care. We were interested in learning whether self-reported healthy behaviors were correlated with how individuals apply discretionary income to health. To determine this, after controlling for the SES variables, we introduced the structural variable of insurance status (any private insurance, only public insurance, or no insurance) for the multivariate models of health promotion behaviors.

In the multivariate models of provider advice, we hypothesized that providers who were well-known to their patients and providers of the same race/ethnicity and gender might have better rapport with their patients and feel more comfortable advising them to stop smoking, eat well, and exercise regularly. Therefore, we included provider characteristics (whether a "regular" provider or not; if regular provider, whether of the same gender, and whether of the same race/ethnicity) in these models.

RESULTS OF ANALYSIS

Smoking Varies by Gender but Not between Racial Groups

Cross-tabulations. More than one-fourth of the men reported that they currently smoke (Table 12.1). Smoking among men did not differ

Table 12.1   Percentage Distribution of Self-Reported Smoking, Eating Habits, and Usual Exercise Level by Race/Ethnicity and Gender

	Smokes		Eats Healthy Diet ≥4 Times/Week		Exercises Hard ≥4 Times/Week	
	Yes	No	Yes	No	Yes	No
African American						
Male	26.2	73.8	42.1	57.9	28.3	71.7
Female	15.6	84.4	51.4	48.6	19.0	81.0
Hispanic						
Male	26.0	74.0	42.5	57.5	33.1	66.9
Female	11.9	88.1	55.7	44.3	16.6	83.4
White						
Male	27.9	72.1	54.6	45.4	34.8	65.2
Female	23.5	76.5	67.0	33.0	17.8	82.2
Asian						
Male	23.6	76.4	46.2	53.8	21.8	78.2
Female	5.2	94.8	70.8	29.2	8.5	91.5

Source: Data from The Commonwealth Fund Minority Health Survey, 1994.

significantly among the four race/ethnicity groups (from 23.6% for Asian men to 27.9% for white men). Women were less likely to self-identify as smokers, although the difference between men and women varied considerably by race/ethnicity group. Asian women reported the least smokers (5.2%), followed by Hispanic women (11.9%), African American women (15.6%), and white women (23.5%) (Table 12.1).

Multivariate model for women. Asian women and men were excluded from all the multivariate models due to the difference in sampling design (see Technical Appendix). We analyzed smoking behaviors separately for men and women, because in preliminary multivariate modeling, gender interacted with several other variables. For women, all sociodemographic variables were associated with self-reported smoking (Table 12.2). African American and Hispanic women were one-half as likely to report being smokers as were white women; married women were one-half as likely to report being smokers as unmarried women; and women less than 65 years of age were more than three times as likely to smoke as the oldest women (Table 12.2).

These associations intensified somewhat when the socioeconomic variables were added, and also when both socioeconomic and structural

Table 12.2   Self-Reported Smoking among Women (multiple logistic regression models)

	MODEL 1		MODEL 2		MODEL 3	
	AOR[a]	95% CI[b]	AOR	95% CI	AOR	95% CI
Sociodemographic						
Race/ethnicity						
African American	0.5	0.31,0.69	0.4	0.29,0.66	0.4	0.27,0.64
Hispanic	0.5	0.32,0.68	0.4	0.27,0.61	0.4	0.23,0.58
Age						
18–39	3.0	1.68,5.46	3.8	1.88,7.73	3.5	1.74,7.14
40–64	3.6	2.02,6.29	4.3	2.19,8.30	3.9	1.98,7.81
Married	0.5	0.32,0.74	0.5	0.33,0.89	0.6	0.35,0.92
Socioeconomic						
Employment status						
Employed			0.9	0.53,1.48	1.0	0.57,1.58
Unemployed			1.6	0.89,3.14	1.5	0.77,2.93
Income						
<$7,500			2.2	1.00,5.02	2.0	0.89,4.63
$7,500–$15,000			1.2	0.53,2.65	1.0	0.45,2.42
$15,001–$25,000			1.6	0.81,3.08	1.5	0.75,2.96
$25,001–$35,000			1.4	0.69,2.84	1.4	0.70,2.87
$35,001–$50,000			1.2	0.58,2.38	1.2	0.58,2.42
Does not own home			0.8	0.53,1.35	0.8	0.50,1.28
Number in household			1.0	1.0,1.0	1.0	1.0,1.0
Education						
<High school			2.4	1.18,4.83	2.3	1.10,4.69
High school/ some college			2.0	1.17,3.38	2.0	1.17,3.38
Structural						
Any private insurance					0.6	0.33,1.15
Only public insurance					0.9	0.40,1.92

Source: Data from The Commonwealth Fund Minority Health Survey, 1994.

Note: Referent categories: white, age >64, unmarried, not in labor force, income >$50,000, owns home, completed college, uninsured.

[a]AOR = adjusted odds ratio (adjusted for other variables in the model).

[b]95% CI = 95% confidence interval.

variables were added. In the full model (model 3, adjusting for socioeconomic and structural variables), African American and Hispanic women were only 0.40 times as likely to smoke as white women; women 18–39 years of age were 3.5 times and women 40–64 years of age were 3.9 times as likely to smoke as women 65 years of age and older; but married women were only 0.6 times as likely to smoke as unmarried women.

After adjusting for sociodemographic variables, the smoking behavior of women was associated with educational attainment (those with less than high school being 2.4 times and those with high school through some college being 2.0 times as likely to smoke as those with a college degree). The other socioeconomic variables—employment status, income, and home ownership—were not significantly associated after adjustment for the sociodemographic variables and education. Insurance status was not significantly associated with smoking status among women, after adjustment for the sociodemographic and socioeconomic variables (Table 12.2).

Multivariate model for men. The sociodemographic characteristics of male smokers were similar to, but not as dramatic as, those of female smokers (Table 12.3). African American and Hispanic men were, respectively, 0.6 and 0.5 times as likely to smoke as were white men, after adjustment for socioeconomic and structural variables. Middle-aged men were the most likely to smoke, followed by younger men, who were 2.7 times as likely to smoke as the oldest men. Marital status was not associated with smoking among men, after adjustment for the other variables.

Unlike women, employment status and income were significantly associated with smoking for men (Table 12.3). Among the men, the employed were twice as likely and the unemployed were almost four times as likely to smoke as male respondents not currently in the workforce. Among men, smoking increased with increasing income to the $25,001–$35,000 range, and then decreased with increasing income to the highest income level. The only significant association was for men in the $25,001–$35,000 income range, who were 1.8 times as likely to smoke as were the wealthiest men. As with women, education was the socioeconomic variable most associated with smoking behavior. Men with less than a high school education were almost six times and men with a high school education or some college were four times as likely to smoke as men with a college degree, after adjustment for sociodemographic and structural variables. Men with private insurance were half as likely to smoke as were uninsured men, after adjustment for sociodemographic and socioeconomic variables (Table 12.3).

Less than One-half Eat a Healthy Diet Regularly

Cross-tabulations. Slightly more than 40 percent of the American adults in the survey reported that they maintain a healthy diet four to seven days a week (Table 12.1). Men were less likely than women to re-

Table 12.3   Self-Reported Smoking among Men (multiple logistic regression models)

	MODEL 1		MODEL 2		MODEL 3	
	AOR[a]	95% CI[b]	AOR	95% CI	AOR	95% CI
Sociodemographic						
Race/ethnicity						
African American	0.8	0.54,1.05	0.6	0.42,0.85	0.6	0.40,0.84
Hispanic	0.8	0.55,1.07	0.6	0.42,0.88	0.5	0.36,0.81
Age						
18–39	3.6	1.96,6.60	2.8	1.29,5.96	2.7	1.26,5.84
40–64	3.6	2.00,6.48	3.2	1.54,6.59	3.3	1.58,6.99
Married	0.7	0.50,0.98	1.0	0.64,1.41	1.0	0.68,1.54
Socioeconomic						
Employment status						
Employed			2.1	1.22,3.66	2.0	1.16,3.63
Unemployed			4.4	1.87,10.51	3.9	1.16,9.32
Income						
<$7,500			1.6	0.72,3.47	1.2	0.54,2.67
$7,500–$15,000			1.6	0.77,3.18	1.3	0.63,2.57
$15,001–$25,000			1.5	0.82,2.66	1.4	0.76,2.45
$25,001–$35,000			1.9	1.08,3.25	1.8	1.02,3.06
$35,001–$50,000			1.3	0.79,2.18	1.3	0.78,2.16
Does not own home			1.2	0.77,1.82	1.2	0.25,1.79
Number in household			0.9	0.77,0.98	0.9	0.76,0.97
Education						
<High school			6.4	3.30,12.51	5.9	2.99,11.78
High school/ some college			3.1	2.61,6.69	4.0	2.48,6.36
Structural						
Any private insurance					0.48	0.28,0.83
Only public insurance					0.70	0.32,1.53

Source: Data from The Commonwealth Fund Minority Health Survey, 1994.

Note: Referent categories: white, age >64, unmarried, not in labor force, income >$50,000, owns home, completed college, uninsured.

[a]AOR = adjusted odds ratio (adjusted for other variables in the model).

[b]95% CI = 95% confidence interval.

port a frequent healthy diet, and there was not much difference among the men by race/ethnicity status. Proportions reporting a frequent healthy diet ranged from 42.1 percent for African American men to 54.6 percent for white men. The range was broader among women, from 51.4 percent for African American women to 70.8 percent for Asian women. However, gender did not interact significantly with other variables in multivariate modeling, so we constructed one model to explore socio-demographic, socioeconomic, and structural characteristics of people who reported healthy eating habits at least four days a week.

Multivariate models. In the multivariate analysis, gender, race/ethnicity, and age were associated with a reported healthy diet (Table 12.4). Women were 1.6 times as likely as men to say that they frequently eat a healthy diet, and this association did not change when adjusted for socioeconomic and structural variables. African Americans were 0.6 times as likely as whites and Hispanics were 0.8 times as likely as whites to report eating a healthy diet. After adjusting for socioeconomic variables, the association between Hispanic ethnicity and diet was still present but no longer statistically significant. The youngest respondents (18–39 years of age) were the least likely to report eating a healthy diet, followed by middle-aged persons (40–64 years of age). The fully adjusted odds ratios were 0.5 and 0.7, respectively, compared with individuals aged 65 and older. Interestingly, marital status was not independently associated with reported healthy dietary habits.

With respect to socioeconomic variables, not being in the labor force and having greater educational attainment were associated with a reported healthy diet, whereas income and home ownership were not associated (Table 12.4). The employed were only 0.6 times as likely to report that they regularly eat a healthy diet as those not currently in the workforce. Those with less than a high school education were 0.4 times and those with high school or some college were 0.7 times as likely to report a frequent healthy diet as college graduates. Insurance status was not statistically associated with eating a healthy diet, after adjustment for the sociodemographic and socioeconomic variables.

Fewer than One-fourth Report Routine Hard Exercise

Cross-tabulations. Only 24 percent of the sample reported that they exercise hard at least four days a week. Men were much more likely than women to respond positively to the question of hard exercise four or more times per week (Table 12.1). Even so, less than one-third of the men reported exercising vigorously and routinely. According to the self-reports, Asian men were the least active men (21.8%), followed by African American men (28.3%), Hispanic men (33.1%), and white men (34.8%) (Table 12.1). Overall, only 18 percent of women reported that they routinely exercise vigorously. Asian women were the least active women (8.5%), followed by Hispanic women (16.6%), white women

Table 12.4   Self-Reported Eating a "Healthy" Diet at Least Four Times a Week (multiple logistic regression models)

	MODEL 1		MODEL 2		MODEL 3	
	AOR[a]	95% CI[b]	AOR	95% CI	AOR	95% CI
Sociodemographic						
Female	1.6	1.29,1.98	1.6	1.22,1.96	1.6	1.23,1.96
Race/ethnicity						
African American	0.6	0.48,0.74	0.6	0.52,0.80	0.6	0.52,0.80
Hispanic	0.7	0.58,0.89	0.8	0.67,1.04	0.8	0.67,1.08
Age						
18–39	0.4	0.27,0.51	0.4	0.31,0.67	0.5	0.31,0.71
40–64	0.6	0.42,0.78	0.7	0.46,1.00	0.7	0.48,1.04
Married	1.0	0.82,1.26	0.9	0.70,1.17	0.9	0.71,1.13
Socioeconomic						
Employment status						
Employed			0.6	0.43,0.81	0.6	0.43,0.81
Unemployed			0.8	0.47,1.31	0.8	0.48,1.28
Income						
<$7,500			0.6	0.40,1.03	0.6	0.39,1.05
$7,500–$15,000			0.8	0.51,1.26	0.8	0.51,1.31
$15,001–$25,000			0.7	0.51,1.06	0.7	0.52,1.08
$25,001–$35,000			0.8	0.53,1.11	0.8	0.53,1.12
$35,001–$50,000			0.8	0.54,1.05	0.8	0.54,1.05
Does not own home			0.9	0.71,1.23	0.9	0.71,1.23
Number in household			1.0	1.0,1.0	1.0	1.0,1.0
Education						
<High school			0.4	0.24,0.56	0.4	0.24,0.55
High school/ some college			0.7	0.54,0.89	0.7	0.54,0.90
Structural						
Any private insurance					1.1	0.76,1.67
Only public insurance					1.2	0.74,2.05

Source: Data from The Commonwealth Fund Minority Health Survey, 1994.

Note: Referent categories: male, white, age >64, unmarried, not in labor force, income >$50,000, owns home, completed college, uninsured.

[a]AOR = adjusted odds ratio (adjusted for other variables in the model).

[b]95% CI = 95% confidence interval.

(17.8%), and African American women (19%). Because of interactions between gender and other variables, the multivariate analyses were separated for men and women.

Multivariate model for women. Among women, marital status was initially the only sociodemographic variable significantly associated with reported physical activity (Table 12.5). Married women were only 0.6 times as likely as unmarried women to report a routine, vigorous physical exercise schedule. This negative association with marriage was masked without adjustment for income, as married women on average have higher household incomes than unmarried women have, and higher incomes were positively associated with regular exercise. After adjust-

Table 12.5   Self-Reported Frequent Exercise among Women ("Exercise Hard" Four or More Days a Week) (multiple logistic regression models)

	MODEL 1		MODEL 2		MODEL 3	
	AOR[a]	95% CI[b]	AOR	95% CI	AOR	95% CI
Sociodemographic						
Race/ethnicity						
African American	1.0	0.70,1.48	1.1	0.72,1.57	1.1	0.74,1.62
Hispanic	0.9	0.64,1.34	1.0	0.66,1.49	1.1	0.70,1.67
Age						
18–39	1.0	0.61,1.75	0.8	0.45,1.52	0.9	0.48,1.69
40–64	0.9	0.54,1.43	0.7	0.39,1.26	0.8	0.42,1.37
Married	0.8	0.54,1.19	0.6	0.40,0.99	0.6	0.39,0.97
Socioeconomic						
Employment status						
Employed			1.3	0.79,2.10	1.2	0.77,2.05
Unemployed			1.0	0.48,2.30	1.1	0.51,2.26
Income						
<$7,500			0.6	0.26,1.30	0.6	0.27,1.30
$7,500–$15,000			0.3	0.11,0.59	0.3	0.12,0.64
$15,001–$25,000			0.7	0.36,1.26	0.7	0.38,1.28
$25,001–$35,000			0.5	0.26,0.93	0.5	0.26,0.92
$35,001–$50,000			0.6	0.33,1.12	0.6	0.33,1.11
Does not own home			0.9	0.56,1.43	0.9	0.59,1.51
Number in household			1.0	1.0,1.0	1.0	1.0,1.0
Education						
<High school			1.0	0.48,2.06	1.0	0.49,2.19
High school/ some college			1.0	0.63,1.62	1.0	0.62,1.60
Structural						
Any private insurance					1.7	0.78,3.58
Only public insurance					1.6	0.65,3.79

Source: Data from The Commonwealth Fund Minority Health Survey, 1994.

Note: Referent categories: male, white, age >64, unmarried, not in labor force, income >$50,000, owns home, completed college, uninsured.

[a]AOR = adjusted odds ratio (adjusted for other variables in the model).

[b]95% CI = 95% confidence interval.

ment for socioeconomic and structural variables, there remained no association between race/ethnicity and vigorous exercise among African American, Hispanic, and white women.

There was also no association with age, perhaps reflecting the nature of the CMHS, in that individuals surveyed were living in households and not in nursing homes or other group settings. After adjustment for the other factors, women with incomes between $7,500 and $15,000 reported routinely exercising vigorously only 0.3 times as frequently as did women with incomes in excess of $50,000; and women with incomes between $25,001 and $35,000 were just half as likely to exercise vigorously as were women with incomes over $50,000 (Table 12.5). Reported vigorous exercise among women in other income brackets was also less than for the wealthiest women but did not reach statistical significance. Surprisingly, educational attainment was not associated with a self-reported routine and vigorous exercise regimen. Insurance status was not significantly associated with vigorous exercise (Table 12.5).

Multivariate model for men. A slightly different picture emerges of men who are physically active (data not shown). First, there is a difference among men by race/ethnicity. African American men reported routinely and vigorously exercising only 0.7 times as frequently as white men did (adjusted odds ratio = 0.7, 95% CI = 0.51, 0.95), whereas Hispanic men were not statistically distinguishable from white men (adjusted odds ratio = 1.1, 95% CI = 0.79, 1.54). Age was not associated with reported hard exercise for men; this lack of association was found among the women as well. Among men, being married was associated with a lesser likelihood of hard exercise (adjusted odds ratio = 0.7, 95% CI = 0.50, 0.94). However, in the full model, the association of exercise with marital status was no longer statistically significant (adjusted odds ratio = 0.7, 95% CI = 0.50, 1.01).

Likewise, the socioeconomic variables characterized the men's exercise patterns differently from the women's. Unlike for women, income was not a statistically significant factor in distinguishing exercising men from non-exercising men. On the other hand, while employment status did not distinguish exercising women from non-exercising women, it was the only socioeconomic variable that was significantly associated with men's reported vigorous exercising. Unemployed men were only 0.3 times as likely to report routinely and vigorously exercising as were men not in the work force (because of retirement, disability, or other reason) (adjusted odds ratio = 0.3, 95% CI = 0.15, 0.83). Employed men were not distinguishable statistically from men not in the workforce.

Providers Give Moderate Advice on Addictive Behaviors

We limited our analyses of health care providers' advice to the 85 percent of the respondents who reported at least one encounter with a health care provider in the twelve months preceding the interview. We also excluded the Asian sample from these analyses. Individuals in the CMHS were asked "During your care in the past year, did the doctor (health professional) talk to you about smoking, or the use of alcohol or other drugs?" This question sought to assess the extent to which health care consumers perceived that they received advice on specific addictive behaviors. Overall, 37.8 percent of the respondents reported receiving such advice.

Cross-tabulations. Responses varied by whether the respondents reported themselves as smokers, who constituted 24 percent of the sample. One would expect that all smokers would have received "quit smoking" advice from their health care providers. However, among smokers, only 69 percent reported hearing advice on addictive behaviors from their health care provider (Table 12.6). Ideally, providers counsel all their patients on addictive behaviors, regardless of whether they believe their patients smoke, use alcohol to excess, or use drugs. However, providers may actually give such counsel only to patients they believe need to change their behaviors. The CMHS did not include questions about alcohol consumption or drug use, so it is not possible to estimate how many self-reported nonsmokers might self-report problems with alcohol or drug use. Among nonsmokers, 28 percent reported receiving counsel on smoking, alcohol, or drugs. This could represent alcohol or drug counseling, or encouragement to continue smoking cessation, or a more generic screening and counseling on addictive behaviors.

Among smokers, there was not a statistically significant difference by race/ethnicity and gender in respondents' receipt of health care provider advice (Table 12.6). However, the smallest percentage was for African American women (57.8%), while the highest percentage was for Hispanic women (78.0%). Likewise, among nonsmokers there were only slight and statistically non-significant differences by race/ethnicity and gender; the smallest proportion was for white women (25.6%), and the largest proportion was for African American women (34.0%).

Multivariate results. The lack of association between gender and health care advice on addictive behaviors held true in multivariate analyses of smokers (Table 12.7) and nonsmokers (data not shown). However, among patients who smoke, and after adjustment for other sociodemographic, socioeconomic, and structural variables, both African Ameri-

Table 12.6   Percentage of Respondents Who Had Received Advice on Addictive Behaviors

	Among Smokers		Among Nonsmokers		Total	
	% Yes	N^a	% Yes	N	% Yes	N
African American						
Male	60.6	43	26.7	123	35.6	166
Female	57.8	34	34.0	185	37.7	219
Hispanic						
Male	58.6	28	29.7	81	37.2	110
Female	78.0	14	31.3	106	36.8	121
White						
Male	68.0	308	29.3	795	40.1	1,102
Female	73.1	319	25.6	1,036	36.8	1,355

Source: Data from The Commonwealth Fund Minority Health Survey, 1994.
Note: Data limited to those who accessed care in the previous twelve months.
[a]Rounded to whole number.

cans and Hispanic Americans were less likely than whites to report receiving counseling. African American smokers were only half as likely, and Hispanic Americans smokers were only 0.8 times as likely, to report having received advice, as were white smokers.

Other sociodemographic variables—age and marital status—did not distinguish smokers who did or did not receive advice. However, among nonsmokers, younger respondents (18–39 years of age) were 1.7 times as likely as the oldest respondents (65 or more years of age) to report receiving advice from physicians on addictive behaviors (adjusted odds ratio = 1.7, 95% CI = 1.02, 2.76).

With respect to socioeconomic variables for smokers, there were no significant associations between employment status, home ownership, or educational level, and reported receipt of advice (Table 12.7). Among nonsmokers, the only significant association between socioeconomic variables and reported receipt of advice was for respondents who did not own their homes (data not shown). Renters were 1.6 times as likely as homeowners to report receiving advice, after adjustment for sociodemographic, the other socioeconomic, and structural variables (adjusted odds ratio = 1.6, 95% CI = 1.13, 2.36).

For structural variables, we chose characteristics of the provider-patient relationship, reasoning that the relationship between consumer

Table 12.7   Provider's Advice about Smoking, Alcohol, or Other Drugs to Patients Who Smoke (multiple logistic regression models)

	MODEL 1		MODEL 2		MODEL 3	
	AOR[a]	95% CI[b]	AOR	95% CI	AOR	95% CI
Sociodemographic						
Female	1.2	0.67,2.18	1.1	0.62,2.14	0.9	0.38,1.94
Race/ethnicity						
African American	0.6	0.38,1.00	0.6	0.36,1.05	0.5	0.28,0.96
Hispanic	0.8	0.49,1.42	0.9	0.48,1.65	0.8	0.43,1.60
Age						
18–39	0.4	0.15,1.17	0.6	0.20,2.06	0.9	0.26,3.19
40–64	0.5	0.18,1.52	0.7	0.22,2.26	0.8	0.24,2.68
Married	0.9	0.50,1.57	0.9	0.43,1.73	1.0	0.50,1.97
Socioeconomic						
Employment status						
Employed			0.7	0.30,1.61	0.7	0.31,1.76
Unemployed			0.4	0.15,1.16	0.5	0.18,1.43
Income						
<$7,500			1.0	0.32,2.95	1.4	0.44,4.49
$7,500–$15,000			1.2	0.39,3.71	1.3	0.43,4.17
$15,001–$25,000			0.7	0.28,1.77	0.9	0.34,2.41
$25,001–$35,000			1.4	0.53,3.56	1.5	0.58,3.99
$35,001–$50,000			0.6	0.25,1.48	0.5	0.21,1.25
Does not own home			1.0	0.53,1.95	1.0	0.51,1.97
Number in household			1.0	0.80,1.20	0.9	0.77,1.15
Education						
<High school			1.3	0.45,3.52	1.4	0.48,3.85
High school/ some college			0.8	0.36,2.03	0.8	0.33,1.82
Structural						
Has regular provider					7.9	3.12,20.24
Regular provider of same race					0.4	0.19,0.75
Regular provider of same sex					1.4	0.62,3.13

Source: Data from The Commonwealth Fund Minority Health Survey, 1994.

Note: Referent categories: male, white, age >64, unmarried, not in labor force, income >$50,000, owns home, completed college, does not have regular provider, regular provider is not of same race, regular provider is not of same sex.

[a]AOR = adjusted odds ratio (adjusted for other variables in the model).

[b]95% CI = 95% confidence interval.

and provider might affect the provider's willingness to give advice and/or the consumer's receptiveness to receiving and recalling the advice received. These variables included whether the respondent had a regular health care provider to whom they go when they are sick or need health care; whether that regular provider was of the same race/ethnicity as the respondent; and whether that regular provider was of the same gender as the respondent. Gender concordance was more frequent among men, because more than 80 percent of regular providers were men. Race/ethnicity concordance was more likely within the white group, as more than 80 percent of the providers for that group were also white; slightly more than one-half of the providers for minority groups were also white (Louis Harris and Associates 1994).

Among smokers, having a regular provider was strongly associated with reported receipt of advice. Respondents with a regular provider were almost eight times as likely to report receiving advice as those without a regular provider (Table 12.7). However, if the regular provider was of the same race, the respondent was only 0.4 times as likely to report receiving advice. Among nonsmokers, the associations between structural variables and reported advice were much less important. Only gender concordance was significantly associated; if the regular provider was of the same gender, the respondent was 1.5 times as likely to report receiving advice on addictive behaviors (adjusted odds ratio = 1.5, 95% CI = 1.02, 2.22).

Two-fifths Did Not Receive Fitness Advice from Providers

Respondents in the CMHS were asked "During your care in the past year, did the doctor (health professional) talk to you about being the right weight, healthy eating, or exercise?" We reasoned that health care focused on health promotion should include such discussion, regardless of the respondent's current fitness level, for the health care provider to assess and advise each individual regarding an appropriate diet and exercise plan. Brief (ten-minute) dietary assessment and advice can be provided in primary care settings by primary care providers (Roe et al. 1994). However, only 59 percent of respondents reported receiving fitness advice from their health care provider; this included 57 percent of the men and 60 percent of the women.

Cross-tabulations. There were some differences in reported receipt of fitness advice between smokers and nonsmokers, among race/ethnicity groups, and between genders within race/ethnicity groups (Table 12.8). The least likely to report receiving advice were Hispanic male smokers (48.8%), and the most likely to receive advice were African American female nonsmokers (68.6%). Smoking status was not associated with receipt of fitness advice. Also, including an adjustment for smoking status in the multivariate models did not affect the association between other variables and receipt of fitness advice (data not shown).

Multivariate results. Race/ethnicity—but not gender—were significantly associated with receiving fitness advice (Table 12.9). After adjusting for the other sociodemographic variables and the socioeconomic and structural variables, African Americans and Hispanics were 1.7 times as likely to report receiving fitness advice as were whites. Surprisingly, none of the socioeconomic variables was significantly associated with the reported receipt of advice. In contrast, individuals who had a regular provider were 2.7 times as likely as those without a regular provider to report receiving fitness advice, and individuals of the same gender as their provider were 1.5 times as likely to have received advice as those of the opposite gender. Concordance by race/ethnicity was not significantly associated with reported receipt of fitness advice (Table 12.9).

Table 12.8   Percentage of Respondents Whose Providers Talked to Them about Being the Right Weight, Healthy Eating, or Exercise

	Among Smokers		Among Nonsmokers		Total	
	% Yes	N^a	% Yes	N	% Yes	N
African American						
Male	57.7	43	63.2	123	61.8	166
Female	52.4	35	68.6	185	66.1	219
Hispanic						
Male	48.8	28	59.5	81	56.7	109
Female	68.1	14	66.6	106	66.8	120
White						
Male	54.9	308	57.9	797	57.1	1,105
Female	55.8	319	60.4	1,041	59.3	1,360

Source: Data from The Commonwealth Fund Minority Health Survey, 1994.

Note: Weighted data, limited to those who accessed care in the previous twelve months.

[a]Rounded to whole number.

Table 12.9 Provider's Advice to All Patients about Being the Right Weight, Healthy Eating, or Exercise (multiple logistic regression models)

	MODEL 1		MODEL 2		MODEL 3	
	AOR[a]	95% CI[b]	AOR	95% CI	AOR	95% CI
Sociodemographic						
Female	1.2	0.92,1.46	1.1	0.89,1.42	1.2	0.91,1.71
Race/ethnicity						
African American	1.4	1.10,1.73	1.4	1.13,1.80	1.7	1.24,2.24
Hispanic	1.3	1.01,1.57	1.3	1.06,1.70	1.7	1.23,2.25
Age						
18–39	0.7	0.47,0.90	0.7	0.47,1.05	0.8	0.53,1.20
40–64	0.9	0.68,1.30	1.1	0.71,1.57	1.2	0.77,1.24
Married	1.2	0.96,1.55	1.2	0.91,1.54	1.1	0.87,1.48
Socioeconomic						
Employment status						
Employed			0.8	0.59,1.15	0.8	0.59,1.17
Unemployed			0.8	0.49,1.41	0.9	0.55,1.62
Income						
<$7,500			1.0	0.60,1.56	1.0	0.64,1.70
$7,500–$15,000			1.2	0.77,1.87	1.4	0.87,2.24
$15,001–$25,000			0.9	0.61,1.29	1.0	0.65,1.40
$25,001–$35,000			1.2	0.83,1.76	1.3	0.86,1.87
$35,001–$50,000			0.9	0.64,1.27	0.9	0.62,1.25
Does not own home			1.0	0.73,1.27	1.1	0.82,1.45
Number in household			1.0	1.00,1.01	1.0	1.00,1.01
Education						
<High school			0.7	0.46,1.05	0.7	0.47,1.10
High school/ some college			1.0	0.79,1.36	1.0	0.79,1.37
Structural						
Has regular provider					2.6	1.71,4.08
Regular provider of same race					1.1	0.81,1.51
Regular provider of same sex					1.5	1.06,2.13

Source: Data from The Commonwealth Fund Minority Health Survey, 1994.

Note: Referent categories: male, white, age >64, unmarried, not in labor force, income >$50,000, owns home, completed college, does not have regular provider, regular provider is not of same race, regular provider is not of same sex.

[a]AOR = adjusted odds ratio (adjusted for other variables in the model).

[b]95% CI = 95% confidence interval.

POLICY IMPLICATIONS

Increase, Target, and Improve Counseling on Addictive Behaviors

Less-educated adults smoke more, irrespective of their race/ethnicity, suggesting that health promotion and smoking cessation programs need to focus more attention on improving success for adults with less than a college education. Among the less-educated smokers, there may be more resistance to accepting the fact that smoking causes disease (Brownson et al. 1992). Coupled with the results that characteristics of providers predict "quit smoking" counseling messages, these findings point to the need for changes in smoking cessation counseling within health care settings. This is especially true for African American and Hispanic smokers who are less likely to report hearing advice. Either messages are not being delivered equally to all socioeconomic, ethnic, and racial groups, or the messages from providers are not being delivered in ways that these individuals perceive and can use to change their behaviors.

One effective intervention is to train medical students how to counsel their smoking patients. A well-tested methodology is the National Cancer Institute program designed to provide clinicians with better skills not only to ask and advise about smoking behavior but also to provide assistance and arrange for follow-up services (Coultas et al. 1994). Another effective intervention to increase provider advice is the insertion of reminders in patients' charts (Chang, Zimmerman, and Beck 1995).

Smokers who have a regular provider were far more likely to report receipt of advice. Perhaps the rapport developed over time permits messages to be given—or conversely, to be heard better when given. It is troubling that the increasing pressure of health care competition is leading to reduced provider time with patients and to providing care in larger, more anonymous practices. These trends may result in even fewer adults being seen by a regular provider who has enough time to give effective "stop smoking" counseling.

Gender concordance was positively associated with provider advice on addictive behaviors to nonsmokers. The direction of the association was the same, albeit not statistically significant, for smokers. As women increasingly join the medical profession, gender concordance may increase and thereby increase comfort levels for providing—and receiving—needed advice on addictive behaviors. We also found that if the regular provider was of the same race, the smoker was less than one-half as likely to report receiving advice. Because the vast majority of race/ethnicity concordance is within the white group, this suggests that regular minority providers give more advice to quit smoking than do regular white providers.

Putting all these factors together, one recommendation to increase effective smoking cessation counseling in large, managed care practices would be to recruit and train peer counselors matched for race/ethnicity and gender with the patients. Peer counselors are individuals who have successfully stopped smoking. Peer counselors should also be matched with clients by educational level. These peer counselors could provide a continuity of service—becoming "regular providers" to smokers—so that they develop the level of trust and rapport needed to deliver an effective "stop smoking" message.

Differences in reported smoking among men and women not currently in the workforce probably represent social class differences not measured by income and education. It may be that men not currently in the workforce include a larger proportion of retired people, and women not currently in the workforce also include stay-at-home mothers and married women choosing not to work. Among women, being married was protective of smoking. Thus, with marital status in the model for females, the relationship between workforce participation and smoking became attenuated because of the correlation between being married and not being in the workforce. Regardless of the reason being employed characterizes male smokers, it is clear that smoking cessation programs should be targeted both within the workplace and among people actively seeking employment, as well as among unmarried women.

The association we found between younger age and greater smoking may be related more to the cross-sectional nature of the sample than to a real effect of increased smoking among younger adults. Decreased life expectancy of smokers means that they would be under-represented in an older, ambulatory group. Nevertheless, the concentration of current smokers among younger men and women suggests that effective "quit smoking" messages can save lives—but that those messages must appeal to young adults.

Eliminating smoking is a key public health goal in its own right. However, eliminating smoking will not eliminate excess morbidity and mortality among minority populations. One of our most striking findings is the confirmation that both Hispanic and African American men and women smoke less than white men and women do, irrespective of their income or educational status or other measures of SES.

This is not a new finding, but it emphasizes the need for policymakers as well as public health researchers to go beyond the "traditional" risk factor of smoking if racial and ethnic disparities in chronic disease incidence and mortality are to be reduced. Why, for example, do African Americans experience the highest death rates from smoking among all groups in this country (Manley 1997)? Are interventions to prevent cardiovascular disease—mainly tested in white populations—applicable to minority populations (Pearson, Jenkins, and Thomas 1991)? Why is nicotine dependence more strongly associated with health problems in African Americans than in whites (Andreski and Breslau 1993)? These are only a few of the research questions which must be answered before fully effective smoking prevention, cessation, and amelioration interventions can be developed and tested.

Routine Health Care Practice Should Incorporate Fitness Counseling

A clear target for reducing the racial/ethnic gap in chronic disease morbidity and mortality would be increasing physical fitness and decreasing obesity in minority populations. Information regarding diet from the CMHS confirms results from other national and regional surveys that few Americans maintain healthy diets (Serdula et al. 1995). African Americans eat less well than whites, and this difference is not explained by differences in SES. Perhaps contextual factors, such as the unavailability of inexpensive fruits and vegetables in neighborhood grocery stores, contribute to poorer diets (Adrogue and Wesson 1996). Conversely, the difference between Hispanics and whites becomes non-significant with adjustment for socioeconomic factors. This suggests that health and diet messages need to be culturally relevant, including desirable foods and food preparation within the cultural context of the racial and ethnic groups.

There is a strong negative association between education and good dietary habits. This may be a combination of knowledge and eating foods that are culturally defined as preferred. It may also reflect the fact that as a cross-sectional survey, this study captures the process of translating health habits from the most to the least educated. The perceived cost of healthy foods can also contribute to less healthy diets among poorer and less-educated people (Cotunga et al. 1992). The association between obesity and low SES is well-documented, but the direction of causation is controversial. That is, it is not clear whether people are obese because they are poor or are poor because they are obese, or are both obese and poor for some other reason related to both factors (Sorensen 1995). For whatever reasons, the least-educated group of

Americans is in need of targeted health promotion to help them achieve healthy dietary habits.

As found in other surveys of dietary habits, more women than men in the CMHS report eating well. Perhaps women have been more exposed to dietary messages through magazines, television, and other media. Even among the women, however, there is much room for improvement. More than one-third still report less-than-optimal dietary habits. Perhaps for different reasons, young adults and individuals in the workforce report having poorer eating habits than others. These segments of the population probably represent "groups on the go," who rely heavily on fast food rather than on having time to prepare food at home. There is a need to explore where, when, and how food is consumed so that fitness counselors can tailor their advice to the realities of individuals' daily lives.

After adjusting for the other sociodemographic variables and the socioeconomic and structural variables, African Americans and Hispanics were almost twice as likely to report receiving fitness advice as were whites. African and Hispanic American adults have a higher prevalence of physical conditions—such as diabetes and hypertension—that are notably affected by diet and fitness. If providers are selectively providing fitness advice to patients whom they perceive to be at highest risk of diet- or exercise-related chronic disease, this may explain the nearly twofold reported higher likelihood that the minority populations are receiving fitness advice.

It is appropriate for people with identified risk factors or chronic health conditions to receive targeted fitness advice. However, only about one-half of American adults report that they eat a diet low in fat and high in fruits and vegetables at least four times a week, and far too few are hearing from their health care providers that they should improve their diet, exercise regularly, and control their weight. All individuals who access health care should be assessed for the adequacy of their diet, weight, and exercise regimen. As they grow older, even the most fit clients need periodic assessments to determine whether their fitness routine is appropriate for their age.

Intensive Health Promotion Campaigns Should Target Sedentary Lifestyles

With respect to vigorous exercise, employed men were not distinguishable statistically from men not in the workforce. This is an interesting finding, in that both unemployed men and men not in the workforce for other reasons (e.g., retirement or disability) theoretically have more time than do men in the active work force to introduce a vigorous exercise routine into their daily life. Unemployed men may be too preoccupied, depressed, or worried to attend to health promotion. Paradoxically, a vigorous exercise program might help them cope with some of their anxieties and better prepare them for re-entry into the workforce.

The results of this survey suggest that a community-based campaign should also address how very busy adults can incorporate routine, vigorous exercise into their hectic lifestyles. Individuals with more leisure time—such as unmarried women, men not in the labor force, and the wealthiest segment of the population—are more likely to report a healthy exercise program. However, these factors are not highly predictive. What is striking is that virtually none of the sociodemographic, socioeconomic, or structural variables we examined explained the diverse patterns of exercise behavior.

More than three-fourths of the adult population in the survey reported that they did not have a strong exercise routine; four out of five women did not exercise hard at least four times a week. These figures point to the need for an aggressive, all-out campaign to change adult behaviors. Now that a sedentary lifestyle is being recognized as a major factor for cardiovascular disease, as well as a contributing factor to chronic depression, it is vitally important that the health community turn its attention to these issues.

To be effective, a pro-exercise campaign must be based on more research that will uncover what motivates adults to exercise and how to motivate those who do not. Messages designed to promote a more active lifestyle will need to be tailored to appeal to each racial/ethnic and gender subpopulation. For this to be successful, targeted behavioral science research must answer questions about what motivates each of these subgroups.

References

Adrogue, H. J., and Wesson, D. E. 1996. Role of dietary factors in the hypertension of African Americans. *Seminars in Nephrology* 16(2):94–101.

Anderssen, N., Jacobs, D. R., Jr., Sidney, S., Bild, D. E., Sternfeld, B., Slattery, M. L., and Hannan, P. 1996. Change and secular trends in physical activity patterns in young adults: a seven-year longitudinal followup in the Coronary Artery Risk Development in Young Adults Study (CARDIA). *American Journal of Epidemiology* 143(4):351–362.

Andreski P, and Breslau, N. 1993. Smoking and nicotine dependence in young adults: difference between blacks and whites. *Drug and Alcohol Dependence* 32(2):119–125.

Anonymous. 1992a. Behavioral risk factor survey of Vietnamese—California, 1991. *Morbidity and Mortality Weekly Report* 41(5):69–72.

Anonymous. 1992b. Behavioral risk factor survey of Chinese—California, 1989. Morbidity and Mortality Weekly Report 41(16):266–270.

Anonymous. 1992c. Cigarette smoking among adults—United States, 1990. *Morbidity and Mortality Weekly Report* 41(20):354–355, 361–362.

Anonymous. 1992d. Cigarette smoking among Southeast Asian immigrants—Washington State, 1989. *Morbidity and Mortality Weekly Report* 41(45):854–855, 861.

Bachman, J. G., Wallace, J. M., Jr., O'Malley, P. M., Johnston, L. D., Kurth, C. L., and Neighbors, N. W. 1991. Racial/ethnic differences in smoking, drinking, and illicit drug use among American high school seniors, 1976–89. *American Journal of Public Health* 81(3):372–377.

Beckman, S. I., Os, I., Kjeldsen, S. E., Eide, I. K., Westheim, A. S., and Hjermann, I. 1995. Effect of dietary counseling on blood pressure and arterial plasma catecholamines in primary hypertension. *American Journal of Hypertension* 8(7):704–711.

Bild, D. E., Jacobs, D. R., Jr., Sidney, S., Haskell, W. L., Anderssen, N., and Oberman, A. 1993. Physical activity in young black and white women. The CARDIA Study. *Annals of Epidemiology* 3(6):636–644.

Boardley, D. J., Sargent, R. G., Coker, A. L., Hussey, J. R., and Sharpe, P. A. 1995. The relationship between diet, activity, and other factors, and postpartum weight change by race. *Obstetrics and Gynecology* 86(5):834–838.

Brink, S. G., Gottlieb, N. H., McLeroy, K. R., Wisotzky, M., and Burdine, J. N. 1994. A community view of smoking cessation counseling in the practices of physicians and dentists. *Public Health Reports* 109(1):135–142.

Broman, C. L. 1995. Leisure-time physical activity in an African-American population. *Journal of Behavioral Medicine* 18(4):341–353.

Brownson, R. C., Jackson-Thompson, J., Wilkerson, J. C., Davis, J. R., Owens, N. W., and Fisher, E. B., Jr. 1992. Demographic and socioeconomic differences in beliefs about the health effects of smoking. *American Journal of Public Health* 82(1):99–103.

Burke, G. I., Savage, P. J., Manolio, T. A., Sprafka, J. M., Wagenknecht, L. E., Sidney, S., Perkins, L. L., Liu, K., and Jacobs, D. R., Jr. 1992. Correlates of obesity in young black and white women. The CARDIA Study. *American Journal of Public Health* 82(12):1621–1625.

Chang, H. C., Zimmerman, L. H., and Beck, J. M. 1995. Impact of chart reminders on smoking cessation practices of pulmonary physicians. *American Journal of Respiratory and Critical Care Medicine* 152(3):984–987.

Clark, D. O. 1995. Racial and educational differences in physical activity among older adults. *Gerontologist* 35(4):472–480.

Cotugna, N., Subar, A. F., Heimendinger, J., and Kahle, L. 1992. Nutrition and cancer prevention knowledge, beliefs, attitudes, and practices: the 1987 National Interview Study. *Journal of the American Dietetic Association* 92(8): 963–968.

Coultas, D. B., Klecan, D. A., Whitten, R. M., Obenshain, S. S., Rubin, R. H., Wiese, W. H., Wilson, B. E., Woodall, G. W., and Stidley, C. A. 1994. Training medical students in smoking-cessation counseling. *Academic Medicine* 69(10 Suppl):S48–S50.

Cox, R. H., Parker, G. G., Watson, A. C., Robinson, S. H., Simonson, C. F., Elledge, J. C., Diggs, S., and Smith, E. 1995. Dietary cancer risk of low-income women and change with intervention. *Journal of the American Dietetic Association* 95(9):1031–1034.

Crespo, C. J., Keteyian, S. J., Heath, G. W., and Sempos, C. T. 1996. Leisure-time physical activity among U.S. adults. Results from the Third National Health and Nutrition Examination Survey. *Archives of Internal Medicine* 156(1):93–98.

Escobedo, L. G., Anda, R. F., Smith, P. F., Remington, P. L., and Mast, E. E. 1990. Sociodemographic characteristics of cigarette smoking initiation in the United States. Implications for smoking prevention policy. *Journal of the American Medical Association* 264(12):1550–1555.

Feigelman, W., and Gorman, B. 1989. Toward explaining the higher incidence of cigarette smoking among black Americans. *Journal of Psychoactive Drugs* 21(3):299–305

Feigelman, W., and Lee, J. 1995. Probing the paradoxical pattern of cigarette smoking among African-Americans: low teenage consumption and high adult use. *Journal of Drug Education* 25(4):307–320.

Felton, G. M., and Parsons, M. A. 1994. Factors influencing physical activity in average-weight and overweight young women. *Journal of Community Health Nursing* 11(2):109–119.

Fiore, M. C., Novotny, T. E., Pierce, J. P., Hatziandreu, E. J., Patel, K. M., and Davis, R. M. 1989. Trends in cigarette smoking in the United states. The changing influence of gender and race. *Journal of the American Medical Association* 261(1):49–55.

Flint, A. J., and Novotny, T. E. 1998. Trends in black/white differences in current smoking among 18- to 24-year-olds in the United States, 1983-1993. *American Journal of Preventive Medicine* 14(1):19–24.

Friedman, C., Brownson, R. C., Peterson, D. E., and Wilkerson, J. C. 1994. Physician advice to reduce chronic disease risk factors. *American Journal of Preventive Medicine* 10(6):367–371.

Gritz, E. R., Prokhorov, A. V., Hudmon, K. S., Chamberlain, R. M., Taylor, W. C., DiClemente, C. C., Johnston, D. A., Hu, S., Jones, L. A., Jones, M. M., Rosenblum, C. K., Ayars, C. L., and Amos, C. I. 1998. Cigarette smoking in a multiethnic population of youth: methods and baseline findings. *Preventive Medicine* 27(3):365–384.

Hurt, R. D., Dale, L. C., Fredrickson, P. A., Caldwell, C. C., Lee, G. A., Offord, K. P., Lauger, G. G., Marusic, Z., Neese, L. W., and Lundberg, T. G. 1994. Nicotine patch therapy for smoking cessation combined with physician advice and nurse follow-up. One-year outcome and percentage of nicotine replacement. *Journal of the American Medical Association* 271(8):595–600.

Lopez, T. K., Marshall, J. A., Shetterly, S. M., Baxter, J., and Hamman, R. F. 1995. Ethnic differences in micronutrient intake in a rural biethnic population. *American Journal of Preventive Medicine* 11(5):301–305.

Loria, C. M., Bush, T. L., Carroll, M. D., Looker, A. C., McDowell, M. A., Johnson, C. L., and Sempos, C. T. 1995. Macronutrient intakes among adult Hispanics: a comparison of Mexican Americans, Cuban Americans, and mainland Puerto Ricans. *American Journal of Public Health* 85(5):684–689.

Louis Harris and Associates. 1994. *Health Care Services and Minority Groups: A Comparative Survey of Whites, African-Americans, Hispanics and Asian-Americans.* New York: Louis Harris and Associates, Inc.

Macera, C. A., Croft, J. B., Brown, D. R., Ferguson, J. E., and Lane, M. J. 1995. Predictors of adopting leisure-time physical activity among a biracial community cohort. *American Journal of Epidemiology* 142(6):629–635.

Manley, A. F. 1997. Cardiovascular implications of smoking: the surgeon general's point of view. *Journal of Health Care for the Poor and Underserved* 8(3):303–310.

Neighbor, W. E., Jr., Stoop, D. H., and Ellsworth, A. 1994. Smoking cessation counseling among hospitalized smokers. *American Journal of Preventive Medicine* 10(3):140–144.

Patterson, B. H., Harlan, L. C., Block, G., and Kahle, L. 1995. Food choices of whites, blacks, and Hispanics: data from the 1987 National Health Interview Survey. *Nutrition and Cancer* 23(2):105–119.

Pearson, T. A., Jenkins, G. M., and Thomas, J. 1991. Prevention of coronary heart disease in black adults. *Cardiovascular Clinics* 21(3):263–276.

Perez-Stable, E. F., Marin, G., Marin, B. V. 1994. Behavioral risk factors: a comparison of Latinos and non-Latino whites in San Francisco. *American Journal of Public Health* 84(6):971–976.

Roe, L., Strong, C., Whiteside, C., Neil, A., and Mant, D. 1994. Dietary intervention in primary care: validity of the DINE method for diet assessment. *Family Practice* 11(4):375–381.

Royce, J. M., Ashford, A., Resnicow, K., Freman, H. P., Caesar, A. A., and Orlandi, M. A. 1995. Physician and nurse-assisted smoking cessation in Harlem. *Journal of the National Medical Association* 87(4):291–300.

Sanders-Phillips, K. 1994. Health promotion behavior in low income Black and Latino women. *Women and Health* 21(2/3):71–83.

Serdula, M. K., Coates, R. J., Byers, T., Simoes, E., Mokdad, A. H., and Subar, A. F. 1995. Fruit and vegetable intake among adults in 16 states: results of a brief telephone survey. *American Journal of Public Health* 85(2):236–239.

Sherman, S. E., and Hershman, W. Y. 1993. Exercise counseling: how do general internists do? *Journal of Internal Medicine* 8(5):243–248.

Shimakawa, T., Sorlie, P., Carpenter, M. A., Dennis, B., Tell, G. S., Watson, R., and Williams, O. D. 1994. Dietary intake patterns and sociodemographic factors in the atherosclerosis risk in communities study. ARIC Study Investigators. *Preventive Medicine* 23(6):769–780.

Sorensen, T. I. A. 1995. Socio-economic aspects of obesity. *International Journal of Obesity* 19(Suppl 6):s6–s8.

Swanson, C. A., Gridley, G., Greenberg, R. S., Schoenberg, J. B., Swanson, G. M., Brown, L. M., Hayes, R., Silverman, D., and Pottern, L. 1993. A comparison of diets of blacks and whites in three areas of the United States. *Nutrition and Cancer* 20(2):153–165.

Wagenknecht, L. E., Burke, G. L., Perkins, L. L., Haley, N. J., and Friedman, G. D. 1992. Misclassification of smoking status in the CARDIA study: a comparison of self-report with serum cotinine levels. *American Journal of Public Health* 82(1):33–36.

Washburn, R. A., Kline, G., Lackland, D. T., and Wheeler, F. C. 1992. Leisure time physical activity: are there black/white differences? *Preventive Medicine* 21(1):127–135.

Wiecha, J. M. 1996. Differences in patterns of tobacco use in Vietnamese, African-American, Hispanic, and Caucasian adolescents in Worcester, Massachusetts. *American Journal of Preventive Medicine* 12(1):29–37.

Winkleby, M. A., Schooler, C., Kraemer, H. C., Lin, J., and Fortmann, S. P. 1995. Hispanic versus white smoking patterns by sex and level of education. *American Journal of Epidemiology* 142(4):410–418.

13

A Look to the Future

Karen Scott Collins, M.D., M.P.H.
Allyson G. Hall, Ph.D.

The U.S population is becoming more ethnically diverse. Nearly 25 percent of the population is currently identified as a racial or ethnic minority, and the number is expected to grow to 40 percent by 2030 (Day 1996). Much of that growth will be among Hispanic and Asian populations, including more recent immigrant groups. Yet, the health care system does not serve minority populations well. Many recent studies document continuing problems in access to primary and specialty care and continued poorer health outcomes for minority groups (Lillie-Blanton, Leigh, and Alfaro-Correa 1996). Providing quality health care to an increasingly diverse population is an important issue facing the U.S. health care system.

The chapters in this book speak to this issue with important information from The Commonwealth Fund Minority Health Survey (CMHS). The researchers' analyses provide greater understanding of the health care challenges of an increasingly diverse patient population—and the extent to which these challenges are compounded by or are attributable to lower income and education. Common themes running throughout all of the chapters point to the health disadvantages experienced by minority populations, particularly with respect to access to health care. Minorities are more likely than others to be uninsured, not to have a regular source of care, to have limited choices in seeking medical care, and to delay seeking medical care. Minorities also are less likely than others to be satisfied with their medical care, are likely to have lower rates of utilization, and are likely to be in poor health, results at least in part due to access difficulties.

The lower socioeconomic status (SES) of minority groups to some extent explains the inability of many minority groups to adequately access and use the health care system. Overall, minorities are less educated and earn lower incomes than their white counterparts. Low-income, less-educated individuals and families tend to be in poorer health and to have a harder time getting needed medical care.

Several chapters point out that discrimination—real or perceived—influences individuals' utilization of and satisfaction with the health care system. This real or perceived discrimination, whether based on race or ethnicity, gender, age, health status, or income level, seems to occur more often in minority groups, particularly among African Americans. However, our findings also demonstrate that when patients are satisfied with the interpersonal skills of and the amount of time spent with their clinicians, the perception of discrimination seems to disappear. The way health care programs are financed and structured also affects patient experiences. Feelings of discrimination appear to be more common among Medicaid beneficiaries and less common among those on Medicare.

This work also highlights the importance of gaining a more complex understanding of minority health in this country. Although there are common themes across groups, the experiences of different subgroups of people often differ in significant ways. For example, reasons for uninsurance differ across the three subgroups of Asian Americans in the survey. Puerto Ricans are more likely to have public insurance than other Hispanic groups, and symptoms of stress differ between Caribbean-born and U.S.-born blacks. Newer immigrant subgroups are not likely to be acculturated to the U.S. health care system, and they encounter significant challenges in accessing that system. Ignoring these subgroup differences will result in ineffective policies to improve access to care and resulting health status.

In the years since 1994, when the CMHS was conducted, the health care system has continued to struggle to find a balance between controlling costs and providing access to quality care. With only small, incremental steps taken by policymakers toward expanding insurance coverage, the problems of the uninsured continue to grow. The current health care environment, unlike that in 1994, is one of managed care and competition. Many providers who have traditionally served minority populations now face uncertain futures, and there is no clear sense of whether other providers will fulfill this mission. Managed care has produced renewed concerns about access, but it also has the potential to shape improvements through quality initiatives. The concerns and experiences of different minority populations must be considered within this changing system.

This chapter will consider the lessons learned throughout this volume, in the context of the current health care system, and discuss those areas of policy and health services improvement that will better meet the needs of a racially and ethnically diverse American population. These areas include improving insurance coverage, maintaining a safety net, assuring access and quality in managed care, strengthening a diverse health care workforce, reducing socioeconomic disparities and racial discrimination, and improving data on minority populations and health.

EXPAND INSURANCE COVERAGE FOR THE UNINSURED

The percentage of our population without health insurance reached 16 percent in 1997—or 43 million Americans (Bennefield 1997). Despite strong economic times, insurance coverage is declining among all groups—especially among those who are low income and were heretofore eligible for Medicaid.

Minority populations remain at higher risk than others for not having health insurance. In 1997, 21 percent of African Americans, 34 percent of Hispanics, and 21 percent of Asians were uninsured (Bennefield 1997). Based on data from the Kaiser/Commonwealth Survey of Health Insurance in 1996 over a two-year period, 37 percent of African Americans and 44 percent of Hispanics were not continuously insured. Both the uninsured and those without continuous coverage describe significantly greater difficulties accessing different types of health services, including primary care and prescriptions (Henry J. Kaiser Family Foundation / The Commonwealth Fund 1997).

Economic disparities are important contributors to the disparities in insurance coverage. Minority populations remain more likely to live in poverty, to have lower education levels, and to be unemployed. Nearly 30 percent of African Americans and Hispanics live below the poverty level. From available national data, nearly one-half of Hispanics have less than a high school education, and unemployment rates for African Americans and Hispanics are twice the rate for white Americans (authors' tabulations of the March 1997 Current Population Survey).

Economic disparities do not explain all health insurance coverage disparities. Minorities are less likely to have insurance coverage regardless of their employment or income level (Hall et al. 1999). For example, 37 percent of Hispanic full-time workers are uninsured, compared to

20 percent of African American workers and 12 percent of white workers. Even within firms that traditionally provide health insurance to their workers, minorities are less likely to have coverage than others. In manufacturing firms, only 71 percent of African American workers and 60 percent of Hispanic workers have employer-sponsored coverage, compared to 85 percent of white workers. Among low-wage workers who earn less than seven dollars an hour, 56 percent of whites and 47 percent of African Americans have employer coverage, compared to 35 percent of Hispanics.

Not surprisingly, then, surveys continue to show that minorities have more difficulty gaining access to care, and they are more likely to use emergency rooms or hospitals for their regular care. In the racially and ethnically diverse population of New York City, minority adults under age 65 have reported greater difficulty getting needed health care compared to whites. Thirty-eight percent of Hispanics, 28 percent of blacks, and 27 percent of Asian Americans have reported having some difficulty getting needed health care, compared to only 19 percent of whites (Sandman et al. 1998).

Minority populations would have much to gain from policies expanding health insurance coverage or making coverage affordable. Because there is no single solution to the problem of the uninsured minority population, several areas of policy must continue to be developed. Short of a national policy of universal coverage, reducing the numbers of uninsured African Americans, Hispanics, Asian Americans, and other minorities will have to be addressed through several types of incremental reforms.

Economic disparities mean that publicly supported or subsidized programs will continue to be a cornerstone of health care access for many minority populations. Building on current public programs through active outreach and enrollment, extending eligibility, or providing ways to "buy in" to programs could assist those with low incomes. By expanding eligibility to include pregnant women and children in the late 1980s, Medicaid now provides insurance and increased access to care for over 30 million adults and children in low-income families (Kaiser Commission on Medicaid and the Uninsured 1998). The current challenges include making sure that those who are eligible for Medicaid have every opportunity to enroll. Three groups require special attention—children, families who have transitioned from welfare to work, and legal immigrants. Diverse minority populations are disproportionately represented within each of these groups. Policies that weaken

Medicaid coverage or benefits, or complicate enrollment, will undoubtedly harm low-income minorities.

The State Child Health Insurance Program (CHIP) enacted in 1997 should insure about one-third of the 11 million uninsured children in the United States (American Academy of Pediatrics 1998). Extending this insurance program to the parents of these children could provide affordable family coverage to those working families who do not qualify for Medicaid, but whose employers do not provide coverage.

As with the overall uninsured population, members of the minority population who are uninsured are typically working—participating in the workforce in some way. For those who own or work in small businesses, such as many Korean Americans, state insurance policies that facilitate purchasing pools can make insurance affordable. As some of the authors in this volume point out, we also need to move beyond affordability to make sure that information about insurance coverage and how it works is communicated clearly in diverse communities.

Along with these important steps toward providing health insurance for the U.S. population, policymakers, legislators and advocates must continue to create broad public will and support for universal coverage. We must also continue our careful analyses to develop long-term financing strategies and study the impact of different policies on different populations. The Commonwealth Fund recently initiated a Task Force on Health Insurance for Working Families that will contribute toward these kinds of activities.

MAINTAIN THE SAFETY NET

With the number of uninsured people growing, and no real solution in sight, it will be critical to maintain providers able and willing to care for the uninsured. Safety-net providers—such as public hospitals, community health centers, and health departments—have traditionally played a large role in caring for ethnically diverse populations and the uninsured across the country. Public hospitals report serving a patient population that is 23 percent African American and 25 percent Hispanic; some 32 percent speak a language other than English (Gaskin and Hadley 1997). Over 70 percent of the inpatient care that public hospitals provide is for Medicaid and self-pay patients. Uncompensated care represented almost 30 percent of gross charges accrued by public hospitals (National Association of Public Hospitals and Health Systems 1997). Similarly, 66 percent of community health center patients are members of minority groups; almost 4 million are uninsured; and another 3.6 million are Medicaid recipients (Hawkins and Rosenbaum 1998). These safety-net providers report growth in their numbers of uninsured patients, and they are seeing long-term patients return to them even after they have been enrolled in managed care plans with other providers.

Safety-net providers have a strong history of developing programs that meet the social and cultural needs of their patients, in addition to providing health care regardless of ability to pay. For this reason, safety-net providers are important resources in many low-income minority communities. A 1997 survey found that public hospitals in New York City were caring for half of the uninsured, working-age adults and one-quarter of Medicaid beneficiaries. The extensive safety-net system has made care more available to uninsured New Yorkers than it is for the uninsured nationally (Sandman et al. 1998).

Increasingly, safety-net providers face many challenges as their ability to cross-subsidize care decreases because of managed care and competition. In the past, much of the uncompensated care was financed from revenues from Medicaid patients as well as direct subsidies from local, state, and national governments, including disproportionate hospital share payments. Now, public financing of these providers is declining as Medicaid managed care plans shift Medicaid patients to non-safety-net hospitals. As a result, safety-net hospitals are experiencing reductions in their Medicaid patients and revenues to support their safety-net missions.

This trend will continue to increase, unfortunately, as states implement the mandatory Medicaid managed care programs stipulated in the Balanced Budget Act of 1997. This Act also reduced disproportionate share hospital payments and the Medicare graduate medical education payments to hospitals; it restricts the reimbursements to federally qualified health centers. These changes will further reduce revenues to safety-net providers, which will affect their ability to care for the uninsured. Changes in payment policies also heighten the importance of making certain that federal and state policies truly reach and reimburse the providers serving disproportionately high numbers of Medicaid, uninsured, and vulnerable populations.

State and local policies to pay for charity care through an uninsured pool—to which health care insurers and providers contribute—make a difference in strengthening the safety-net providers. Massachusetts is an example of such an uncompensated care pool, supported primarily by a provider tax on acute care hospitals (Chapman and Johnson 1998). This is one way that safety-net providers could continue to provide care to the uninsured.

States such as Massachusetts also strengthen safety-net providers through Medicaid policies that help safety-net providers participate in Medicaid managed care. Community health centers automatically qualify as providers in MassHealth, the Medicaid managed care program in Massachusetts (Chapman and Johnson 1998). The California Medi-Cal program has also developed policies to increase the inclusion of traditional providers in managed care networks. More mainstream health plans have received Medicaid contracts based on the extent to which they include traditional community providers. As a result of these requirements, many traditional providers have been able to participate in managed care arrangements (Coye and Alvarez 1998).

The safety-net providers themselves also have to respond to the real changes in the health care system. Issues of quality reporting on performance and accountability are receiving increased attention, especially within managed care. Health care providers must show they can provide quality care within a cost-conscious environment. More efficient ways of providing care and competing will mean different kinds of mergers for some. Others will create their own managed care plans. All will require careful strategic management and leadership.

THE SHIFT TO MANAGED CARE: ASSURE ACCESS, QUALITY, SATISFACTION, AND CULTURAL COMPETENCE

As with the overall insured population, minorities with insurance coverage are now more likely to be in a managed care plan. The number of Medicaid beneficiaries in managed care has grown substantially over the last six years. In 1991, 2.6 million beneficiaries (or 9.5% of the total Medicaid population) were enrolled in some form of managed care. By 1997, 15.3 million Medicaid beneficiaries, representing 47.8 percent of the Medicaid population, were enrolled in managed care plans (Health Care Financing Administration 1998). Medicaid managed care should continue to grow substantially because the Balanced Budget Act of 1997 permits mandatory enrollment of Medicaid beneficiaries into managed care.

Increases in managed care enrollment for employer-sponsored insurance are also occurring. In 1993, only 32 percent of individuals and families covered by employers were in managed care (defined as preferred provider and health maintenance plans). By 1997, this number had increased to 64 percent (KPMG Peat Marwick 1998). The Commonwealth Fund analysis of the Medical Expenditure Panel Survey shows that in 1997, 62 percent of commercially insured African Americans, 65 percent of Hispanics, and 51 percent of whites were in managed care (authors' tabulation). This transition to managed care in both the public and private sectors has become an important policy issue in minority health because of concerns about the health plans' capacity to care for the special needs of vulnerable, culturally diverse populations.

Minority Patient Experiences with Managed Care

We have limited information on minority experiences with managed care. Early concerns have included further limitations on access to care for minorities, or a perpetuation of discriminatory practices, such as the creation of care barriers through enrollment procedures or separate provider networks for Medicaid beneficiaries (Rosenbaum et al. 1997). Very little analysis has been conducted on the impact that managed care has on the health services received by minorities. Work contained in this volume and documented elsewhere shows that minorities often receive different and poorer care than whites. Consequently, managed care utilization restrictions can have a greater negative impact on the availability and quality of care delivered to minorities than to others.

The literature is mixed on how managed care has affected the accessibility and quality of care delivered to enrollees and the population at large. Early studies suggest that managed care plans deliver care that is comparable to care provided under fee-for-service arrangements for general populations, but that some populations, such as those in poor health, minorities, and low-income people, may fare worse in managed care (Lurie et al. 1992; Wagner and Bledsoe 1990; Ware et al. 1986). Data from the Medical Outcomes Study suggest that enrollees in HMOs in poor health will have worse health outcomes compared to individuals in poor health who are in fee-for-service arrangements (Ware et al. 1996). A recent analysis of low-income individuals in five states found that managed care enrollees, whether in Medicaid or private insurance programs, report that they have had more problems obtaining health care and are more likely to be dissatisfied with their health plans than those in fee-for-service plans (Lillie-Blanton and Lyons 1998).

Changing patients to managed care has often meant disrupting patterns of care and changing physicians when enrolling in health plans (Davis et al. 1995). Lack of a regular provider appears to be greatest among individuals who have joined their health plans recently. However, a significant number of Medicaid and managed care enrollees in health plans for two years or more do not have a regular physician either (Lillie-Blanton and Lyons 1998). The chapters in this volume highlight the importance of established relationships with a regular health care provider. Patient experiences with the health care system, including feelings of discrimination or dissatisfaction with a physician's interpersonal skills, are linked to being less able to identify a long-term source of continuous care. Managed care, with its limits on provider choice and pressures to shorten physician visits, may very well hinder the development of long-term relationships between patients and providers.

Patient experiences, including satisfaction, are important aspects of quality of care. Surveys measuring satisfaction with health care often find lower rates among minority groups. The contributions in this volume highlight that significant factors related to satisfaction include no barriers to access, having a choice of providers, and having time with the physician. Because minority groups are less likely to experience these factors, this situation leads to greater levels of dissatisfaction. However, these factors can be remedied within policies related to access and coverage. It is also noteworthy that for some minority groups, particularly African Americans, satisfaction increases when they have a physician of the same race. Perceptions of trust, being able to talk about feelings of discrimination, and health provider understanding of cultural background are some aspects of patient-physician relationships that may explain increased satisfaction.

Because of sample size limitations, the CMHS could not be used to compare the health care experiences of managed care enrollees to individuals in fee-for-service plans across specific racial and ethnic categories. Nevertheless, comparisons between minorities and non-minorities indicate that more individuals in managed care have a regular provider compared to those in fee-for-service plans. For example, in the survey 28 percent of minority fee-for-service respondents did not have a regular provider, compared to 16 percent of managed care enrollees. Among white respondents, 18 percent had a regular provider in fee-for-service versus 11 percent in managed care. These results must be interpreted with caution, however. In 1994 when the CMHS was conducted, many managed care arrangements required enrollees to select a primary care physician to act as a "gatekeeper" to other more specialized services. Thus, at any point in time, managed care enrollees may be able to name a specific doctor who is in charge of their care. However, because

health plans change providers, patients change health plans, and beneficiaries cycle on and off Medicaid, it is unclear whether this identified
provider is actually a regular, continuous source of care.

Plans unaccustomed to serving Medicaid patients may not be totally
dedicated to the special needs of Medicaid patients. For example, health
plan enrollment and referral processes often become significant barriers
to care for minority low-income populations, especially among Medicaid
beneficiaries. Studies show that many Medicaid beneficiaries lack sufficient information to effectively navigate the managed care system (Molnar et al. 1996). As a result, many of these patients are auto-enrolled
into health plans and assigned to providers outside their neighborhoods.
Medicaid managed care plans may offer an inadequate number of primary care physicians and traditional safety-net providers who are accustomed to caring for these populations in their networks. Also, providers
included in plan networks may not accept new patients or may have long
waiting lists for appointments.

Complicated referral procedures can also restrict access to special-
ists. Medicaid beneficiaries who are new to managed care commonly do
not understand that a visit to a specialist often requires a referral from
their primary care physician. Thirty-three percent of minority managed
care enrollees in the CMHS said they had no access to specialty care.
Among whites in managed care, 24 percent reported no access to spe-
cialists.

In addition to providing insufficient education, some plans can be
faulted for marketing abuses such as intentionally misinforming beneficiaries about managed care and misrepresenting plan benefits. To perma-
nently prevent marketing abuses, states have begun to contract with enrollment brokers to enroll and educate Medicaid beneficiaries in an
unbiased manner.

There is an emerging consensus that community-based organizations
are an important resource for educating Medicaid beneficiaries who are
enrolled in managed care. Approximately half the states with Medicaid
managed care programs have or intend to contract with community-
based organizations to assist with education (Kenesson 1997). Many of
these agencies have developed culturally and linguistically appropriate
services, and they employ staff that mirror the populations they serve.
The Community Service Society (CSS) of New York has developed a
community-based model to educate Medicaid beneficiaries enrolled in
Harlem and South Bronx. The CSS curriculum consists of a low-literacy
handbook and participatory workshops, that engage Medicaid beneficia-

ries in dialogues about managed care. The curriculum focuses on teaching Medicaid beneficiaries how to choose a health plan that meets their family's needs, how to obtain services in a managed care system, and what to do when a problem arises. The program was initially implemented in New York City and has expanded to Los Angeles and Philadelphia.

Cultural Competence and Managed Care

Cultural competence has been defined as the "demonstrated awareness and integration of three population-specific issues: health-related beliefs and cultural values, disease incidence, and prevalence and treatment efficacy" (Lavizzo-Mourey and Mackenzie 1996). Many of the chapter authors highlight cultural competence as an important aspect of any discussion of quality of care for minority populations. Experiences and expectations related to patient-physician communication, perceptions of discrimination, health education, and patient understanding of insurance coverage information are some key areas where cultural competence plays a role. Research on the importance of cultural competence on health outcomes, while in the earliest stages, clearly demonstrates its benefits (Carrese and Rhodes 1995; Blackhall et al. 1995).

Managed care plans must strive to become culturally competent systems of care. System-wide cultural competence can occur at three levels: (1) ensuring that racially and ethnically diverse physicians, nurses, and other allied professionals make up the health workforce; (2) developing and supporting training programs that guarantee that all workers meet some minimal standard of cultural competency; and (3) collecting epidemiologic and survey data to better understand morbidities and health outcomes of various racial and ethnic groups (Lavizzo-Mourey, Mackenzie, and Taylor 1997).

Health Plan Initiatives and Public Policy

Health plans can undertake a number of initiatives that can improve the quality of health care their minority populations receive. Provider panels can be configured to enhance continuity of care by including providers who have experience with and typically care for low-income and racially and ethnically diverse populations. In particular, community health centers, minority health care providers, and physicians located in minority and low-income neighborhoods should be included in Medicaid managed care plans. Also, plan-wide systems to increase the use of preventive services can improve outreach and use of these services (Heiser and St. Peter 1997). Targeting these systems to populations still at risk for not receiving these services, and assessing their effectiveness, should be incorporated into health plan operations.

While time with physicians is being squeezed, particularly in managed care, this is critical to patient experiences (Collins, Schoen, and Khoransanizadeh 1997). For patients with different language or cultural backgrounds, this time builds trust and can facilitate educating patients about their health conditions. Where physician time cannot be extended, plans may have to explore additional ways of effectively educating patients.

We also need to assure quality services in health plans through public policy and practice. We must better target efforts to monitor the quality of care delivered by plans to their minority populations. Current health plan performance measures can miss key quality-of-care issues for minorities. For example, a plan's aggregate measure of diabetic control for all patients may miss problems in control among African American or Hispanic patients. Similarly, measuring the overall stage of breast cancer at diagnosis in a health plan may be a good level for women in general, but it could miss the fact that a large number of African American women have late-stage cancers at time of diagnosis. As an increasing number of minorities become enrolled in managed care, reliable and valid measurement tools must be in place to assess the quality of care delivered to these populations. With support from The Commonwealth Fund, Henry Ford Health Systems is developing a set of performance measures that would assess the quality of care provided to minority patients in managed care plans.

States can help shape the health care services for low-income minority Medicaid beneficiaries through their contracts with plans participating in Medicaid. States now have greater opportunity to specify expectations—and hold plans accountable—for the delivery of health services, including the participation of safety-net providers, access to providers within the community, and culturally competent care. The George Washington University Center for Health Policy Research team of policy and legal analysts has been working to develop specific contract language and to assist states in incorporating that language into their agreements with plans. As Medicaid managed care further develops, some health plans are questioning whether to participate. State contracts will also have to address protections for patients and communities as plans sign up for and then pull out of Medicaid.

Medicaid and Medicare programs can also encourage the widespread reporting of quality information, including analysis by race and ethnicity, by requiring this information of the plans participating in the public programs. Medicaid state agencies should also begin to adopt exemplary community-based educational programs for implementation on a statewide basis. Similarly, the Health Care Financing Administration could begin to think about how such programs can be adopted nationally.

INCREASE DIVERSITY IN THE HEALTH CARE WORKFORCE

There are several ways in which the health care system can respond effectively to a culturally and ethnically diverse population. Efforts to support a diverse health care workforce are central. Minority physicians are more likely to work in minority and low-income neighborhoods and serve Medicaid and uninsured patients (Komaromy et al. 1996). Many patients feel more comfortable with physicians and other providers who are similar in terms of language and background. Yet, only 6 percent of physicians are black, Hispanic, or Native American, and another 9 percent are Asian (American Medical Association, 1997/1998). The nation has entered a period of rethinking affirmative action policies that have helped increase under-represented minorities in medicine. Despite benefits described by many, this backlash is reflected in declining numbers of under-represented minorities in medical school. Between 1994 and 1997, there was a 7.1 percent decline in minority entrants to medical school (Council on Graduate Medical Education 1998).

The need to increase diversity among medical school students and faculties continues, and public and private programs can provide critical support. Programs that must be sustained include educational and training opportunities bringing minorities into the sciences from the earliest grades, as well as support of the development of medical faculty and physicians engaged in policy and public health. Dynamic, committed health policy leaders can translate research findings and assure that minority health policy issues are at the forefront of the national, state, and local policy agendas. The Commonwealth Fund currently supports a Harvard University program that prepares physicians for leadership positions in minority health and public policy. It is hoped that the program will develop a cadre of leaders that will make a significant impact on policy and programs related to minority health.

In addition to physicians and other health professionals, community health workers can contribute through their ability to provide language translation (Coye and Alvarez 1998), health education, and outreach to populations difficult to bring in for care (Rosenthal 1998). Programs incorporating such workers into health centers and health plans serving low-income minority populations could be tested for effectiveness in improving appropriate use of services, quality of care, and health outcomes.

ADDRESS ISSUES RELATED TO SOCIOECONOMIC STATUS AND DISCRIMINATION

Emphasized throughout this volume is the relationship between SES, race, access to health care, and health status. Minorities are more likely to be uninsured, often because they are more likely to be poor, unemployed, or hold part-time jobs. Mostly as a result of not having the financial means to obtain care, the uninsured—and therefore a significant percentage of minorities—are less likely than others with insurance to utilize health care services.

Improving the socioeconomic circumstances of minority populations is obviously a challenging societal endeavor. Nevertheless, without economic equity, health equity may not be possible. Significant public action must be taken to reduce the income and other socioeconomic inequities that are so pervasive throughout our society. On a broad level, communities must improve public education systems so that, as students graduate, they are better able to seek higher education and earn higher incomes. In addition, specific early childhood interventions may help lessen the excess mortality linked to lower SES. Such interventions could improve family interactions and child development, thereby mitigating some of the effects of poverty (Williams 1998). More immediately, income tax credits could be used to equalize the income of poorer families.

Lack of access to health care services can explain some but not all of the difference in health status across racial and ethnic groups. There are other social determinants, including education, poverty, social status, and real or perceived discrimination that can adversely affect health status. Persons in lower socioeconomic strata will have exposure to a range of psychosocial elements that are predictive of increased mortality and morbidity (Chapter 11; Lantz et al. 1998). Persistent poverty, for example, has been shown to be directly related to mortality for persons under the age of 65 (McDonough et al. 1997). Similarly, studies in this book and elsewhere show that lower levels of education and income in some— but not all—racial or ethnic groups are associated with increased risky behavior, including smoking, being overweight, and physical inactivity (Chapter 12; Lantz et al. 1998). Also, minorities are more likely to experience real or perceived discrimination. The experience of feeling racial or other bias can increase levels of stress which in turn can affect both mental and physical health (Chapter 11; Krieger et al. 1993; Strogatz 1997). On the part of providers, the race and sex of a patient has been found to influence how physicians manage symptoms (Chapter 10; Schulman et al. 1999).

Issues related to racism and discrimination are perhaps even harder to eliminate than SES differentials, because they have to do with attitudes and beliefs of individuals. However, provider training to increase awareness and decrease overt discrimination could change some behaviors. Patients' perceptions of discrimination may decrease with improved SES, increased access to care, and heightened cultural sensitivity on the part of providers.

IMPROVE DATA AND RESEARCH ON DIVERSE POPULATIONS

One of the key findings from analyses of the CMHS is the need to understand the diversity of experiences within the broader groupings of "minority," or "black", "Latino", and "Asian." Continuing to "lump together" peoples from varying ethnic backgrounds into broad groups without any systematic understanding of the variations within these groups can lead to a gross misinterpretation of the health and well-being of different populations. For example, 25 percent of the total Asian sample in the CMHS reported that they were in excellent health. However, of this sample, only 13 percent of the Vietnamese considered themselves to be in excellent health; failure to subcategorize findings into more specific ethnic groupings would lead to erroneous conclusions about the health of Vietnamese immigrants. Collecting and analyzing data by race and ethnic subcategories would help to identify the differential impact of diseases and experiences on different populations.

National health care data are rarely available with the level of detail that allows for information on separate groups. This is due in large part to the expense associated with such an effort. Minority ethnic groups and subgroups are not evenly distributed throughout the United States and are small relative to the overall size of the population. Thus, to assemble large enough numbers suitable for statistical analysis, oversamples of specific groups must be collected. For the CMHS, the oversample of Asians was collected using a nationwide list of Asian surnames compiled from telephone directories. The problem with incorporating this approach into larger national surveys is that the different sampling methodologies employed limit the ability to perform statistical comparisons across groups. Alternate methods for oversampling are available, but they are likely to increase survey costs and the overall size of the sample.

The growing field of patient satisfaction surveys will also have to consider collecting and analyzing satisfaction data by race and ethnicity, and incorporate questions that reflect the experiences of different minority groups. In addition, analyses of health plan claims and encounter data can begin to answer questions about the quality of care delivered to diverse populations. However, to discern trends across groups, health plans and providers must collect data that include racial and ethnic identifiers of patients.

Beyond assuring that we collect adequate survey and epidemiologic data on racial and ethnic groups and subgroups, we need to incorporate results and findings into health policy development. Methodologically, we need sound health services researchers interested in minority health issues to move the field of inquiry forward. Areas for further research include: evaluation of state programs attempting to expand coverage for low-income families; options for maintaining a regular provider and continuity of care within a changing managed care system; the relationship between culturally competent care and health outcomes; and tracking the impact of changes in the safety net on access to and utilization of health care. Social scientists should extend their research to contribute a greater understanding of the special needs of different populations within minority populations and how to reach them and to effectively remove nonfinancial barriers to care, such as lack of knowledge about health care services.

CONCLUSIONS

Early in 1998, a presidential radio address and a Department of Health and Human Services report drew national attention to the continuing racial and ethnic disparities in health status (U.S. Department of Health and Human Services 1998). The report focused on the significant disparities in heart disease, cancer, diabetes, infant mortality, immunizations, and HIV/AIDS. Other health conditions could be added to that list. Continued leadership from federal agencies, along with states, community organizations, and private foundations will be necessary for definitive progress to be made toward eliminating these disparities. Improving access and continuity of care, removing significant financial barriers, assuring that managed care plans are held accountable for quality care to diverse populations, and maintaining commitments to a diverse health care workforce and research base are all necessary pieces of solving these disparities. However, the significant roles of limited educational and employment opportunities, poverty, and discrimination cannot be ignored. Better-informed health care policy will have to be linked with social and economic policies in all of these areas so that all Americans have real opportunities to live healthy and productive lives.

References

American Academy of Pediatrics. 1998. *Analysis of 1994 to 1997 March Demographic File. Current Population Survey and 1998 State Population Projections by Single Year of Age, Sex, Race, and Hispanic Origin.* Series A. U.S. Washington, D.C.: U.S. Bureau of the Census.

American Medical Association. 1997/1998. *Physician Characteristics and Distribution in the U.S.* Chicago, Ill.: American Medical Association.

Bennefield, R. L. 1997. Health insurance coverage. *Current Population Reports.* Washington, D.C.: U.S. Bureau of the Census.

Blackhall, L. J., Murphy, S. T., Frank, G., Michel, V., and Azen S. 1995. Ethnicity and attitudes toward patient autonomy. *Journal of the American Medical Association* 274:820–825.

Carrese, J. A., and Rhodes L. A. 1995. Western bioethics on the Navaho reservation. Benefit or harm? *Journal of the American Medical Association* 274: 826–829.

Chapman, T., and Johnson, K. 1998. The urban health issues for low-income, minority communities. Unpublished report prepared for The Commonwealth Fund.

Collins, K. S., Schoen, C., and Khoransanizadeh, F. 1997. Practice satisfaction and experiences of women physicians in an era of managed care. *Journal of the American Medical Women's Association* 52(2):52–64.

Council on Graduate Medical Education. 1998. *Minorities in Medicine.* Rockville, Md.: U.S. Department of Health and Human Services.

Coye, M., and Alvarez, D. 1998. *Medicaid and Managed Care and Cultural Diversity in California and New York.* New York: The Commonwealth Fund.

Davis, K., Collins, S. K., Schoen, C., and Morris, C. 1995. Choice matters: enrollees' views of their health plans. *Health Affairs* 14(2):99–112.

Day, J. C. 1996. Population of the United States by age, sex, race and hispanic origin: 1995–2050. Washington, D.C.: U.S. Bureau of the Census, Current Population Report Series P25–1130. 131 pp.

Gaskin, D., and Hadley, J. 1997. Population Characteristics of Safety Net Hospitals and Other Urban Hospitals' Markets. Unpublished report prepared for The Commonwealth Fund.

Hall, A. G., Collins, K. S., and Glied, S. 1999. *Employee-Sponsored Health Insurance Coverage: Implications for Minority Workers.* New York: The Commonwealth Fund.

Hawkins, D., and Rosenbaum, S. 1998. The challenges facing health centers in a changing healthcare system. In S. Altman, U. Reinhardt, and A. Shields, eds., *The Future of the U.S. Healthcare System: Who Will Care for the Poor and Uninsured?* Chicago, Ill.: Health Administration Press.

Health Care Financing Administration. 1998. *National Summary of Medicaid Managed Care Programs and Enrollment.* Washington, D.C.: U.S. Department of Health and Human Services. http://www.hcfa.gov/medicaid/trends.htm.

Heiser, N. A., and St. Peter, R. F. 1997. Improving the delivery of clinical preventive services to women in managed care organizations: a case study analysis. *Joint Commission Journal on Quality Improvement* 23(10):529–547.

Kaiser Commission on Medicaid and the Uninsured. 1998. *Medicaid Program at a Glance.* Washington, D.C.: The Kaiser Foundation.

The Henry J. Kaiser Family Foundation and The Commonwealth Fund. 1997. *The Kaiser/Commonwealth 1997 National Survey of Health Insurance.* Washington, D.C.: The Kaiser Foundation.

Kenesson, M. 1997. *Medicaid Managed Care Enrollment Study.* Princeton, N.J.: Center for Health Care Strategies, Robert Wood Johnson Foundation.

Komaromy, M., Grumbach, K., Drake, M., Vranizan, K., Lurie, N., Keane, D., and Bindman, A. 1996. The role of black and Hispanic physicians in providing health care for underserved populations *New England Journal of Medicine* 34(20):1305–1310.

KPMG Peat Marwick. 1998. *Health Benefits in 1998.* Montbale, N.J.: KPMG Peat Marwick.

Krieger N., Rowley, D. L., Herman, A. A., Avery, B., and Phillips, M. T. 1993. Racism, sexism and social class: implications for studies on health, disease and well-being. *American Journal of Preventive Medicine* 9(Suppl.):82–122.

Lantz, P. M., House, J. S., Lepkowski, J. M., Williams, D. R., Mero, R. P., and Chen, J. 1998. Socioeconomic factors, health behaviors and mortality. Results from a nationally representative sample of US adults. *Journal of the American Medical Association* 279(21):1703–1708.

Lavizzo-Mourey, R., and Mackenzie, E. 1996. Cultural competence: essential measurements of quality for managed care organizations. *Annals of Internal Medicine* 124:919–921.

Lavizzo-Mourey, R., Mackenzie, E., and Taylor, L. 1997. *Cultural Competence in Managed Care: Physicians Recognize the Need.* Unpublished report prepared for The Commonwealth Fund.

Lillie-Blanton, M., Leigh, W., and Alfaro-Correa A., eds. 1996. *Achieving Equitable Access: Studies of Health Care Issues Affecting Hispanics and African Americans.* Washington, D.C.: Joint Center for Political and Economic Studies.

Lillie-Blanton, M., and Lyons, B. 1998. Managed care and low-income populations: recent state experiences. *Health Affairs* (Millwood) 17(3):238–247.

Lurie, N., Moscovice, I. S., Finch, M., Christianson, J. B., and Popkin, M. K. 1992. Does capitation affect the health of the chronically mentally ill? Results from a randomized trial. *Journal of the American Medical Association* 267(24):3300–3304.

McDonough, P., Duncan, G. J., Williams, D., and House, J. 1997. Income dynamics and adult mortality in the United States, 1972 through 1989. *American Journal of Public Health* 87(9):1476–1483.

Molnar, C., Soffel, D., and Brandes, W. 1996. *The Knowledge Gap: What Medicaid Beneficiaries Understand and What they Don't—About Managed Care*. New York: Community Service Society of New York.

National Association of Public Hospitals and Health Systems. 1997. *Preserving America's Safety Net Health Systems: An Agenda for Action*. New York: National Association of Public Hospitals and Health Systems.

Rosenbaum, S., Serrano, R., Magar, M., and Stern, G. 1997. Civil rights in a changing health care system. *Health Affairs* (Millwood) 16(1):90–105.

Rosenthal, L. E. 1998. *Summary of the National Community Health Advisory Study*. Tucson: University of Arizona.

Sandman, D., Schoen, C., Des Roches, C., and Makonnen, M. 1998. *The Commonwealth Fund Survey of Health Care in New York City*. New York: The Commonwealth Fund.

Schulman, K. A., Berlin, J. A., Harless, W., Kerner, J. F., Sistrunk, S., Gersh, B. J., Williams, S., Eisenberg, J. M., and Escarce, J. J. 1999. The effect of race and sex on physicians' recommendations for cardiac catheterization. *New England Journal of Medicine* 340(8):618–625.

Strogatz, D. S., Croft, J. B., James, S. A., Keenan, N. L., Browning, S. R., Garrett, J. M., and Curtis, A. B. 1997. Social support, stress and blood pressure in black adults. *Epidemiology* 8(5):482–487.

U.S. Department of Health and Human Services. 1998. *Racial and Ethnic Disparities in Health*. Washington, D.C.: U.S. Department of Health and Human Services.

Wagner, E. H., and Bledsoe, T. 1990. The RAND health insurance experiment and HMOs. *Medical Care* 28(3)191–200.

Ware, J. E., Jr., Bayliss, M. S., Rogers, W. H., Kosinski, M., and Tarlov, A. R. 1996. Differences in 4-year health outcomes for elderly and poor, chronically ill patients treated in HMO and fee-for-service systems. Results from the Medical Outcomes Study. *Journal of the American Medical Association* 276(13):1039–1047.

Ware, J. E., Jr., Brook, R. H., Rogers, W. H., Keeler, E. B., Davies, A. R., Sherbourne, C. D., Goldberg, C. A., Camp, P., and Newhouse, J. P. 1986. Comparison of health outcomes at a health maintenance organization with those of fee-for-service care. *Lancet* 1(8488):1017–1022.

Williams, R. B. 1998. Lower socioeconomic status and increased mortality. Early childhood roots and the potential for successful interventions. *Journal of the American Medical Association* 279(21):1745–1746.

Technical Appendix

Allyson G. Hall, Ph.D.

Allyson G. Hall, Ph.D.

SAMPLING DESIGN

The following is a description of Louis Harris and Associates' National Telephone Sample. This description was provided by Louis Harris and Associates (February, 1996).

The Louis Harris and Associates, Inc., National Telephone Sample is based on a methodology that is designed to produce representative samples of persons in telephone households in the 48 continental United States. The Harris National Telephone Sample makes use of random-digit selection procedures which assure sample representation of persons in households which are "listed" in telephone directories, as well as persons in households which are "unlisted" in telephone directories.* The sample design is also explicitly designed to assure proper representation of households in central city, suburban, and rural areas within each of the 48 continental states.

The Harris National Telephone Sample is selected by a three-stage, stratified sampling process. The ultimate result of this process is a set of

---

*Some households are "unlisted" as the result of a request for an unlisted number by the telephone subscriber. Other households are "unlisted" in the published directory because the telephone number was assigned after the publication date of the directory. Samples that are restricted to directory-listed numbers only may contain serious sample biases because of the exclusion of the various types of unlisted households.

sample selections (phone numbers). In order to assure that the maximum degree of sample control is maintained, the basic sample design has been set up to produce cross-sectional national samples in increments of 500, 1,000, or 1,250 sampling points (i.e., households).

First Stage: Selection of 144 Strata and PSUs

In preparation for the first stage of sample selection, the entire United States is divided into 144 first-stage basic strata. The U.S. Census classifies all areas within the U.S. into three urbanization groupings. These groupings are central city, suburban, and rural.* On the basis of this classification, three basic strata (central city, suburban, and rural) are defined within each of the 48 continental states. This produces a total of $144 = 3 \times 48$ first-stage basic strata.

The process of determining how many sample elements (households) should be selected from each stratum is known as sample allocation. The Harris National Telephone Sample is allocated among the first-stage basic strata on the basis of 1988 population estimates prepared from U.S. Census data by National Planning Data. The process is carried out as follows: Each of the 144 strata accounts for some fraction of the total population of the 48 continental states. The fraction of the total sample allocated to each stratum is proportionate to the stratum size in the population. For example, the stratum consisting of rural (non-MSA) counties in New York State accounts for 0.7069% of the total 48 continental states' population (i.e., 0.007069 as a proportion). As a result, for the cross-sectional sample design consisting of 1,250 telephone households, the rural New York State stratum receives an allocation of nine households. $[1,250 \times 0.007069 = 8.83 = 9$ (rounded)]. Each stratum, in turn, receives an allocation of households in direct proportion to the amount of population contained within its borders relative to the population of the continental U.S.

The term primary sampling unit (PSU) is used to describe the actual units that are selected in the first stage of sampling. In the Harris Na-

---

*Suburban areas are defined as those portions of standard metropolitan areas (MSAs) that are not part of central cities. Rural areas are defined as county or non-MSA county balances that are not included within MSAs.

tional Telephone sample, PSUs are defined as either entire counties or portions of entire counties.*

The appropriate number of PSUs are selected within each of the 144 basic strata on the basis of the population allocation discussed above. This sample selection is carried out with probabilities proportional to the population of each PSU within the stratum. For example, a PSU with a population of 500,000 persons would be given a selection probability that is twice that of a PSU with 250,000 persons.

Second Stage: Selection of Telephone Exchanges and Banks

For PSUs selected in the first stage of sampling, there is a corresponding second-stage sample selection. The second stage involves the selection of actual hundreds-banks of telephone numbers. This is accomplished as follows.

For each county or county part that is selected in the first stage of sampling (i.e., the selected PSU), all the telephone directories that have listings in that county or county part are obtained by the Harris Sampling Department. By inspection of these directories, a listing of directories and page numbers is prepared so that each telephone listing within the selected county or county part appears once and only once on the list.** This effectively creates a single list of all directory listings within the selected PSU.

Following the creation of this single list, a systematic sample of 80 directory listings is obtained for each selection within the PSU. For each

---

*It should be noted that central cities do not necessarily follow boundaries of entire counties. For example, the city of Chicago is located within Cook County, Illinois, but some portions of Cook County are not located within the city of Chicago. In these instances, the portion of the county covered by a central city would be included in the central city stratum, while the portion of the county that is not within the central city stratum is included in the suburban stratum.

It should also be noted that in New England, this additional complexity may extend to entire MSA. More specifically, an MSA may cover only some portion of an entire county. In this case, a single county may have a portion that is classified as central city, a portion that is classified as suburban (MSA but not central city) stratum, and a portion that is classified as rural (non-MSA).

**This step which often involves unduplication, is necessary since certain listings may be duplicated in telephone directories for adjoining areas.

selected listing, the 3-digit exchange (prefix) and the first two digits in the 4-digit suffix are recorded.

It should be noted that this step in the sampling process does not select the actual telephone numbers of listed households. If this were the case, the sample would only include households with listed telephone numbers. Instead, this second stage of sampling results in the selection of banks of 100 numbers. For example, if one of the 80 directory listings has the number 343-4589, this actually selects all 100 potential telephone numbers in the range 343-4500 through 343-4599. This range may be expected to include both listed as well as unlisted numbers.

Third Stage: Selection of Telephone Numbers

In the third stage of selection, the actual telephone numbers that will be contracted are selected. Depending upon the size of the final project, either the sample consisting of 500, 1,000, or 1,250 primary selections may be used. For larger samples, appropriate combinations of these basic samples are employed.

For each selection in the first stage, the corresponding second stage of sampling resulted in the selection of 80 banks of 100 potential numbers. In the third stage of selection, 10 of these 80 banks are randomly selected, and a 2-place random number is appended separately to each of these banks. This produces a sample of 10 different, full telephone numbers for each first stage selection.

Thus, for a standard cross-sectional sample based on the first stage selection of 1,250 PSUs, there will be a full final selected sample of $12,500 = 1,250 \times 10$ telephone numbers. For standard cross-sectional samples based on 1,000 and 500 PSUs, the numbers of generated telephone numbers are 10,000 and 5,000, respectively.

In the process of conducting interviews, an attempt is made to contact the first telephone number selected for each PSU. If it is determined that the number is not a working telephone number, or if the telephone household refuses to participate in an interview, an interview attempt is made at the next selected number associated with the selected PSU. In the case of "no answer" at the selected number, the specific study specifications will dictate the number of different attempts that are made prior to replacement with the next generated number for the PSU. In general, the replacement process continues within each selected PSU until a successful interview is completed.

APPLICATION OF THE NATIONAL TELEPHONE SAMPLE
FOR THE CMHS

Oversamples of African Americans and Hispanics were obtained by screening additional cross-sections and interviewing only members of these groups until satisfactory sample sizes were achieved. The final national cross-sectional sample included 1,114 whites, 1,048 African Americans and 1,001 Hispanics (Louis Harris and Associates 1994).

An attempt was made to contact the first number selected from each list. If this telephone number was not working, or the household would not participate, an attempt was made with the next telephone number on the list. Up to four attempts were made to contact each household. If a callback was arranged, a fifth attempt was made.

Respondent selection within households was based on the "Frankel-Goldstein" grid procedure. It is known that women are more likely than men to respond to telephone surveys because they are more likely to be at home when the interviewer calls. Also, more men than women refuse to be interviewed. To assure adequate male participation, the male/female designations for the cross-section were assigned a 65/35 ratio so that completed interviews represented a 48/52 ratio of males to females. Different gender ratios applied to minority samples: a 60/40 ratio for the Hispanic oversample, 70/30 for the African American oversample, and 50/50 for the Asian oversample.

Initially, households were screened to determine if an individual over the age of 18 lived at that location. Once this was ascertained, all individuals in a household were rostered by sex. Using sample cards and the respondent selection grid, interviewers would ask to speak with a male or female member of the household. If that household contained more than one adult of the specified sex, then the respondent selection grid specified which adult to interview.

For example, using the grid below, if three women lived in a household, the interviewer would speak with the eldest. However, if five women lived in that household, the youngest would be interviewed.

Sample Respondent Selection Grid

# of Adults	1	2	3	4	5	6
Oldest	1	1	1	3	5	1

Referrals, designees, or other eligible respondents were not interviewed in place of the designated respondent.

The method for collecting the Asian subsample was different from the random sampling methodology described above. A separate sample of the Asian American population was collected, using a nationwide list of Asian (Chinese, Korean, and Vietnamese) surnames compiled from telephone directories by Survey Sampling, Inc. Survey interviewers included 632 Asian Americans, of which 205 were Chinese, 201 were Korean, and 205 were Vietnamese. Because of the different sampling methodology, this group was not included in the detailed survey analyses conducted on the entire sample.

SAMPLING RESULTS

The sampling process yielded 3,789 interviews. An overall response rate of 60 percent was obtained based on the following formula:

$$\text{Response Rate} = \frac{\text{Completed interviews} + \text{screen outs}}{\text{Completed interviews} + \text{screen outs} + \text{refusals} + \text{terminated interviews}}$$

"Screen outs" are the number of potential respondents who were willing to participate in the survey but were ineligible because they did not belong to a relevant minority group. "Refusals" represent the number of respondents who indicated that they were unwilling to participate in the survey, multiplied by the "screen-in" incidence. The screen-in incidence was calculated by dividing the number of eligible and willing participants by the sum of eligible and ineligible willing participants. "Terminated interviews" refers to the number of instances in which eligible respondents began an interview but did not complete it.

The survey's complex multistage sampling design affects the estimation of standard errors. Consequently, the analyses used SUDAAN (Shah, Barnwell, and Hunt 1996) or Stata (Stata Corporation 1997) statistical software, which adjust for the complex sample design. These analyses require at least two observations for each stratum for the calculation of sample variances. Because some strata in the sample contained only one sampled unit, postsampling combinations of selected strata were conducted. Within a given race/ethnicity sample, a stratum with one sampled household was combined with another stratum within the same state or an adjacent state. Rural and urban strata were combined, but these strata were not combined with suburban strata because of perceived commonalties (such as access issues) between inner-city and rural areas and perceived differences between those areas and suburban PSUs.

WEIGHTING AND TELEPHONE BIAS

Telephone interviewing is often criticized because the sample is limited to households with phones. This is particularly critical with respect to the CMHS, because households without phones may be more likely to be poorer and therefore less likely to have adequate access to health care. As shown in this section, this is indeed the case with the CMHS.

To correct for some of this bias, all respondents, including the Asian sample, were assigned postsampling weights based on March 1993 Current Population Survey (CPS) distributions. The CPS is a household sample survey conducted monthly by the United States Census Bureau. The CPS sample is selected using a multistage procedure, designed to represent the total U.S. population. The sample is not limited to households with telephones. Postsampling corrections by Louis Harris and Associates, weighting the CMHS respondents by the 1993 CPS distributions, resulted in a weighted CMHS sample similar to the 1993 CPS population estimates with respect to (1) insurance status within race and ethnicity, (2) age by sex within race and ethnicity, and (3) education.

CMHS survey analysts demonstrated the effect that weighting has on the CMHS sample and compared the weighted CMHS distributions to the March 1994 CPS estimates. The March Supplement CPS provides population estimates of various demographic characteristics such as age, sex, race, and marital status (United States Census Bureau 1996). After the weighting procedure, the CMHS is similar to the U.S. population, with the exception of income (Table A.1). This is not unexpected, given that the CMHS sample consists only of households with telephones.

The exclusive use of households that have telephones does create a bias toward respondents with higher socioeconomic status (SES). The potential effect of SES-related bias was examined in more detail (Tables A.2, A.3, and A.4). Overall, respondents to the CMHS were more educated, wealthier, and more likely to be employed than the respondents in the sample reported in the 1994 CPS.

The CPS reports a higher percentage of individuals who have not completed high school compared with the CMHS (19% vs. 15%). Within African American and Hispanic groups, the differences between the CPS and the CMHS are more pronounced. CPS responses indicate that 27 percent of the sample did not complete high school. The CMHS

Table A.1   Percentage Distribution Comparisons between the 1994 Commonwealth Fund Minority Health Survey (Unweighted Sample), Commonwealth Minority Health Survey (Weighted Sample), and the 1994 Current Population Survey

	CMHS Unweighted Sample	CMHS Weighted Sample	March 1994 CPS
Sex			
Male	51	48	48
Female	49	52	52
Age			
18–29	21	24	24
30–44	39	34	34
45–64	28	27	26
≥65	12	15	16
Educational attainment			
Less than high school	16	15	19
High school graduate	29	40	34
Some college	26	25	26
College graduate	19	13	14
Postgraduate	9	6	7
Not sure	1	1	
Employment status			
Self-employed	9	10	
Full-time worker	50	45	
Part-time worker	8	9	
Total employed	67	64	62
Retired	13	17	
Unemployed	5	5	
Student	5	4	
Total unemployed	23	26	38
Other[a]	10	10	
Marital status			
Single	23	22	23
Married[b]	57	56	58
Widowed	8	10	7
Separated	4	4	3
Divorced	8	8	9
Race and ethnicity			
Hispanic	26	8	9
White	30	74	76
African American	27	11	11
Asian	16	3	3
Native American	0.5	2	1
Other	0.6	2	c

(continues)

Table A.1 (*Continued*)

	CMHS Unweighted Sample	CMHS Weighted Sample	March 1994 CPS
Income			
<$7,501	10	11	30
$7,501-$15,000	11	13	21
$15,001-$25,000	16	17	19
$25,001-$35,000	16	15	12
$35,001-$50,000	17	17	10
$50,001-$75,000	11	11	5
$75,001-$100,000	5	5	2
>$100,000	4	4	
Not sure	10	7	

Source: Data from the Commonwealth Fund Minority Health Survey (CMHS), 1994; and U.S. Census Bureau, 1996, *CPS Annual Demographic Survey*.

[a]Includes homemaker, not looking, and unsure.

[b]For CMHS data, this includes living as a couple.

[c]Negligible.

reports that only 19 percent of African Americans did not graduate from high school. Similarly, 45 percent of CPS Hispanic respondents did not complete high school, while only 25 percent of the CMHS Hispanic sample did not graduate (Table A.2).

The CPS sample is shown to have lower incomes than the CMHS sample, a finding that is consistent throughout all racial groupings (Table A.3). Overall, 30 percent of the respondents in the CPS earned less than $7,501 a year, compared with 11 percent reported in the CMHS. Similarly, 21 percent of the CPS sample earned between $7,501 and $15,000, and 13 percent of the CMHS sample earned between $7,501 and $15,000.

People in the CPS sample have higher rates of unemployment, particularly among African American and Hispanic ethnic groups. Some 44 percent of the African American CPS sample were unemployed, versus 36 percent of the African American CMHS sample. Among Hispanics, 40 percent of the CPS sample were unemployed, while 32 percent of the Hispanic CMHS sample were unemployed (Table A.4).

The CMHS reports that a higher percentage of African Americans were married (43%), compared to the CPS data, which indicate that only 36 percent of African Americans were married. Correspondingly,

Table A.2   Percentage Distribution of Education by Race and Ethnicity among Respondents in the 1994 Commonwealth Fund Minority Health Survey and the March 1994 Current Population Survey

Race	Less Than High School CMHS	CPS	High School Graduate CMHS	CPS	Some College[a] CMHS	CPS	College Graduate CMHS	CPS	Postgraduate CMHS	CPS
White	12	15	41	35	25	28	14	15	7	7
African American	19	27	40	36	24	25	10	9	6	3
Hispanic	25	45	36	27	26	20	9	6	3	2
Asian	26	15	26	23	13	25	22	26	9	11
Total	15	19	40	34	25	26	14	14	6	7

Source: Data from The Commonwealth Fund Minority Health Survey (CMHS), 1994; and the U.S. Census Bureau, 1996, *CPS Annual Demographic Survey.*
[a]Includes two-year vocational training.

29 percent of African Americans in the CMHS had never married, while 39 percent of African Americans in the CPS had never married (data not shown). White and Hispanic ethnic groups differed between the data sets in marital status by four percentage points; the CPS reported that 62 percent of the white and 54 percent of the Hispanic groups were married, while the CMHS reported 58 percent married for both groups. Marital status for Asians was reported as 63 percent in both surveys.

On other indicators, the CMHS and the CPS produced similar findings. For example, the weighted age distribution between the two studies is comparable (Table A.5). The CPS and the weighted CMHS have the same gender distributions (data not shown).

Insurance status is also fairly similar, except that among African American and Hispanic groups the CPS sample had higher percentages of people on Medicaid, with correspondingly fewer people on Medicare, compared with the CMHS sample (Table A.6).

IMPUTATION OF INCOME

Information on income was missing for 345 respondents in the CMHS. Because of the importance of this variable to all analysts, imputed values were provided for the missing data. All analyses in this book reporting information by income use this imputed variable.

Table A.3 Comparison between the 1994 Commonwealth Fund Minority Health Survey (Weighted) and the March 1994 Current Population Survey: Percentage Distribution of Income by Race and Ethnicity, Adults Age 18 and Older

Race	≤$7,500		$7,501–$15,000		$15,001–$25,000		$25,001–$35,000		$35,001–$50,000		$50,001–$75,000		$75,001–$100,000		>$100,000	
	CMHS	CPS	CMHS	CPS	CMHS	CPS	CMHS	CPS	CMHS	CPS	CMHS	CPS	CMHS	CPS	CMHS	CPS
White	9	27	12	20	17	20	16	13	18	10	11	6	5	2	5	2
African American	16	42	16	22	21	18	14	9	12	6	8	2	3	0.5	2	0.25
Hispanic	13	43	14	25	22	17	15	7	15	5	8	2	3	0.5	1	0.5
Asian	10	36	13	15	11	18	16	11	17	9	9	6	4	2	4	2
Total	11	30	13	21	17	19	15	12	17	10	11	5	5	2	4	1

Source: Data from The Commonwealth Fund Minority Health Survey (CMHS), 1994; and the U.S. Census Bureau, 1996, *CPS Annual Demographic Survey.*

Table A.4   Comparison between the 1994 Commonwealth Fund Minority Health Survey (Weighted) and the March 1994 Current Population Survey: Percentage Distribution of Employment Status by Race and Ethnicity, Adults Age 18 and Older

Race	Unemployed[a]		Employed	
	CMHS	CPS	CMHS	CPS
White	37	37	63	63
African American	36	44	64	56
Hispanic	32	40	68	60
Asian	37	39	63	61
Total	35	38	65	62

Source: Data from The Commonwealth Fund Minority Health Survey (CMHS), 1994; and U.S. Census Bureau, 1996, *CPS Annual Demographic Survey.*
[a] Includes retired individuals, students, and homemakers.

Respondents with missing data on income were sorted by race/ethnicity, gender, age (18–20, 21–29, 30–39, 40–49, 50–64, 65+, and unknown), educational attainment (< high school, high school graduate, > high school), and marital status (single, married, divorced, widowed, living together as a couple). People with known income were likewise sorted and matched with those whose income was unknown. When more than one individual with known income was matched to one with

Table A.5   Percentage Distribution of Age by Race and Ethnicity among Adults Age 18 and Older in the 1994 Commonwealth Fund Minority Health Survey (Weighted) and the March 1994 Current Population Survey

Race	Age 18–19		Age 30–44		Age 45–64	
	CMHS	CPS	CMHS	CPS	CMHS	CPS
White	20	21	33	33	28	28
African American	29	29	35	36	25	23
Hispanic	34	35	36	35	25	21
Asian	26	27	39	38	26	25
Total	23	24	33	34	27	26

Source: Data from the Commonwealth Fund Minority Health Survey (CMHS), 1994; and U.S. Census Bureau, 1996, *CPS Annual Demographic Survey.*

Table A.6   Percentage Distribution of Insurance Status by Race and Ethnicity among Respondents in the 1994 Commonwealth Fund Minority Health Survey (Weighted) and the March 1994 Current Population Survey, Adults Age 18 and Older

Race	Employer-Based and Other Private Insurance		Medicaid		Medicare		Uninsured	
	CMHS	CPS[a]	CMHS	CPS	CMHS	CPS	CMHS	CPS
White	63	66	4	5	21	17	12	12
African American	50	49	9	18	16	10	24	23
Hispanic	48	44	7	15	7	6	37	34
Asian	61	64	6	8	9	5	22	22
Total	60	61	5	8	18	15	16	16

Source: Data from The Commonwealth Fund Minority Health Survey (CMHS), 1994; and U.S. Census Bureau, 1996, *CPS Annual Demographic Survey.*
[a]Includes CHAMPUS.

unknown income, the imputed income was chosen at random among those who matched, using a table of random numbers.

A total of 271 of the 345 were matched on all five variables. Of the remaining 74, six were matched on four variables and "neighbor matched" on the fifth, which was educational status. In all of these instances, people with less than a high school education were matched with those who had a high school education. These were African American females who were unmarried and were 30 to 39 or 50 to 64 years of age. An additional 40 respondents were matched on the first four variables (i.e., with marital status "collapsed"). Another 14 were matched on a different set of four variables: race/ethnicity, gender, age, marital status, but not education. Finally, nine were matched on three variables: race/ethnicity, gender, age, but neither education nor marital status.

After imputation, five individuals were still classified as "missing income." They could not be matched on all three demographic variables of race/ethnicity, gender, and age.

ASSESSMENT OF THE QUALITY OF THE SAMPLE

Common methods for collecting health status and health care experience information from respondents include personal face-to-face interviews, self-administered questionnaires, and telephone interviews. Although there are certain disadvantages associated with collecting data in this way, telephone interviewing does produce data comparable to that collected by other means and at lower cost (Aday 1996). Concerns have also been raised about whether telephone respondents under-report health events and illnesses. However, because telephone surveying affords a greater sense of anonymity, the respondent may be more likely to report socially undesirable responses such as ill-health or substance abuse. Aday (1996) reports that a large study conducted by the University of Michigan concluded that there was little or no difference in the reporting of health events in telephone surveys compared to in-person surveys. Similarly, in a study done by the Research Triangle Institute, researchers found that the reporting of health events over the telephone was equivalent to or more accurate than data collected in person (Weeks et al., 1983). However, these results are contrary to what other researchers comparing telephone and in-person interviewing have found (McHorney et al. 1994).

Studies comparing survey data with medical records provide mixed results. One study that measured the reliability of patients' accounts versus medical records in determining whether certain services were performed concluded that patient self-reporting is fairly accurate (Brown and Adams 1992). Another study of cancer screening found that concordance between self-reported data and medical records was greater for procedures that generated a test report (mammogram, Pap smear, fecal occult blood test, and sigmoidoscopy) than for those generating a physician's note (clinical breast examination and digital rectal examination). This suggests that self-reported data may overestimate the percentage of the population that has been screened and underestimate the interval since the last cancer detection procedures (Gordon et al. 1993).

The differences between the CMHS and the CPS suggest caution in interpreting overall survey findings primarily because poor and unemployed individuals are underrepresented in the CMHS. The poorer health status and lack of access to health care services experienced by minorities can in part be attributed to their lower SES. Therefore, overall differences in findings across racial and ethnic groups are likely to be muted because of the association between poverty, unemployment and race/ethnicity, health status and access to and utilization of health care services.

However, multivariate analysis permits examination of racial and ethnic differences within SES categories. This type of analysis has an added advantage, in that it permits comparisons across groups without concern about undersampling the poor and unemployed, assuming that nonrespondents in these groups would report similarly to respondents. Because all the authors in this book controlled for SES in multivariate analyses, their findings and conclusions related to the complex interrelationships between ethnicity and health care access, availability and utilization should not be unduly affected by the overall sample biases.

For these reasons, the editors feel confident that the results reported here are relevant and may be useful in the public policy debate about providing adequate health care for minority populations in the United States. This conclusion does assume that the samples within ethnicity and socioeconomic subgroups are representative of the populations from which they were sampled. With an overall response rate of 60 percent, this assumption can be challenged. On the other hand, when results of the CMHS are compared to results of other national surveys for Hispanics, African Americans, and whites, there is considerable consistency in findings. Information for Asian Americans is unique in this survey and therefore potentially quite valuable.

References

Aday, L. A. 1996. *Designing and Conducting Health Surveys: A Comprehensive Guide.* San Francisco: Jossey-Bass.

Brown, J. B., and Adams, M. E. 1992. Patients as reliable reporters of medical care process. Recall of ambulatory encounter events. *Medical Care* 30(5): 400–411.

Gordon, N. P., Hiatt, R. A., and Lampert, D. I. 1993. Concordance of self-reported data and medical record audit for six cancer screening procedures. *Journal of the National Cancer Institute* 85:566–570.

Louis Harris and Associates. 1994. *Health Care Services and Minority Groups: A Comparative Survey of Whites, African-Americans, Hispanics and Asian-Americans.* New York: Louis Harris and Associates, Inc.

Louis Harris and Associates. 1996. *Louis Harris and Associates National Telephone Sample.* Memo to the Commonwealth Fund, February 1. New York: Louis Harris and Associates.

McHorney, C. A., Kosinski, M., and Ware, J. E., Jr. 1994. Comparisons of the costs and quality norms for the new SF-36 Health Survey Collected by Mail versus Telephone Interview: Results from a National Survey. *Medical Care* 32(6):551–567.

Shah, B. B., Barnwell, B. G., and Hunt, P. N. 1996. *SUDAAN Users Manual: Professional Software for Survey Data Analysis for Multi-stage Research Designs.* Research Triangle Park, N.C.: Research Triangle Institute.

Stata Corporation. 1997. *Stata Statistical Software: Release 5.0.* College Station, Tex.: Stata Corporation.

United States Census Bureau. 1996. *CPS Annual Demographic Survey.* March Supplement. www.bls.census.gov/cps/ads/1995/ssampdes.htm. Last modified: September 25, 1996.

Weeks, M. F., Kulka, R. A., Lessler, J. T., and Whitmore, R. W. 1983. Personal versus telephone surveys for collecting household data at the local level. *American Journal of Public Health* 73(12):1389–1394.

Author Index

Subject Index

Library of Congress Cataloging-in-Publication Data

Minority health in America: findings and policy implications from the
    Commonwealth Fund minority health survey / edited by Carol J. R.
    Hogue, Martha A. Hargraves, Karen Scott Collins.
        p.   cm.
    Includes bibliographical references and index.
    ISBN 0-8018-6298-1 (alk. paper).—ISBN 0-8018-6299-X (pbk.:
alk. paper)
    1. Minorities—Health and hygiene—United States.   2. Health
surveys—United States.   I. Hogue, Carol J. R.   II. Hargraves,
Martha A.   III. Collins, Karen Scott.   IV. Commonwealth Fund.
RA448.4.M566   2000
362.1'089'00973—dc21   99-30914
                                                            CIP